VETERINARY HANDBOOK
for CATTLEMEN

VETERINARY
Handbook
for
Cattlemen

By

J. W. BAILEY
D.V.M.

Fourth Edition ■

SPRINGER PUBLISHING COMPANY, INC.

NEW YORK

Fourth Edition

First Printing, June 1972

Second Printing, June 1973

Third Printing, January 1975

Third Edition
First Printing, August 1963
Second Printing, February 1967
Third Printing, March 1970

Second Edition
First Printing, May 1958
Second Printing, April 1962

Copyright © 1972
SPRINGER PUBLISHING COMPANY, INC.
200 Park Avenue South, New York, N. Y. 10003

International Standard Book Number: 0-8261-0284-0
Library of Congress Number: 70-161129

Printed in U.S.A.

PREFACE TO
THE FOURTH EDITION

During the eight years since this book was last revised there have been many changes and discoveries which we have incorporated in this fourth edition. Virus diarrhea and mucosal disease have been shown to be the same disease. Effective vaccines have been developed for the prevention of such diseases as virus diarrhea, vibriosis, and red nose. The definite diagnosis of certain diseases has been made easier and faster through laboratory aids such as the fluorescent antibody test. An effective test for the identification of anaplasmosis carrier animals has been demonstrated. Two completely different possible causes of "crooked calf disease" have been discovered. New agents like thiabendazole and organic phosphates have been developed for the control of internal parasites. Such drugs as tylosin and new broad-spectrum antibiotics are now available for the treatment of various diseases. Several old diseases as well as new ones have been discovered as being caused either wholly or in part by psittacosis-granuloma (PL) agents and myxovirus parainfluenza-13. Overnight, intercontinental movement of cattle by air has increased the danger of introducing into the United States such foreign diseases as rinderpest and contagious pleuropneumonia, so these are being covered in this book for the first time. Mycoplasma, polyarthritis, aspergillosis, tumors, and coccidioidomycosis, diseases that were not considered important enough to mention in previous editions, have now become important and warrant inclusion in this fourth edition. The same is true of various poisonings, for example, those caused by urea and kerosene. Additional information has become available about some of the older diseases such as grass tetany, shipping fever, and foot rot, and that too has been included. Several new illustrations have been added. We hope that this handbook will continue to be helpful to cattlemen,but it is not intended to take the place of a veterinarian. It will always be best to get professional help in making a diagnosis before spending money for treatment that may do no good. In addition, early recognition of a contagious disease can often prevent its spread and consequent extensive losses.

Springfield, Illinois   *J. W. Bailey*

PREFACE TO
THE FIRST EDITION

THERE ARE SEVERAL REASONS why a book like this one can not be expected to replace a veterinarian. A caesarean section or an operation to remove hardware from a cow's stomach requires skill and instruments not possessed by the average owner. The correct dosage of medicines can often be determined only through careful examination of animals by a trained observer. Efficient treatment may require something like adrenalin or special serums not available on the farm. Most important of all is the fact that the same symptoms are often those of several different troubles. Consequently, the personal attendance of a veterinarian is often the only way in which a correct diagnosis can be obtained so that appropriate treatment can be started.

On the other hand, there are times when a veterinarian can not be obtained in a hurry, and there are sections of the country where veterinarians aren't available at all. Under such conditions emergency treatment by an owner may save animals that otherwise might die. Then, too, there are often minor troubles that do not warrant calling a veterinarian, and which can be satisfactorily treated by owners. It is hoped that this book will provide useful information and advice while serving as a guide that will help cattlemen to take care of their stock in times of need.

We wish to caution readers against using remedies unless they know what is wrong with animals. Such practice runs into money pretty fast without yielding any returns. After all, sulfas and penicillin and other "wonder" drugs won't cure every animal disease, so don't expect too much from them. In addition, the wrong medicines can make animals sicker instead of better, so you'd better use the old motto when you're doctoring sick cattle, "Be sure you're right, then go ahead."

CONTENTS

1.

PRACTICAL
POINTERS FOR OWNERS

Breaking Heifers To Milk

It is highly important that heifers are not hurt or frightened when they are first milked. Otherwise, they are likely to associate milking with unpleasant experiences, and will either fight the procedure or fail to "let down" their milk. Slow movements and a reassuring voice are always desirable, and petting or scratching the animals at milking time will often help. If such measures are not successful, there are others that may be used.

A nose lead with three or four feet of rope attached to it is quite effective when properly used. Once fastened in the nose, a heifer is pulled forward until her shoulders are snug against the stanchion. Her head is then swung sharply to the right and the rope is tied with a single bow knot around the top of the next stanchion. Turning the head to the right generally causes the heifer to swing her hind end to the left so a milker has plenty of room at her right side. In such a position the animal can't kick without hurting her nose and losing her balance, so she usually learns quickly that it pays to stand still while being milked. The bow knot is desirable so it can be instantly released in case of an emergency.

About six feet of quarter inch rope with an eye splice in one end can also be used to good advantage for breaking heifers to milk. The plain end of the rope is thrown over the cow's back in front of the hip bones and brought under her belly just ahead of the udder. It is then run through the eye splice and drawn up extremely tight so the animal is fastened in a noose. The free end of the rope is then fastened with a knot squarely on top of the backbone. Any attempts to kick are painful to the cow and are usually discontinued within a short period. If they aren't, the rope may be drawn still tighter around the body.

Some dairymen favor tying up a hind leg when heifers are violently opposed to being milked. We're always a little afraid the practice will cause a cow to break a leg or dislocate a joint, but it's widely used with few accidents. The only required piece of apparatus is a quarter inch rope about ten feet long with a running noose or "lasso" in one end. A loop about one foot in diameter is thrown on the floor by the right hind foot and the cow is forced to step in it. An alternative method consists of making a bigger loop and hanging it over the hind end of the animal so that it touches the ground on the right side. Regardless of how it is accomplished, once the cow has stepped into the loop it is tightened around the pastern. The free end of the rope is thrown over a beam so the

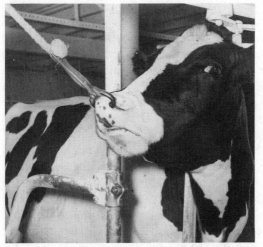

A nose lead with a few feet of rope attached to it is effective in breaking heifers to milk.

foot can be raised and drawn back until the toes barely touch the ground to supply balance. Such an arrangement practically puts the animal on three legs and helps to keep her quiet.

A short length of rope with a noose in one end can also be used for tying the hind legs together to keep a heifer quiet. The noose is first placed around one leg just above the hock, and the free end is then carried around the other leg and back in a figure eight fashion that draws the legs close together. The pattern is continued until several turns have been taken around both legs above the hocks, after which the rope is tied in a single bow knot.

There are also several different kinds of so-called "anti-cow kickers" available on the market which act on much the same principle as the figure eight of rope around the hocks. These are usually effective after a brief period of trial by heifers, but severe falls are often suffered before they learn to respect the devices. Regardless of what is used in breaking heifers to milk, use of the device is best discontinued as soon as possible.

Breaking the Kicking Habit

The methods just described for breaking heifers to milk can also be effectively used on kicking cows. However, a natural "kicker" is seldom reformed and is apt to be respectable only so long as some means of restraint is used. With her hind feet left unhindered she is likely to start kicking again at any time. Consequently, anti-kicking devices are best regarded as insurance against injuries rather than remedies for a dangerous habit.

An Emergency Halter

An emergency halter can be made in a few seconds from a short piece of rope. A running noose is made in one end and this is slipped over the animal's head. The rest of the rope is then doubled to form another noose which is shoved through the first

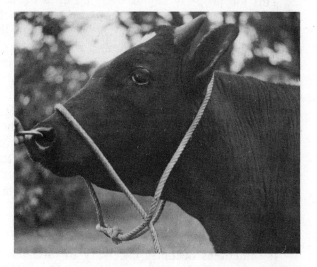

An emergency halter.

one from the side next to the shoulders. The second loop is then carried forward and up over the nose. A pull on the free end of the rope and a little adjusting will result in a halter that is easily removed, but still won't slip off or choke the animal.

A less desirable type of emergency halter can also be made from the same rope. The noose is slipped over the animal's head as before but drawn up snugly and a half-hitch then taken around the animal's nose. However, pulling on the end of the rope has a tendency to make the half-hitch slip off so a critter is held by nothing but a loop around the neck.

Breaking Animals To Stand When Tied

It is perfectly natural for cows and calves to "pull back" when they are tied up for the first time. The tendency can be remedied by proper tying. An emergency halter is made as described above from a rope ten or twelve feet long. With it the animal is pulled up close to a manger or board fence. The rope is then passed over the manger top and returned through the tie hole, or in the case of a fence it is passed around a post and returned over the top of a board at shoulder level. Slack is taken up in the rope and it is tied to the pastern of a front foot. Any attempts at "pulling back" will jerk a foot off the ground, and most animals soon learn that it's best to stand still where they have been tied.

Breaking Animals To Lead

This job properly begins by tying up a beast as just described and letting it stand for a few hours at a time until it has learned the meaning of restraint. When leading is actually started, a surcingle with a ring in it and another rope will be desirable in addition to the regular halter. A slip-knot is made in one end of the extra rope, and a noose is placed on the animal so that the knot rests on the backbone just in front of the hip bones. The surcingle is put on just back of the front legs, with the ring arranged so that it also rests on the backbone. The free end of the rope is brought forward through the surcingle ring and on out to the animal's head. The trainer carries a rope in each hand, and the loin rope is jerked a few times whenever the animal refuses to lead. Most pupils soon learn that it is better to follow the halter rope than to have their middles pinched.

An Emergency Sling for Raising Hind Quarters

It sometimes becomes necessary to raise the hind quarters of animals that are unable to stand up without help. In such cases an emergency sling may be made with a few feet of strong rope. A running noose is made in one end of the rope and slipped over a hind leg until it is close against the body. The free end of the rope is then carried under the belly just in front of the udder location, and a second running noose is made and slipped over the other hind leg. When it has also been drawn up close to the body, a wire stretcher or tackle is fastened overhead and hooked through both nooses at the backbone. Loops fastened only around the legs will cause the legs to be pulled out back of the animal. A rope around the body alone will permit the legs to work forward under the patient. Consequently, a combination of the two methods can be expected to give better results.

An Emergency Sling for Raising Entire Animals

The same kind of a rope can be made into an emergency sling for raising entire animals instead of just the hind quarters. After determining the mid-point of the rope, it is placed just in front of the animal's shoulders and the ends brought down and crossed just

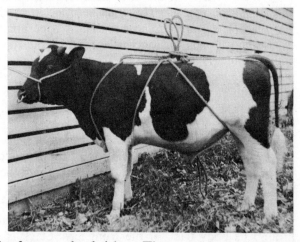

A rope sling for raising entire animals.

in front of the forelegs at the brisket. They are then continued between the forelegs, up over the sides and crossed again about the middle of the back. After that they are brought down over the flanks and back between the hind legs, one on each side of the udder or scrotum as the case may be. The ends are then carried up over the buttocks on each side of the tail and passed forward under themselves where they crossed on the back. A pause is made here while the ropes are tightened so they fit snugly against the body at all points, after which the ends of the rope are fastened to its middle at the point of the shoulders. The hook of a block and tackle is inserted under all four ropes at the crossing place on the back for raising the critter.

Moving Paralyzed Animals

Every once in a while cattle become paralyzed and go down in driveways or other places from which they have to be moved. The easiest way out of such a situation is to drag the poor brutes out of the way with a tractor or team of horses. However, this procedure is not permissible under any conditions, since the dragging will cause painful and serious skin injuries for animals. A better method consists of rolling the paralyzed beast onto a stoneboat and then moving it. If a stoneboat isn't available, something like an old barn door or binder canvas will serve as a means of transportation.

"Throwing" Cattle

For one reason or another cattle frequently have to be "thrown" or cast on the ground. This may be done in two somewhat similar ways with no more equipment than a rope about forty feet long.

One way calls for looping an end of the rope around the animal's shoulders in the form of a loose-fitting collar. The lower part of the loop should fall across the brisket and it should be tied at the withers with a non-slipping knot so the beast won't be choked when pulling is started. If the animal has horns, a running noose may be slipped over them instead of making the loop around the shoulders. Depending on where the loop is placed, the end of the rope will come from either the top of the shoulders or the back of the head. It is then carried back a foot behind the shoulders, where it is dropped to the ground, passed under the belly, back up the other side and under the rope where it was dropped to the ground in the first place. The animal is then caught in a loop that passes around its body back of the front legs. Slack is taken up and the rope is carried back to a point just in front of the hip bones where a second loop is made around the body in the same way that the first one was formed. If the animal is a cow, care must be used to make sure that this second loop does not touch the udder. If a bull, the bottom part of the loop is best padded with a sack to avoid injuring the penis when the rope is tightened. After slack has been taken up again, the rope is ready for use. However, the animal must be haltered and tied to a post or fastened in a stanchion before pulling is started or it will be drawn backward. With the head suitably anchored a steady pull straight back on the rope will cause the beast eventually to collapse on its belly.

An alternative method consists of doubling the rope into two equal lengths. The middle of the rope is then hung on the animal's withers and the free ends are brought down between the forelegs from the front. They are crossed at this point and carried up and around to the small of the back where they are crossed again. They are then brought down and passed between the hind legs from the front, one on each side of the udder or testicles as the case may be. The head must be fastened as before, and a steady backward pull on both ropes will cause the animal to go down as in the first case. Extra pull on one rope or the other will help to throw animals

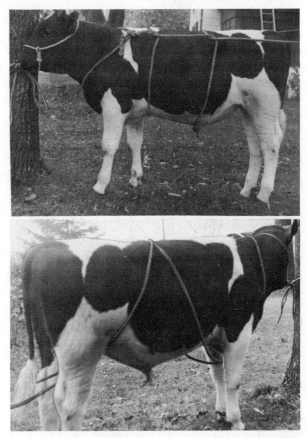

Two methods of throwing cattle.

on the desired side. This method has the advantage of being unlikely to injure either the penis of males or the udder and milk veins of females. A disadvantage lies in the fact that two rope ends require pulling instead of a single one.

Moving Calves

Since calves are notoriously stubborn by nature, it's sometimes quite a job to get them moved from one place to another around the barn. Leading doesn't work so well, since the animals usually brace themselves and pull back. A better plan consists of turning them around and backing them into the desired location. If the calf will suck, it will sometimes follow a finger that is placed in its mouth and slowly drawn away in the right direction.

Laying Down Calves

Larger animals are best thrown by use of a rope arrangement described earlier in this section. However, calves up to three hundred pounds are easily laid down with the hands. Standing on the right side of the calf, the left hand is passed over the back to grasp the lower edge of the left flank. The right hand is passed under the neck, and the calf is suddenly lifted off the ground at the same time that the left knee is used as a boost to swing the legs outward. With the legs out of the way, a calf can be gently laid on its side before a struggle can be made. With the left flank grasped in one hand and the neck doubled back towards the shoulder with the other, the calf can be held down without much trouble.

Keeping Animals Down

Once cattle have been cast, they may be kept down in any one of three common ways. When ropes have been used for casting, continued pull on them will serve to do the job. As an alternative, the animal may be haltered and a long lead rope attached to it. This is used to draw the head as close as possible to a hind leg where it is tied above the hock. The rope is then continued on up over the body and across the shoulders and is tied to something beyond so the animal can't roll over on its head. The third method consists of doubling up the hind legs at both the hock and pastern joints and tying them in that position. The front legs are similarly tied after being doubled up at the knees and pasterns. The hind legs can also be tied together with the figure eight knot described earlier for breaking heifers to milk. This type of restraint is particularly useful on animals that are unable to stand up but may cripple themselves by doing a "split" while struggling to gain their feet.

Raising a Front Foot

A single long rope can be used for raising a cow's front foot. The animal's head is first tied fairly high with an emergency halter made in one end of it. The other end is carried just back of the withers, down the side, between the front legs, and back up in

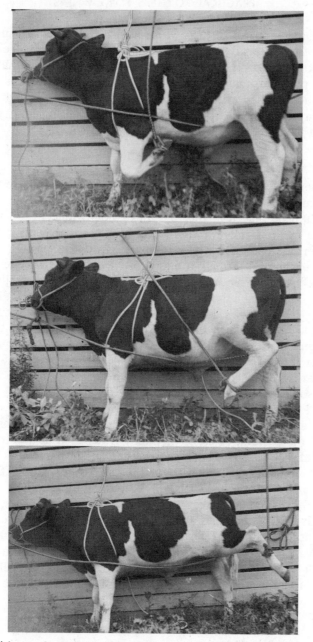

Top: Raising a front foot after loop around shoulder and side line are in place.

Center: Raising a hind foot forward.

Bottom: Raising a hind foot backward.

front of the shoulder to the withers again. Here it is tied in a non-slip knot to form a large loop which is fastened above the animal to support the cow. If the loop is made large enough so that it will stay in place around the point of the shoulder, the foot can be lifted and handled without much trouble. A second and shorter rope may be looped around the pastern for raising and tying up the foot if desired.

Raising a Hind Foot

When a cow's hind foot is to be raised, it is desirable to have the animal in a stanchion or tied with a halter. Whenever possible she should be placed against a wall or board fence.

One method calls for the use of a single rope with a running noose in one end. The noose is placed around a pastern and the free end is passed through a pulley or clevis that is fastened above and a couple of feet behind the animal. It is then brought down and secured with a half hitch just above the hock of the same leg. The foot is next raised to the desired height and slack is taken up in the rope between the pastern and hock. After that the rope is continued along the side of the animal and tied with a single bow knot at shoulder level. Running the rope along the side is important, for it keeps the animal from swinging around.

A somewhat similar method also calls for the use of a single rope with a running noose in one end. In this case the noose is placed about half way between the hock and fetlock instead of around the pastern. A clevis or pulley is fastened at a point above the middle of the cow's back and the free end of the rope is brought along the side and through it for the purpose of raising the foot. A single bow knot in the rope will serve to hold the foot in position.

A third method makes use of two fairly long ropes, one of which is tied at each end and runs along the animal's side to hold it against the wall or fence. A slip knot in one end of the other rope is then placed just above the hock, and the free end is run through a pulley or clevis fastened above and slightly behind the cow. This allows more freedom of the leg than the last method mentioned, but has the advantage of making it easier to work on the bottom of a foot.

Bandaging a Foot

Foot bandages for cattle can be easily made by cutting gunny sacks into strips about two inches wide. It is best to use a layer of cotton over the entire foot under bandages to avoid trouble due to interference with circulation of blood. After raising the foot and cleaning it, bandaging can be started by dividing one end of a strip for three or four inches and tying a knot at that point to prevent further tearing. The divided end is then tied loosely around the pastern to serve as an anchor. After that the free end is brought through the cloven hoof, around one of the toes, up over the heel, and back to the front of the hoof again. It is again brought down through the cleft, but is continued around the opposite toe the second time. This figure eight sort of bandage winding is continued until the foot is adequately protected. The end of the bandage is then split and tied snugly around the pastern. A few stitches taken through the bandages with heavy thread will help to hold them in place for a longer time.

A bandage can be made out of an old inner tube to protect cattle with sore feet or foot rot. The foot is first cleaned and trimmed, after which a suitable remedy is applied and covered with cotton held in place by gauze. About 16 inches is cut off an inner tube and four or five hog rings are set like belt loops around one end.

This end is drawn up over the foot and fastened with twine passed through the hog rings to be tied fairly tightly above the fetlock. The other end is

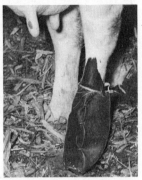

Inner tube bandage.

folded over from one side, brought across the bottom of the foot and up the opposite side of the leg. More hog rings are then used to fasten the edges of the folded-over end. Such a bandage will keep infected feet clean and will stay on the foot for a long time.

A less elaborate bandage may be used for simple cuts and cracks between the toes. The job is started with one end of the bandage tied loosely around the pastern as before. However, the bandage is brought straight between the toes from front to back. At this time it may again be split and tied around the pastern. An alternative consists of drawing the bandage through to a point above the fetlock and then doubling it back between the toes again, this time from back to front. Here the doubling may be repeated, and several layers of bandage inserted between the toes while the doubled ends are held in the free hand. When completed, one end of the bandage may be tied around the pastern to hold the packing in place. As before, a few stitches with heavy thread will make the job last a little longer. Appropriate remedies may be used on feet under both types of bandages.

Breaking Fence Jumpers

A so-called "poke" is probably the best known device for controlling fence-jumping cattle. It is usually nothing more than a couple of pipes or light poles with the animal's head stuck between them. Crossbars above and below the neck on the uprights keep them fastened to the animal. Commercial products consist of single metal bars perpendicular to the ground and welded to a collar worn by the fence-jumper. The devices not only discourage jumping, but they also make it difficult for beasts to crawl through fences.

Another arrangement calls for a short metal strap carrying a ring and buckle, a short chain, and a halter. The strap goes around a forefoot at the pastern and is buckled. The chain runs from the ring on the strap to the one on the lower part of the halter, and is adjusted so that the head can't be raised for jumping.

Jumping over electric fences can often be stopped by placing an ordinary bull ring in the animal's nose and suspending a short length of chain from it. When the head is extended over the fence for jumping the chain touches the "hot" wire and gives the critter a shock in the nose.

Care of the Bull

Bulls should be fed so they stay in thrifty condition without growing fat. In addition, young animals will need extra feed to take care of their growth requirements. Considerable care must be used in regard to feeding roughages since too much of these may cause a bull to become paunchy and consequently slow and clumsy at service. Silage is particularly likely to put a big middle on a bull, so it's generally recommended that this feed be held down to not more than 10 to 15 pounds daily for sires. When hay is fed alone, 15 to 20 pounds daily will usually be needed, with the amount dependent on the size of the bull.

Although the amount will be determined largely by his size and amount of service, a bull fed good roughage can usually be kept in desirable breeding condition on 4 to 6 pounds of grain daily. The percentage of protein needed in the ration will of course depend on the kind and quality of roughage available. Most authorities advise a concentrate mixture such as recommended for dry cows and heifers since a bull doesn't need nearly so much protein as a high-producing cow.

With the exception of unusually cold sections of the country, a bull is best kept in an open shed the year around. This should be furnished with an outdoor run where he can exercise, since it is essential that these animals aren't penned up too much. Confinement in small quarters is to blame for many ugly-dispositioned and impotent herd sires. A breeding pen can be built into the bull pen with good advantage, for the bull can then be used without danger of injury to anyone.

Bulls kept in these outdoor quarters stay in the best of health, but they often become shaggy and unkempt in appearance so some breeders prefer to keep the animals in box stalls inside a warm barn. When bulls are kept in such quarters they have little chance to wear their feet down, so hoofs will require trimming at regular intervals to avoid serious trouble.

Ringing the Bull

The bull should first be tied up with a halter and crowded against a wall to prevent struggling. With the thumb in one nostril and the forefinger in the other, a thin place can be located in the cartilage that divides the nostrils, and this is the place where the ring should go. A trocar and canula such as are used for "tapping" bloated cows is handy for the piercing job. Both are thrust through the thin place in the nose, after which the trocar is removed while the canula is left in place. The sharp end of the ring is then placed in the canula and is pushed on through the nose at the same time the canula is removed. The ring can be snapped shut after that and a screw inserted to keep it closed. It is well to hold an old hat under the ring until the screw is well started or a sudden jerk of the animal's head may cause it to be dropped and lost.

Some farmers like a hook such as is used for handling baled hay to pierce the nose, while others use an ordinary pocket knife. Still others get along without instruments of any kind by using "self-piercing" rings. Ringing should be done when the bull is about six months old and fairly easy to handle. It is best not to lead or tie by the ring for several days after it has been inserted. Rings should be changed every year since they wear thin by being dragged. A great deal of such wear can be prevented by slipping a one inch piece of rubber tubing over the lower part of the ring.

Handling the Bull

It is best to keep bulls in pens fitted with gates opening into breeding chutes so that they don't have to be handled at all. If the brutes do have to be handled, we consider leading a bull to be a job for two men. One walks in front, holding a bull staff that has been snapped into the ring. The other follows, carrying one

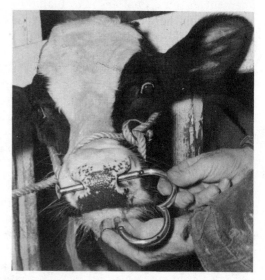

Inserting sharp point of bull ring in small end of canula just before it is pushed through the nose.

end of a strong rope that passes between both the hind legs and the front ones, with the other end attached to the ring. Each man is then in a position to protect the other in case the bull should attack his handlers. When it is absolutely necessary for one man to lead a bull, he should do it with a staff, for a charging bull can't be pushed back very far with a strap or rope. And don't think that rules of safety won't need to be followed because your bull is "gentle as a kitten," either. Tame bulls are always the ones that kill people, probably because chances aren't taken with those that advertise themselves as dangerous. *Be careful!*

Telling When a Cow Is in Heat

Cows sometimes have "quiet" heats which are almost impossible to detect. Generally, though, the commonest sign of heat is attempted "riding" of other animals. A cow that is in heat will "ride" other cows and also permit them to "ride" her. One that is not in heat will "ride," but refuse to let other cows mount her. Other indications of heat may include bawling, decreased milk production, restlessness, and even attempts to "ride" human beings. In most instances mucus greatly resembling egg white is discharged from the vulva, particularly when "riding" is attempted. Careful watching of cows for fifteen or twenty minutes right after they're turned out of a barn will usually indicate any that may be in heat. Cows that have "quiet" heats may have to be turned in with a bull each day in order to detect their periods.

Collecting Semen from Bulls

Some kind of a dummy for the bull to mount will be needed, and on the average farm it is most convenient to use a cow that is in heat. An artificial vagina, some kind of vegetable oil, and a thermometer will also be needed. An old sack is tied over the hind end of the cow and she is tied or stanchioned in a place where there is good footing for the bull behind her. If a breeding chute is available, the collector can work through a "cutaway" side and be completely separated from the bull at all times. Without such protection, the bull should be led on a staff by a man who stands on the left side of the cow.

The vagina is prepared for use by filling it about two thirds full of water that has a temperature of 110 degrees Fahrenheit. Complete filling is not advised, as a little extra space will prevent the vagina from being torn apart by the force of the bull's leap. With the water in it, the inside of the vagina is lubricated with the vegetable oil. A vegetable product is preferred since rubber is easily destroyed by mineral oil and substances like vaseline.

Now ready for use, the vagina is held in the right hand of the collector who stands on the right side of the cow. When the bull mounts for service, the man places his left shoulder in the flank, grasps the sheath in his left hand and steers the penis into the vagina. Following ejaculation, the vagina is left on the penis until the bull dismounts. It is then turned with the open end up so the semen runs down into the glass collection tube attached to the other end. It will be advisable to have this tube covered with several thicknesses of paper held in place by a rubber band. Aside from protecting the tube against breakage, the paper will also protect the semen against direct sunlight and sudden changes of temperature which are likely to kill the spermatazoa in it. Left-handed collectors should stand on the left side of the cow.

Semen can also be collected by massaging the genital organs of the bull through the wall of his rectum while a tube equipped with a funnel is held beneath the sheath. Since this procedure calls for special training it is not likely to be practical on the average farm and will not be discussed here.

Storage of Semen

Semen can be stored raw, frozen, or diluted with egg yolk and various types of "buffer" solutions intended to prolong life of spermatazoa. In any case it must be remembered that semen deteriorates and becomes of progressively poorer quality as it grows older. Consequently, it is doubtful if storage and the use of buffers is practical on farms with only a few cows. Fresh semen would seem more desirable in the interest of increasing breeding efficiency and rate of conception. If semen must be stored, we recommend that it be left in the original collection tube and placed in a glass of milk-warm water. Glass and all is then set in a refrigerator where the temperature is constant at about five degrees above freezing. Keeping the semen in water serves two purposes; providing for gradual cooling and later protecting it against sudden changes in temperature when doors are opened. It is impossible to predict how long semen can be stored. Pregnancies have followed the use of semen well over one hundred hours old, while in other cases spermatozoa have all been dead in semen less than twenty-four hours old.

Artificial Breeding

We suggest that readers first study the anatomy of the cow's genital tract as found in this book at the beginning of the section devoted to reproductive troubles. It will also be a good idea to list paper towels, a small table, a 2 cc. glass syringe, and either glass or plastic inseminating tubes with rubber connections as being necessary for this work.

Actual insemination of the cow should start with placing the table and equipment conveniently close behind the animal. One cc. of semen is then drawn into the syringe through an inseminating tube and both are laid on the table. The left hand is next lubricated with soap and introduced into the rectum of the cow. When the cervix has been located and picked up, one or more of the paper towels can be used to clean off the vulva. The syringe is then picked up again and the inseminating tube is manipulated through the cervix where the semen is deposited. The above procedure can be reversed if the inseminator is left-handed. It is not desirable to use more than one cc. of semen, since the introduction of added amounts means that there will be just that much more for Mother Nature to clean up in the uterus. If glass inseminating tubes are used, they should be cleaned, disinfected, and dried between services to prevent the spread of disease. The plastic tubes have the advantage of being cheap enough so they can be thrown away after being used a single time.

Another method of artificial insemination is much the same except for the fact that a speculum and electric light are used to locate the cervix. The speculum is a hollow tube of glass, metal, or plastic which is introduced into the vagina. Light is then directed through it to aid in finding the cervix. Once seen, the inseminating tube is introduced through the speculum and into the cervix where the semen is deposited as before.

Using a Small Bull on Big Cows

It is sometimes desirable to use young bulls on big old cows that are hard for them to reach. This can be made fairly easy by standing the hind feet of the female in a shallow hole in the ground or backing her up into the gutter inside the barn. In either case the hind end of the cow is lowered so breeding can be accomplished.

Bleeding after Breeding

Some owners believe that bleeding a day or two after service indicates that a cow has failed to "settle." This is probably because pregnant females aren't supposed to menstruate. Other owners take the opposite view and consider the bleeding a proof of conception. As a matter of fact, both beliefs are wrong, for the bleeding has no significance as regards conception in cattle. Cows do not really menstruate, and bleeding may or may not occur after service.

When Should Heifers Be Bred?

There is no such thing as a definite age at which dairy heifers should be bred for the first time. Instead, the time is properly dependent on size, and this will vary somewhat according to the breed. If heifers are well-fed and properly cared for, most of them will be big enough to breed at about fifteen months of age so they can freshen at two years and start paying off their board bill. However, many heifers will be too small at that age.

Some of these will be naturally small for their age, but most of them will be under-developed because of poor feeding. It is regrettable, but true, that a great many dairy heifers are weaned and then more or less forgotten until they are about fifteen months of age. Then they are bred, turned to pasture again, and forgotten until they reach calving time.

At that time they try to deliver a good-sized calf from an under-developed reproductive tract, and the job may be physically impossible for them. As the best and most humane way out of such a situation, most veterinarians will perform a caesarean operation. As an alternative, the calf may be cut up inside the heifer and taken out in pieces. In a few cases we have known animals to be hopelessly crippled by having calves pulled out with a tractor or block and tackle. No matter what is done, trouble at calving time may leave the heifer as a nonbreeder and poor milk producer. Considering these risks in addition to lowered resistance to disease, it just doesn't pay to breed heifers too soon.

Repeated reference to size naturally brings up the question of how an owner is to know when heifers are big enough to breed. The following list shows recommended weights and ages:

Breed	Weight at First Breeding	Age in Months
Jersey	500 to 600 lbs.	14 to 17
Guernsey	550 to 650	15 to 18
Ayrshire	600 to 700	16 to 19
Holstein	800 to 900	16 to 20
Brown Swiss	800 to 900	17 to 20
Aberdeen-Angus	900 to 1000	19 to 23
Hereford	900 to 1000	19 to 23
Shorthorn	900 to 1000	19 to 23

If the heifers have been well fed and properly cared for, the ages and weights will be pretty closely related.

In case there is any doubt about the weight, an owner can get the right answer within a few pounds by using a tape measure on the heifers. This is placed around the body just back of the front legs to get the heart girth. Be sure to get a tape intended for your breed, since they are made for both beef and dairy cattle.

Gestation Table for Cows

The gestation period of cows is subject to considerable variation, and is likely to be dependent upon heredity, environment, and breed. The average period of gestation is 282 days. The following table, based on averages, is generally used, and a few days, give or take, can be accepted as reasonably accurate.

Service Date		Approx. Birth Date		Service Date		Approx. Birth Date		Service Date		Approx. Birth Date	
Jan.	1	Oct.	10	May	7	Feb.	13	Sept.	10	June	19
	8		17		14		20		17		26
	15		24		21		27		24	July	3
	22		31		28	March	6	Oct.	1		10
	29	Nov.	7	June	4		13		8		17
Feb.	5		14		11		20		15		24
	12		21		18		27		22		31
	19		28		25	April	3		29	Aug.	7
	26	Dec.	5	July	2		10	Nov.	5		14
March	5		12		9		17		12		21
	12		19		16		24		19		28
	19		26		23	May	1		26	Sept.	4
	26	Jan.	2		30		8	Dec.	3		11
April	2		9	Aug.	6		15		10		18
	9		16		13		22		17		25
	16		23		20		29		24	Oct.	2
	23		30		27	June	5		31		9
	30	Feb.	6	Sept.	3		12				

Currently, based on breed differences, the American Dairy Science Association recommends the following table as being more accurate than the 282-day period:

Breed	Days
Ayrshire	278.7
Brown Swiss	290.8
Guernsey	284.0
Holstein	278.9
Jersey	279.3

It is suggested that the table be reduced by two days for all first-calf heifers.

Preventing Calving Troubles in First-Calf Heifers

Most calving troubles in first-calf heifers can be prevented if owners will do these five things:

1. Use size instead of age as a basis for deciding when to breed heifers for the first time. This is important because some heifers will be naturally small at the generally accepted age for breeding, no matter how well they have been cared for. Many others will be under-developed at that age because of poor care and feeding.

2. Control the birth weight of the calf through planned feeding of the dam. This is a pretty touchy problem. The heifers

can't be starved through their first gestation period, for they are still growing. Restriction of feed to an extreme degree would reduce the size of the calves, all right, but expected results would also include such things as abortions, weak calves, and lowered fat reserves which would decrease potential milk-producing ability.

An ideal ration would provide for complete maintenance and normal growth without providing many excess nutrients to encourage the development of a big calf. In the case of beef cattle, at least, a couple of California cases indicate that a satisfactory ration is within reach of every cattleman. When the heifers on these ranches were kept on hay in the feed lot until after calving, instead of being routinely turned to pasture in the spring, they had very little trouble in delivering their calves. If similar results can be secured in other sections, they can be taken as pretty definite proof that first-calf heifer calving troubles can be largely prevented by keeping the heifers on a ration of good hay until after freshening.

3. Eliminate blood lines that carry a trait for a small pelvic inlet or "birth canal" from the herd. The advisability of such a program was demonstrated at the Fort Robinson Beef Cattle Research Station. Workers determined that the size of the pelvic opening varied considerably, ranging from 190 to 360 square centimeters. They advanced the opinion that the size of the calf might have little to do with delivery trouble, since even a small calf would not have sufficient room for passage through one of these extremely narrow pelvic inlets. The workers noted that certain blood lines showed a tendency to continue this undesirable feature.

4. Breed heifers of the dairy breeds to Angus bulls. In our own dairy practice we have never hesitated to recommend this type of mating. The Angus-cross calves are considerably smaller than other calves. A shorter gestation period may also be favorable. The average gestation period for the Angus is reported as being ten days less than that of the Hereford, and about five days less for cross-breds.

5. Breed heifers to yearling bulls. A review of calving records over a period of several years has definitely indicated that calves from older bulls are larger than those from yearling bulls. This has been found regardless of the age of the dams.

How Much Service for Bulls?

Bulls vary greatly in regard to their capacity for breeding, so it is impossible to prescribe an exact number of services for each individual animal. However, there are certain limits within which bulls can be used with little risk of making them sterile through over-use. To be safe, you may want to follow these rules:

1. Bulls under a year old should never be put in service.
2. Bulls should not be allowed to run loose with cows; instead, services should be restricted to a single leap.
3. Services should be distributed throughout the year as evenly as possible.
4. Under such conditions, bulls between one and two years old may be used on 10 to 15 cows per year.
5. Bulls between two and three years old may be used on 20 to 25 cows per year.
6. Bulls between three and four years old may be used on 30 to 35 cows per year.
7. Bulls over four years old may be used on 40 to 50 cows per year.

Telling Age by Teeth

The age of cattle can be closely estimated by examining the eight front teeth which are all in the lower jaw. Calves are born with two or more "baby" teeth, and within the first month all eight of the first teeth usually have appeared.

At about two years of age the center pair of "baby" teeth are crowded out by a bigger permanent pair. At three years another permanent tooth usually crowds out the one on each side of the central pair, making a total of four. In another year an additional permanent tooth appears on each side of the last pair to make six, and by five years the last pair of baby teeth has been crowded out on the corners to give the animal a full set of eight permanent teeth.

After that, age is estimated by the wear and general appearance of the teeth. At six years the central pair of teeth is likely to be worn level, both pairs next to them are partly leveled, and the corner teeth show only a little wear. This is what would be expected, considering the different periods the respective pairs have been used. Differences in wear are noticeable until about ten years of

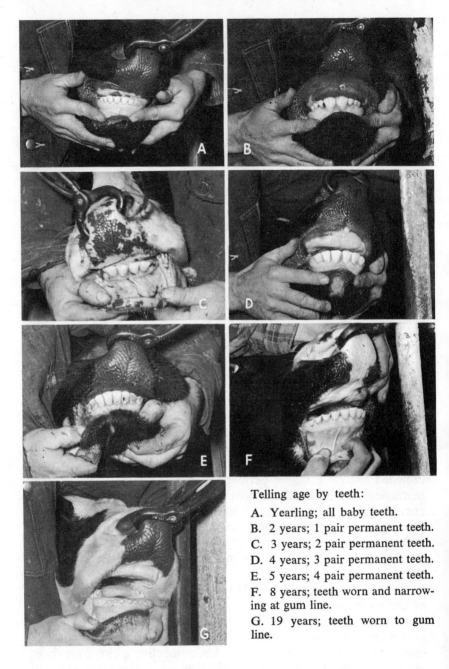

Telling age by teeth:

A. Yearling; all baby teeth.

B. 2 years; 1 pair permanent teeth.

C. 3 years; 2 pair permanent teeth.

D. 4 years; 3 pair permanent teeth.

E. 5 years; 4 pair permanent teeth.

F. 8 years; teeth worn and narrowing at gum line.

G. 19 years; teeth worn to gum line.

age, when all of the teeth are considerably worn down. The arrangement of teeth in the jaw gradually changes, too. At first they form an arc or horseshoe pattern in the mouth, but with age they assume more and more of a straight line. Since the crowns of the teeth are the biggest, the teeth become smaller and further apart as they grow out and become worn down to the narrow roots. This accounts for their pinched appearance at the gums which often causes them to be called "peg teeth."

What Horns Tell

The rings on a cow's horns will tell her age, but they don't always tell the truth. On the other hand, they are pretty dependable records of past breeding efficiency. This is because a cow's horns naturally grow thicker and heavier for some time before and after calving, this being the actual reason why the rings appear. If a cow has a calf every year, the rings will come pretty close to telling how old she is. However, they are reliable only when evenly spaced, since a cow may go more than a year between calvings. When spaces between rings are uneven and show wide differences, it's a pretty safe bet that the cow has experienced considerable breeding trouble and is apt to do so again. You'd better be careful about buying such animals.

Drying Off Cows

There are three generally recognized methods of "drying off" cows, with the so-called "intermittent milking" probably being the commonest one. Under this system the cow is milked with increasing intervals between milkings as long as necessary. Thus she may be milked once a day for a while, then every other day for a while, and then every third or fourth or fifth day until she finally goes dry.

A second is the so-called "incomplete milking" method which consists of leaving about half the milk in the udder at milking time. This system is usually combined with intermittent milking in one form or another.

Under the third method, milking is simply stopped. The cow is milked completely dry one last time, the udder and teats are carefully washed and dried, and that's all there is to it. As a safety measure a dab of collodion can be applied to the end of each teat. This dries in a few seconds, leaving a protective film over the openings to effectively seal off the udder against bacterial invasion.

We personally feel that this last method is the best for cows that have sound and healthy udders. The udder will probably fill up and appear hard and swollen for a few days, but back pressure in the organ will soon stop the secretion of milk. The average udder will then gradually become flabby to appear completely empty and dry within a couple of weeks' time. In addition to saving time and bother over the other two methods of drying off cows, there's no "bad" milk to take care of in some way or another while the job is being done. This method has repeatedly been demonstrated as being safe, even when cows are producing up to 20 pounds of milk daily. Experiments have also shown that it has no effect on bacteria count, test, or amount of milk produced during a cow's next lactation period. However, the method isn't recommended for animals with bad or diseased udders.

Whatever method is used for drying off cows, animals shouldn't be abused by taking away part of their feed or water, since such a practice really defeats the purpose of the dry period. Starvation not only keeps a cow from laying up stores of body reserves, but it causes her to draw on the few that remain after months of heavy milk production. It is doubtful if the practice is ever really necessary, anyway.

It is sometimes a good idea to take away a cow's grain for a few days and to shut her up in a box stall where she can't steal from her neighbors. However, she should be allowed plenty of good quality roughage and given all the water she wants. Whenever she is dry the grain feeding can be resumed.

Taking Care of the Pregnant Cow

A dry period is probably the most important requirement for a pregnant cow. Such an interval of rest will allow the animal to store up body reserves of fat, minerals, protein, and vitamins so she can milk well after calving. The amount of those reserves is pretty apt to be in direct proportion to the length of the cow's vacation, but if a dairyman is to make any money he has to set some kind of a limit on the length of time his cows can stand dry. This should be determined by the physical condition of the animals.

The average good cow will need a six-weeks' vacation. However, hard-working animals that have milked themselves down to skin and bones will need a longer one of up to ten weeks or even more. A cow thin at freshening time certainly isn't going to milk at her full capability. By way of contrast, those that have a suitably long dry period so they're in good rig at calving time will generally pay owners well for giving them a little time off.

Next to a dry period, the matter of feeding is quite important for the pregnant cow. During the winter a suitable ration consists of silage, good legume hay, and grain. Silage isn't available on all farms, and may be replaced with root crops or even omitted entirely with no particular harm to dry cows. The story is considerably different in regard to supplying legume hay and grain.

Legumes are especially important because they represent the best source of vitamin D among the farm feeds. They furnish plenty of other things, too, but vitamin D is the one that makes possible the use of phosphorus and calcium to replace what was lost in making milk during the previous lactation. Most authorities agree that pregnant cows should get all of such roughage they will eat without waste. Cows on good pasture probably won't need any other feed, but grain is often needed for supplying protein during the dry period.

The percentage of protein a grain ration should contain is dependent on the type and quality of roughage being fed. When good legume hay is fed alone, cows will get along pretty well on a half and half mixture of ground oats and corn or barley. When the good hay is partly replaced by silage or corn fodder, a 12 per cent grain ration is recommended. If poor quality roughages are fed, the grain ration should contain at least 16 per cent protein, and possibly even more. A good ration for feeding with poor roughage can be made by mixing equal parts of bran, linseed meal, ground oats, and ground corn or barley.

The amount of grain actually needed will depend on the cows themselves. Those in good condition at drying off time will usually do all right on two to four pounds of grain daily, while thin ones may need 8 or 10 or even 12 pounds per day. There's no infallible rule, so owners will have to use their eyes and good judgment in regard to how much grain their dry cows should get. A good idea calls for feeding the animals so they gain steadily all through the dry period without being actually fat at calving time.

Besides adequate grain and roughage, pregnant cows will need salt and probably some minerals, too. Some owners mix both compounds with the regular grain ration, but this may not be enough for some cows. Consequently, it's usually a good idea to supply the salt and minerals free-choice in separate boxes so animals can help themselves to whichever they like. If salt is furnished alone, it should be of the trace-mineralized variety to prevent any possible deficiencies of such elements.

Taking Care of the "Fresh" Cow

A recently "fresh" cow should be blanketed whenever possible. One that has just given birth to a calf has used up considerable energy in the process. Since energy is little more than another word for heat, she may be a bit chilly afterward, particularly if the blessed event has occurred in the middle of a cold winter night. With possible chilling in mind, it's also a good idea to furnish the cow with a warm bran mash as soon as possible after calving. Besides supplying heat, the bran will also act as a mild laxative and furnish easily digestible nutrients at a time when they may be badly needed. Since dry bran is fairly bulky, four or five pounds will make a pretty big meal even when it's mixed with water to make a fairly thick "soup." The water should be quite hot when added, since it will cool considerably when stirred into the bran. A watertight basket or big pail makes a good mixing bowl, and the cow can eat out of such a container, too. When bran isn't available the cow should be given all the warm water she'll drink.

There are two reasons why this procedure is recommended. First of all there's the matter of heat as mentioned before. A fresh cow is usually thirsty and will drink water if she has a chance. However, cold water will require warming to body temperature and this will use up precious body heat so the cow may be left cold and shivering. On the other hand, warm water may be a few degrees above body temperature and even replace a few calories that were lost at calving time.

Then there's an angle concerned with space, for a certain amount of shock is likely to follow the sudden removal of 60 to 90 pounds or more from the inside of a cow. We've always contended that a few gallons of warm water inside a fresh cow helps a little to lessen shock by partly filling that space recently vacated by the calf. Right or wrong, most fresh cows seem to feel better if they get the warm water shortly after calving, so it certainly doesn't do them any harm.

The next thing to consider is the matter of milking. When the udder is healthy we favor the part-milking plan, with the cow not being milked entirely dry for three days after calving. This procedure has two points to recommend it. In spite of what some of the experts say, we contend that milk fever attacks may be invited when high-producing cows are milked completely dry shortly after calving, so we've always advised against it. Secondly, there's a good chance that incomplete milking serves to discourage milk production a little. This is desirable because a fresh cow is best considered as a sick cow, and we don't like the idea of putting her to work right away after calving. Accordingly, we favor anything that will help bring her gradually into full milk production.

During the three-day period of incomplete milking it is best to feed the cow a light, bulky, laxative diet. Bran is good from this standpoint, and a little molasses may be added to advantage. The animal can have all the good quality hay she wants, but it's wise to feed silage and grain rather lightly for a while. A couple of pounds of grain and 10 or 12 pounds of silage daily is plenty for the first week after calving. When the week is up the diet can be gradually changed and increased until the cow is eventually on "full feed" and milking at her normal level of production.

Pregnancy Diagnosis

Pregnancy in the cow is most commonly determined by "bumping" a calf in the right flank, but the animal is usually six or seven months "along" before this can be done. A pregnancy diagnosis can be made much earlier by feeling the genital organs through the wall of the rectum. We suggest a review of the anatomy of the genital tract as given under the heading of Reproductive Troubles.

The hand may then be lubricated with soap and inserted in the rectum, but it may be necessary to remove considerable manure before the reproductive organs can be felt. In case the rectum is "ballooned" with air and made so hard that exploration is impossible, the hand is held motionless until relaxation occurs. Feeling along the lower wall of the rectum will eventually result in finding the uterus and ovaries.

Pregnancy diagnosis primarily depends on feeling the calf or a uterus enlarged with fluid. Unless twins are being carried, one horn of the uterus is generally larger than the other. The ovary on the same side carries a growth that is known as a "yellow body" or corpus luteum of pregnancy. The uterine arteries of the pregnant horn are also larger and have a stronger pulsation than those on the other side. All of these indications are apt to change and become more apparent as pregnancy advances. For example, a calf at thirty days is a vesicle little larger than the end joint of a finger, while at three months it is as large as a rat and surrounded with fluid which makes it seem much larger in the uterus. Along the same line, an artery little larger than a knitting needle on the thirtieth day of pregnancy may be as big as a lead pencil when the uterus contains a ninety-day calf.

Practice and experience are the only things that will qualify a man to make accurate pregnancy examinations, for mistakes are easily made by the beginner. An accumulation of pus or some kind of a tumor may enlarge a uterus. Uterine arteries may increase in size and pulsation because of infection in the genital tract. A corpus luteum may persist on an ovary because of a mummified calf in the uterus or some kind of a hormone deficiency. The sense of touch must be developed so the abnormal can be told from the normal, and plenty of practice affords the only way of doing it. At the present time there is no satisfactory way of diagnosing pregnancy in the cow by means of urine tests

It is possible to diagnose pregnancy definitely as early as the twenty-sixth day by using the method described by Wisnicky and Casida of Wisconsin in 1954 (Paper at the Wisconsin Veterinary Medical Association annual meeting.) This consists of feeling the uterine horns with the thumb and forefinger for the amnionic vesicle. It will slip away as it is palpated, and this "slipping action" is enough for a positive diagnosis of pregnancy. Although there are exceptions, the amnionic vesicle is usually located in the uterine horn on the same side as the ovary carrying the corpus luteum of pregnancy.

Delivering Calves

The first thing to do is to make sure that the calf is coming in the correct position. This is done by disinfecting the hand and arm, lubricating it with oil, and inserting it in the vagina. Regardless of which end is coming first, a calf should come through the birth canal on its belly. This is primarily because the canal is shaped like a keystone, and is wider at the top than the bottom just like a calf's body. A little later on another reason will be given for delivering calves on their bellies. Anyway, any that are coming upside down or on their sides are best turned before attempting delivery or both cow and calf may be seriously injured. With the body in proper position, both legs are brought straight out, regardless of which end is coming first. If front feet come first, the head must be turned so that it rests squarely on top of them. Sometimes the feet must be pushed back inside the cow before the head can be brought into proper position. With everything in order, ropes or obstetrical chains can be attached to the pasterns of the presented feet. Calves that have become dry can be delivered easier if they are thoroughly greased with mineral oil or unsalted lard. If plenty of help is available the calf may be "pulled" by hand,

and if not a wire stretcher or block and tackle may be used for the purpose. In either case pulling is best done only when the cow strains and should be down and under in the direction of the dam's heels. This particular direction of pull is important, since calves lying on their bellies are delivered in a sort of arc that is made possible by the natural bending of the back. Pulling toward the heels completes the arc and helps to deliver the calf in a natural fashion. This fact further explains why it is desirable for a calf to come belly-down, for delivery in any other position doesn't permit bending of the body in the right direction.

It must be realized that all calves can't be delivered through the vagina by simply applying enough power. Sometimes they are simply too big for passage through the birth canal. At other times they may be hopelessly twisted, deformed, or twins grown together in Siamese fashion. In such cases the calves must either be cut up and delivered in pieces or in entirety by means of a caesarean operation. Jobs of this kind are best left to a veterinarian who has the skill and instruments to get the calf without killing the dam.

Getting a Urine Sample from Cows

Dairymen often need urine samples from cows in order to test the animals for acetonemia. Urination can usually be induced by taking a handful of straw and briskly rubbing the skin with it a short distance below the vulva. If this doesn't work, a cupful of warm water may be allowed to trickle down over the vulva before rubbing is repeated. Urine can be collected only when there is some in the bladder, of course, so the best time to get it is after a cow has been lying down and undisturbed for an hour or so. If a sample isn't collected within a short time, the cow is best left completely alone for a few minutes and then tried again.

Transplanting Cuds

It's a fairly easy job to take a cud from one cow and give it to another. An animal that is chewing its cud is approached from the right side, the left knee is placed under the jaw, and the left arm is laid over her nose so the fingers can be stuck in the side of her mouth. If done quietly, the cow will stop chewing her cud, but won't swallow it. Using the fingers of the left hand to open the mouth, the right hand can be inserted from the front. Swelling will show which cheek the cud is being carried in, and it will be found outside the back teeth at that point. The left hand can be used to prevent biting while the cud is removed with the right.

When giving cuds to other animals, the same approach is used and the mouth opened with the left hand. The right is then used to place the cud well back over the base of the tongue so that it is automatically swallowed by reflex action of throat muscles.

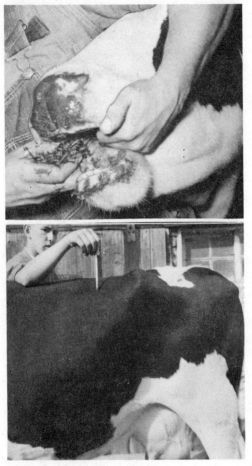

Transplanting a cud.

Correct location to "tap" for bloat.

"Tapping" for Bloat

As a last resort cattle are sometimes "tapped" for bloat. This means puncturing the first stomach to release gas. The correct spot for "tapping" is high up in the left flank about half-way between the hip bone and last rib. If time permits some of this area can be shaved and disinfected before the puncture is made. A trocar and canula are especially made for this job, but an ordinary knife may be used in an emergency. Since the skin is tough, it may be desirable to cut completely through it with a sharp knife as the first step. After that, the trocar or knife should be driven downward and forward in a single powerful stroke to pierce the stomach wall. The resultant wound may take weeks to heal, since the escaping gas can be expected to carry stomach contents with it to cause extensive infection.

Restraint by the Tail

The tail offers an effective means of restraining cattle while teats are being removed, castration performed, sore teats treated, or other things done that may encourage kicking. The job is done by raising the tail straight in the air with one hand so that it can be grasped near the base with the other. Forcing it toward the animal's head has a restraining effect because the feet can't be raised for kicking without hurting the back.

Removing Extra Teats

Extra teats are best removed when heifers are six to eight months old. The job is most easily done by putting the animals in stanchions and applying tail restraint as just described. After pulling out a bit on the ends, extra teats can then be snipped off close to the udder with a pair of heavy scissors. The resultant wounds can be daubed with iodine to prevent infection and healing usually occurs in a few days.

Extra teats can be removed bloodlessly by placing rubber bands around them close up against the udder. They will drop off in a week or ten days leaving a completely healed wound behind them.

Breaking the Self-Sucking Habit

No single method can be expected to break all cows of self-sucking, but those given here have all been effective at times and one of them may work on your particular cow.

An old one consists of fastening a double wire or longitudinally divided metal bit in the cow's mouth. In a few days she is supposed to become used to the bit and be able to eat while being prevented from sucking herself. Instead of the double or divided bit, a single large hollow one may be used. Such a bit should have a fair-sized slot in the middle that extends clear through and connects with the hollow interior. A similar one can be made by boring several holes in a length of quarter-inch pipe. Theoretically, such bits cause the cow to suck air when she tries to milk herself.

They require daily cleaning to keep them from being plugged and changed into solid round bits.

Different kinds of harnesses have also been used to break the self-sucking habit. One consists of a web belt with a ring in it, a halter, and a strong stick about four feet long. The belt goes around the cow just back of the shoulders, with the ring placed on the bottom of the chest. One end of the stick is fastened to this ring and the other is attached to the halter, leaving the stick

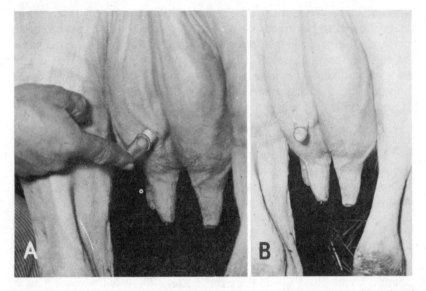

Removing extra teats: A. Half-ounce gelatin capsule carrying rubber band is being slipped over unwanted teat. B. Capsule is withdrawn leaving rubber band in place so teat will drop off in about ten days.

between the front legs. Such an arrangement makes it hard for the cow to get her head around to the udder for sucking.

Another device consists of two hoops of wood or metal, one resting on the shoulders like a horse collar and the other fitted around the body back of the shoulders. The hoops are connected with a straight piece of wood on each side of the neck, and this is also designed to keep a cow from turning her head.

A modification consists of two double wire hoops, one of which is fitted around the neck just back of the jaws and the other larger one just in front of the shoulders. Several straight pieces of wood are used to connect the hoops, and the cow's neck is then surrounded by what looks like a cut-off cone made out of snow fence that is supposed to prevent turning of the head.

Sticks, wires, and bull rings are also frequently placed in the noses of animals to break the self-sucking habit. These may be used alone or serve as hangers for additional rings, sections of metal, strips of leather, lengths of board, or pieces of chain that hang

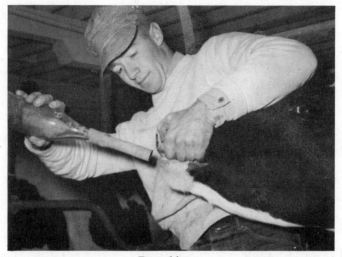

Drenching.

down over the mouth. A ring with a piece of chain attached to it can also be used to break animals of jumping over electric fences as mentioned under the heading, "Breaking Fence Jumpers." Sometimes nails or sharp pieces of metal are welded to rings so that the udder is jabbed whenever sucking is attempted. In addition to home-made devices, a great many different kinds of factory made muzzles are available on the market for preventing self-sucking.

A rather brutal practice consists of setting hog rings in the under side of the tongue to prevent its being cupped around teats for sucking. Two rings are ordinarily used, with one being set just in front of the "string" under the tongue and the other a little closer to the tip of the tongue. If the rings are set too deeply they will slough out before they have had a chance to do much good.

"Drenching" Cattle

Pouring liquids down the throats of animals is a practice known as "drenching." It must be done carefully or part of the liquid may go down into the lungs to cause gangrene and death. Oil is particularly dangerous, since it won't evaporate like water when it goes in the wrong place. To minimize danger, the following suggestions are given for drenching cattle:

1. Elevate the nose until it forms a straight line with the neck.
2. Don't raise the head too high for such a position interferes with swallowing.
3. Don't give more than two ounces of liquid at a time.
4. Allow about a minute for swallowing and breathing before giving the next two ounces.
5. Free the head any time coughing starts so that it can be lowered to help the escape of liquid from the lungs.
6. Don't pull the tongue out of the mouth; it needs to be free for swallowing.
7. Hold animals for drenching as described under transplanting cuds in this section.
8. When more than a pint of liquid must be given, allow ten minutes rest between bottles.

Dehorning Cattle

Cattle are best dehorned as calves, and caustic potash is an old favorite for use on animals under three weeks old. The hair is first clipped around the "buttons" and one end of the caustic stick is wrapped in paper or rubber to prevent burning the fingers. The other end is then applied to the buttons with a rotary motion that is continued until bleeding starts. A ring of vaseline is applied around each eye so that the caustic won't run down and cause blindness. The animals are best stanchioned for a couple of hours to prevent scratching and rubbing of the treated horns. Caustic potash won't work in this manner after horns have broken through the skin and are pretty well hardened. However, a satisfactory job can be done if the tips of such horns are cut off with a knife and the caustic applied to the cut surfaces. Numerous commercial pastes and liquids are now available on the market for dehorning calves, too.

Calves that have become too old for chemical dehorning may be dehorned with heat. Irons may be heated in a fire, or an electrical device can be used. In either case, specially shaped cups are fitted over the horns and kept there for a few seconds until a copper-colored ring has been burned around the base of the horns.

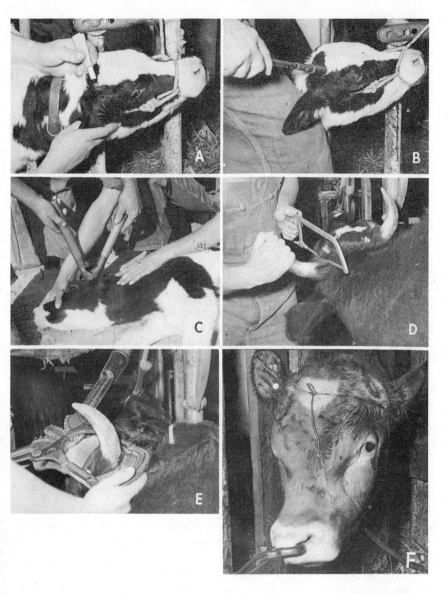

Dehorning cattle: A. With caustic potash stick. B. With electric dehorner.
C. With "gouge." D. With saw. E. With clippers. F. String tied tourniquet-
fashion around head below cuts to prevent bleeding after dehorning.

They will then drop off a month or so later without any bloodshed and will leave a completely healed wound. Various types of gouges and scoops are also available for removing horns from calves that have grown too old for chemical dehorning.

The horns of animals over six months old should be removed with clippers or a saw, the animals first being tied up securely so that work can be done fast and accurately. Horns should always be cut low enough so that an inch-wide collar of hair comes off with each horn. Otherwise "scur" horns are likely to grow out a year or so later. When cut low enough, bleeding can be controlled by grasping spurting vessels with forceps and either pulling them out or twisting them off. If arteries can't be removed, bleeding can often be stopped by tying binder twine tightly around the poll just below the dehorning wounds. Such strings can't be safely left on for more than a couple of hours at a time, since they cut off circulation of blood in the top of the head.

Strings can also be used to accomplish what is practically bloodless dehorning. The animal's head is first fastened and a strong piece of cord or twine about eight inches long is laid across the poll so it extends well down between the eyes. A running noose is made in one end of a second cord that is about two feet long, and the loop is slipped over the horns so it encircles the poll and lays on top of the first cord. The loop is worked down until it fits snugly in the groove found under the hair at the base of each horn, after which it is drawn up as tightly as possible and tied. It is tightened even more by tying the first cord around it so the middle part of the loop is drawn together. The second cord then acts as a tourniquet on the arteries that bring blood to the horns and dehorning can be done with little bleeding. Similar results can be obtained by using a strong rubber band around the head below the horns, and some owners have sliced rings off old inner tubes for such a purpose. This method has the disadvantage of preventing the removal of horns at a desirable depth, so "scurs" and stub horns may grow out at a later date.

The use of substances like flour and cobwebs is to be avoided, since they really do little to stop bleeding. On the other hand, they are very likely to cause infection of wounds. While on the subject of infection it should be mentioned that disinfection of instruments between animals is desirable to prevent it as well as the spread of some disease like anaplasmosis. Animals that are kept in barns may have the dehorning wounds covered with cotton or strainer pads to keep dirt and chaff from falling into the exposed sinuses. Cattle that have been fed heavily on sweet clover are poor dehorning risks, since failure of blood to clot may cause animals to bleed to death.

Castrating Bulls

Like dehorning, this job is best done on calves. It is easiest done on standing animals after they have been confined in stanchions and restrained by the tail as described in another part of this section. Some owners prefer to use the so-called "elastrator" and slip a rubber band around the base of the scrotum after the testicles have been forced well down into the end of it. Scrotum and testicles then drop off together a few weeks later, leaving a completely healed wound behind them. Another method consists of cutting off the end of the scrotum with a sharp knife, squeezing out the testicles and in turn cutting them off. A similar method calls for making a cut on each side of the scrotum for removal of the testicles. The Burdizzo pinchers or emasculatomes act on the same principle as the elastrators, since they destroy the testicles without actually

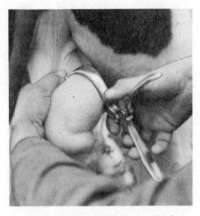

Castrating with Burdizzo pinchers or emasculatomes.

removing them. When the testicles are pulled down into the scrotum, a cord can be felt that leads from each one back up into the body. The pinchers are applied to these cords to crush the contained nerves and blood vessels without breaking the skin over them. When properly done the testicles then shrivel up and completely disappear in a few weeks time. Castration is best done from directly behind the animal for vision is better and danger from kicks is less in that position.

Disinfecting Barns

Disinfection of barns properly begins with a thorough cleaning. Dust and cobwebs should be swept away, manure should be cleaned out, and rotten boards removed and replaced with sound ones. Prolonged soaking with water may be needed before dried and hardened filth can be scraped away. Once cleaned up, all surfaces should be scrubbed with a suitable disinfectant solution. A cheap and efficient one can be made by adding a pound can of lye to every fifteen gallons of scalding hot water. This solution is effective against practically all germs except those of tuberculosis which are covered with a waxy shell to give them special protection These germs will require use of a coal tar disinfectant or one of the newer quaternary ammonium products.

Whitewashing Barns

Once a barn has been cleaned up and disinfected, it may be desirable to whitewash it. Several ready-made whitewash prepara-

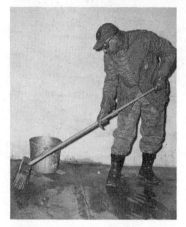

tions are available that require only the addition of water, and they are probably easiest to use. One can be made at home by mixing 50 lbs. of hydrated lime with 8 gallons of boiling water and then adding 6 gallons of boiling water that contains 10 lbs. of ordinary salt and one pound of alum. After thorough stirring of the two mixtures, 5 lbs. of Portland cement is added and mixed in.

When scrubbing with lye solution, rubber gloves, boots, and goggles should be worn.

Whenever whitewash is mixed up at home, a few facts are worth remembering. An ounce of alum or powdered glue added to each gallon of whitewash will help to keep it from rubbing off. A pint of molasses or corn syrup added to every five gallons of whitewash will increase solubility of the lime and permit deeper penetration of wood by the preparation. A pound of soap dissolved in a gallon of hot water and added to every five gallons of whitewash will help to give it a glossy finish. Whitewashing may be done by hand with a brush, but a faster and better job can be accomplished with a power sprayer.

Building Dry Concrete Floors

Concrete floors are often accused of causing pneumonia in calves. This isn't surprising, for the concrete acts like a blotter and allows soil moisture to come up through it to make the floor wet. The University of Arizona offers a suggestion for making the floors safer.

In making the floor, first put down from four to six inches of gravel fill. Then top off the gravel with a mortar coat of cement, using just enough concrete to cover the gravel.

Next lay a single layer of heavy asphalt building paper on top of this thin layer of concrete. Be sure to overlap the edges of the paper, and let it extend up the walls for the thickness of the floor you plan to pour.

Finally, pour the concrete on top of the paper, being careful not to punch any holes in the paper so that moisture can then come on up through the floor. Finish the floor in any preferred manner, and you can depend on it for remaining dry the year around.

Drinking Cups instead of a Tank

An arrangement of drinking cups can sometimes be used to replace a water tank in the barnyard. It is best to set them up against a wall of the barn. A framework of pipe to carry the cups is built first, with the perpendicular pieces being set in concrete to give strength to the structure. A water pipe is brought through the barn wall and the water cups hooked onto the framework and connected with the water pipe in the usual manner. A valve will be needed inside the barn to turn off the water, and a plug in the end of the outside pipe to allow draining so freezing is prevented during the winter months. Although such a structure can be set up anywhere, arrangement along the barn not only makes piping water a little easier, but also minimizes danger of damage to it. The cups can easily be removed for storage when they are not being used. Although units of any size can be used, five cups will furnish drinking space equal to the average tank.

Over a period of years the cups will probably prove better than a tank because of the following advantages:

1. Colder and cleaner water is furnished during the summer.
2. No watching or floats are required to prevent running over and the formation of a mudhole.
3. No supervision is needed to insure a constant supply of water, for the cups never go dry.
4. There is no danger of cattle being shoved into a tank.
5. The tank is eliminated as a drowning hazard for small children.

A Built-In Salt Box

In some cases it will be possible to have a combined salt and mineral box built into the side of a shed or other building which adjoins the barn yard. After cutting a rectangular opening in the wall, it is connected with a good-sized box which is constructed inside the building. A wide board is set in on a slant at the front of the box and raised about an inch and a half at the bottom to provide an outlet on the order of a self-feeder. A narrow board across the front of the opening at the bottom keeps material from being licked out on the ground, and a division through the middle of the box makes it possible to fill it with minerals on one side and

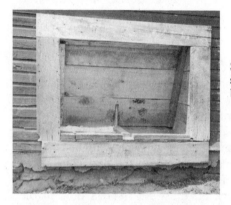

Salt box built in so that supply of salt and minerals can be kept under barn cover.

salt on the other so cattle can eat whichever they like. The box is fitted with a lid which can be closed to keep out barn dust and dirt between fillings. This sort of an arrangement makes it easy to supply salt and minerals while they're protected against the weather at all times to prevent waste.

A Foldaway Barn Table

A writing table in the barn is particularly appreciated by the cow tester at milking time, and it often comes in handy on other occasions, too. A handy one can be built anywhere along a barn wall, with hinges allowing it to be folded up out of the way when it is not in use. Some light boards are cut to a suitable size and mounted on cleats along the top and the two sides. A fourth cleat is nailed to the wall at the desired height, and the boards are fastened to this by means of a hinge at each of the lower corners. A third hinge is fastened at about the middle of the under side of the boards, and the other end of the hinge is fastened to one end of a narrow board that is just long enough to reach the barn wall when the table is dropped down to a convenient writing angle. A cleat is nailed on the barn wall so it furnishes a rest for the free end of the narrow board, thus providing a strong brace for the lower part of the table. The boards can be covered with something like old linoleum so that a smooth writing surface is available. When not in use, the table can simply be raised, folded back against the wall, and held there with a metal hook or wooden button. A more elaborate table can be made by first building a box on the barn wall and then hinging the door at the bottom so it acts as a foldaway table in the same way. This box can be provided with shelves for the storage of herd records, medicines, and equipment like electric clippers.

A Restraint for Drenching

Cattlemen who remember being thrown around while drenching animals may appreciate this method of making the job a little easier. Take a piece of light rope or sash cord about 8 feet long and double it in the middle. Poke the two ends through the resulting loop to form a running noose. Slip this over the animal's upper jaw work it well back in the mouth, and draw tight.

The head can then be raised and fastened in position by tying the ends of the rope to the stanchion top at one side or the other.

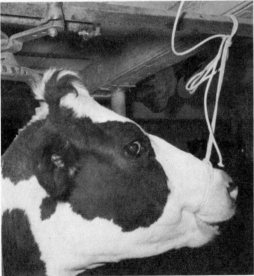

Upper jaw held up by rope, as a help while drenching cattle.

In addition to immobilizing the head, the rope in the cow's mouth causes the cow to keep her mouth open and make constant chewing movements. These help her to swallow medicine with less danger of breathing it down in her lungs.

If one is available, a nose lead can also be used for raising the head and restraining an animal whille it is being drenched.

An Aid in Drenching Cattle

Owners can use either a short piece of rubber hose or an old milking machine inflation to extend an ordinary short-necked bottle while using it for drenching cattle. The added length allows liquids to be placed well back in the mouth so they are sure to be swallowed, and at the same time avoids any danger of the bottle neck being broken off between the back teeth.

An Aid in Reading Tattoos

Owners often find it hard to locate and read tattoo marks of Bang's vaccination and identification, especially in the case of Holsteins, Angus, and other dark-eared cattle. In such cases the tattoo marks can be shown up clearly by holding a flashlight back of the ear, and then examining the ear from the front against the light.

Using Milker Vacuum in Removing Extra Teats

If you have ever used a rubber band to remove extra teats from heifers, you have probably had trouble getting them placed exactly where you wanted them. The vacuum of a milking machine can be used to get around this difficulty. Attach one end of the milking machine air hose to the stall cock. In the other end of the air hose, insert a short piece of glass tubing carrying a rubber band wound fairly tight. Place the end of the glass tube over the extra teat, turn on the vacuum, and allow the teat to be drawn into the tube. The rubber band can then be slipped off at the desired place on the teat. A glass tube is desirable so that the entire teat can be seen during the operation.

Gate to Keep Chickens out of the Barn

Chickens are raised on many dairy farms, and if given a chance they will get into·the cow barn through the summer months. Rather than close the barn with regular doors during hot weather, one can easily be built out of woven wire. It is fitted with a couple of strap iron hangers which have rollers attached to the upper end that fit the regular door track. If the track is extended, this gate can be used to close off the entire driveway, or any part of it, with the regular barn door then being pulled shut to close off the rest of it. When cold weather comes, the gate is rolled off the end of the track and stored away in the machine shed until needed again the next year.

Gate to keep chickens out of barn while allowing for adequate ventilation in summer.

Sacks Prevent Wire-Cut Calves

Most dairymen are aware of the danger when calves are turned outdoors for the first time. Serious injuries are often inflicted when the wildly running calves crash into unfamiliar wire fences which they apparently do not see at all.

A few empty gunny sacks may be hung up on fences to avoid such accidents. Although the wires may escape notice, the sacks are easily seen and running calves will usually veer away from them before it is too late to stop and avoid serious wire cuts.

This procedure is made even more effective by turning the calves out with quiet, older cattle for a few minutes the first time they are freed in a lot. Under such crowded conditions they won't be able to run very far before having to change directions in order to avoid running into other animals. The shorter the run, the less danger there is of a calf crashing into a fence.

When You Buy a Bull

There are at least a dozen things you can do when you go out to buy a bull. You can:

1. Buy him from someone you know pretty well so you get truthful answers to questions. Among other things, you'll want to know: Has the bull been used before? Does he

have any calves in the herd? If previously used, what kind of a conception record does he have? How does he compare in price with other bulls for sale on the farm? Why is there a higher or lower price on him?

2. Buy a proven bull. If you can't afford a proven bull, your next best bet will be the son of a proven bull.

3. Check the bull for physical defects, including blindness. The mouth can be checked for bad teeth and infection. He can be moved about to show up lameness and stiff joints, while the skin can be examined for signs of mange and other troubles. Type should be considered, too, even though you're not interested in showing him. Undesirable traits like a sloping rump and wing shoulders and weak legs can be transmitted in your herd for years by his descendants.

4. Examine his genital organs. Blisters and sores on the penis may be a sign of vaginitis which can be spread to any cow he serves. A crooked penis or growths on it may be due to tumors or ruptured blood vessels. Both testicles should be of the same size, and if they are shrunken or enlarged, injury or dangerous infection may be indicated.

5. Check the production records of female ancestors to see if they are transmitting the things you want from your bull. While on this subject, remember that several records are much better than one.

6. Check the reproductive records of female ancestors to see if there is any tendency to breeding troubles. This is important because fertility or a lack of it are both largely inherited.

7. Check the conception record of the bull if he has been in service. Too many repeat services may indicate sterility or infection with some contagious disease like trichomoniasis.

8. See that the bull can pass tests for Bang's and tuberculosis.

9. Check the health status of the herd he comes from, and play safe by getting him from a herd that is certified as being free of both Bang's and tuberculosis. If it isn't certified, you can find out when the herd was last tested and the results of the test. In addition, you can review the herd history and see if past troubles are suggestive of contagious disease outbreaks that may have left the bull as a dangerous recovered carrier of pinkeye or vibriosis or leptospirosis.

10. Inquire where the bull has been in recent months. If he's been to fairs or shows or sales barns, he may have been exposed to some kind of contagious disease like shipping fever, so he's in the "coming-down" stage at sale time. This can happen even when the herd of origin is above question as a source of infection.
11. Find out whether or not the bull has been protected by vaccination against diseases like blackleg and malignant edema and shipping fever. If so, you can find out if he was injected with bacterin or a serum that gives him protection for a much shorter time.
12. Ask the owner if he'll let you take the bull on trial as a breeder. If not, you can find out if he'll return your money or replace the bull within a reasonable length of time in case the animal proves incapable of settling your cows.

When You Buy a Cow

When you go out to buy a cow there are at least eight things you can do. You can:

1. Get her from some one you know pretty well who can be depended on to answer your questions truthfully. Why is the cow for sale? Is she a kicker or fence jumper? Does she come down with milk fever or acetonemia every year? Does she suffer from recurring mastitis attacks? Does she suck herself or other cows? Was she calfhood-vaccinated against Bang's disease? Then you might ask if you can have your pick of cows in the herd for the price quoted on a certain animal. Most owners have no objection to telling why some of their cows are more valuable than others.
2. Examine her for various physical defects, especially any that involve the feet or udder. You can find out if she has a "light" quarter or if she's a hard milker or a "leaker" from one or more teats. You can feel the udder for lumps of scar tissue that are evidence of damage from past attacks of mastitis. It will pay to look in her mouth to see if she has good teeth, and you'll do well to be alert for symptoms of mange and other skin troubles. It's a good idea to consider type to some extent, too, whether or not you're interested in show possibilities. Undesirable traits like crooked legs and a weak back and a poorly attached udder can be inherited and may be continued in your herd for years by her descendants.

3. Ask for production records, for the best judges can't look at a cow and accurately predict her performance in a milking line or the kind of calves she will produce. Several records are better than a single one, too, and you'd better look for consistent, year-after-year performance as shown by her calves and the herd books. Several records will help in another way, too, for they'll indicate whether or not the cow was bothered with breeding troubles. If she's had a calf approximately once a year, she's settled without much difficulty in the past.

4. Check the reproduction records of her relatives, since fertility or a lack of it are generally regarded as being largely inherited. You can also check on the service record of the bull your cow was bred to the last time. A large number of "repeat" services to him may be a sign that he has had a chance to infect your cow with some contagious disease like trichomoniasis or vibriosis.

5. Be sure that the cow is able to pass a blood test for Bang's disease. Depending on the herd history and location, it may be advisable to test for other ailments like Johne's disease and leptospirosis and tuberculosis. Remember, though, that a clean test doesn't show up possible exposure that may allow a cow to come down with disease weeks or months after you've brought her home.

6. Investigate the health status of the herd she comes from. You'll do well to buy only out of herds that are certified as being free of Bang's and tuberculosis. In addition, you can ask about past outbreaks of diseases like anaplasmosis and pinkeye in the herd which may have left your cow as a dangerous recovered "carrier."

7. Recognize the possibility that your cow may have been exposed somewhere other than the home farm. This is true if she's been away to fairs or shows so she has a chance of being in the "coming-down" stage at sale time. Accordingly, it may be a good idea to ask some questions about recent movements of your prospective purchase.

8. Make sure to what extent the owner will back up his statements regarding the cow. In short, will he return your money within a reasonable time if she doesn't prove to be all he claims she is?

False Teeth for Cattle

This title is a bit misleading, for the "false teeth" are really caps or crowns that are placed over each of the eight front teeth. They are made of stainless steel, a metal which does not tarnish or wear away, and has the faculty of hardening with use. After a period of use, these crowns are reported to develop a strength of 1,000 times that of tooth enamel. They are used to protect badly worn teeth and to prevent excessive wear on normal teeth that may eventually reduce animals to "gummers" and doom them to either starvation or slaughter. Teeth may become badly worn either because they are abnormally soft or because of considerable sand in forage that acts as a grindstone on them.

The teeth of an animal should not be capped until all of the permanent teeth have erupted, and in sandy areas where experience has demonstrated that excessive tooth wear must be expected, the crowns should be applied soon after this time, or at about the sixth year of life. Although the crowns will not make a young animal out of a "gummer," they will extend the useful life of one which already has badly worn teeth. Such teeth may be so sensitive that they can no longer be used for biting and pulling off pasture plants.

The steel crowns are made in ten sizes to fit snugly over all kinds of teeth. The dentistry requires three main steps:

1. Measuring the tooth to determine the proper crown for use.
2. Placing dental cement in the cap to act as an insulator and to hold it in place.
3. Applying the crown to the tooth and crimping it to make it fit exactly.

At the time of this writing the cost of the crowns is estimated at between $15.00 and $20.00 per animal. They can be secured through a Nebraska corporation, called Bovine Crowns, Inc., and are best applied by veterinarians.

Rubber Mats for Dairy Cow Stalls

In recent years many dairymen have turned to rubber mats in their cow stalls as an aid in cutting the cost of bedding. Three different types of these mats are generally recognized.

1. *Foam rubber*. These are 1-1½ inches thick, completely

enclosed in a fabric-reinforced rubber jacket, and at the
time of this writing cost about $78.00 per stall.

2. *Solid all-rubber corrugated mats.* These are made in Holland,
   are ⅝ inch thick, come in 22 different sizes, and cost from
   $24.00 to $35.00 each.

3. *Corrugated hard rubber mats.* These are ¼-½ inch thick
   and are made from reclaimed rubber. They come in 13
   different sizes, and sell from $24.00 to $46.00 each. Since
   they contain fiber, they are somewhat harder than all-rubber
   mats.

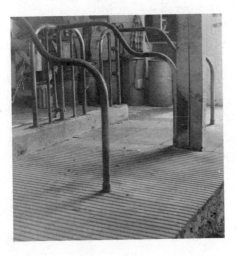

Rubber mats like these may be
both the cheapest and best bedding for dairy cows in stalls.

All of these different types weigh about 100 pounds each and
most of them are furnished with a 10-year guarantee. One user
recommends that owners measure each of their cow stalls before
buying mats, for three or four different sizes may be needed in a
barn where all of the stalls appear to be the same size. Ordering the
proper size will eliminate the need for trimming, and will of course
save money.

Although the initial cost is high, savings on bedding over a 10-
year period may actually make the mats a bargain. For example,
with bedding at $20.00 per ton and allowing a ton of bedding
annually per cow, the yearly cost of bedding for a 50-cow herd
would be an even $1000.00. At $35.00 per stall, the total cost of
mats for this same herd would be $1750.00. However, allowing
for a life of 10 years, this investment would figure to a yearly cost
of $175.00, or a difference of $825.00 per year in favor of the mats.

This figure is slightly misleading, for the mats can't be expected to completely replace bedding. Most owners find it desirable to keep a liberal sprinkling of straw in the gutter to absorb urine and prevent splashing of tails by cows. Even when this is done, it will still be possible to save about two-thirds of the bedding formerly used. Owners will also save the time spent in spreading and shaking up bedding, and will find the stalls easier to keep clean. Other advantages that have been claimed include less mastitis, less slipping, and the prevention of swollen hocks and knees caused by bruising on concrete floors.

How to Trim the Hoofs of Cattle

The hoofs of cattle often grow out too long when they are stabled or running on soft ground. These overlong hoofs can cause trouble in two different ways. First, they can break off and tear down into the sensitive underlying soft tissues to pave the way for foot rot and other infections. Second, they can cause lameness because they place an abnormal strain on tendons and ligaments and muscles when feet are tipped back so animals are forced to walk almost on their fetlocks.

In addition to growing out too long in front, hoofs may become abnormal on the bottom. Sometimes the sole merely becomes so thick that the animal walks on "rockers" instead of flatfooted in a normal manner. In other cases the sole remains practically normal, but the outside edges of the hoof grow in and fold over, much like an ingrown toenail in human beings. These outer edges really support the foot, and under normal conditions wear down about as fast as they grow out. If they continue to grow, the weight of the animal tends to force the edges inward so that they fold over the bottom of the foot. The sole isn't bothered much because it is hard enough to withstand considerable gouging. Instead, the bulbs of the heel are affected, which are normally high enough so there is little pressure on them when animals stand and walk. If the toes also happen to be overlong, the feet are tipped backward to put even more weight on the bulbs. These bulbs are quite sensitive, and pressure on them causes considerable pain and swelling. In addition, the folded hoof edges form a catch-basin for filth which then serves as a good living place for bacteria that can cause infection after hoof edges have cut into the heel bulbs.

Methods of restraining animals for hoof trimming vary considerably, and some owners have specially built chutes for such work. Others prefer to cast animals and tie them up before touching the feet, and still others put the animals in stanchions and then raise the feet with ropes, as described elsewhere in this book. Regardless of the method used to expose the bottom of the foot, hoof trimming should always be considered a two-men job, with one man helping to hold the foot in the desired position while the other does the actual trimming.

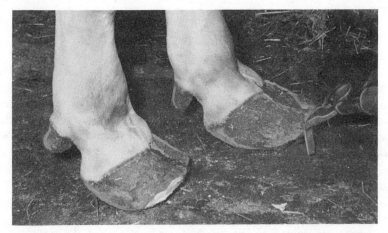

One hoof has been trimmed; trimmers are in place on other hoof.

It sometimes happens that hoof edges turn in so badly that the entire sole is covered, and a bad hoof may have to be examined pretty closely before trimming can be started. After the edges of the overlapping hoof walls are located, they can be carefully cut away while making sure that the sole of the foot and bulbs of the heel aren't injured. When these walls have been trimmed off, the bottom of the hoof may need to be pared away so that the foot sets squarely on the ground with no turned-up "sled runner" appearance in front.

Regular long-handled hoof trimmers can generally be used to cut back hoofs that have grown out too long, but hoofs are sometimes so hard and thick and misshapen that they almost resemble "club" feet. These problem hoofs are usually seen on cattle that have been "foundered" at some time or other, but some blood lines seem to carry an inherited tendency toward them. The trimmers are entirely useless on such feet, and so is a knife. Instead of these instruments, an ordinary hand saw can be used.

The animal is first tied or stanchioned, and the foot to be trimmed is placed on a short length of plank. The toe of a hoof is sawed off at the desired angle, and the process is then repeated on the other hoof. The plank serves two purposes, for it raises the hoof to make sawing easier at the same time that it prevents sawing into the floor. When animals are confined in stanchions, the manger curb may interfere with sawing on the front feet. In such cases one end of the plank can be placed on the curb. Most animals will require no restraint, for the sawing is painless unless the cut is made too far back in the hoof. If necessary, the head can be drawn to one side with a nose lead, or an anti-kicking device can be applied to the lumbar region of the back.

Regardless of how the hoofs are trimmed down, they should be cut down until the two halves of each foot balance each other in size and shape. No definite rule can be given in regard to how much should be trimmed off the toes and sides, since cattle vary considerably in foot structure. To be on the safe side, only a little should be taken off at a time. Evidence of pain or the appearance of blood are indications that cutting has been too deep, and this knowledge can then be used in trimming the other hoofs, for they will all be pretty much the same on a single animal.

Although hoof trimmers can be used to do a great deal of the heaviest trimming, a hoof knife will be desirable for finishing off the sole and edges. These are made in both right and left-handed styles, and one of each will be found handy. Otherwise, an owner will have to be ambidextrous in order to get good results with a hoof knife on all four feet. We also recommend wearing heavy canvas gloves while trimming, for those sharp hoof edges can easily injure hands if a knife slips or an animal kicks at the wrong time.

How to Feed Milk to Calves

Most authorities believe that milk should be fed to calves at a near-body temperature (100 degrees), and at regular intervals. They also believe that Jersey and Guernsey milk should be diluted because milk from these breeds may be so high in butterfat that it may cause indigestion and scouring. However, research work at the University of Arkansas casts a great deal of doubt on these beliefs.

The matter of temperature was tested by feeding 5.4% Jersey milk to Jersey and Holstein calves between 14 and 42 days of age, at the rate of 10 pounds per cwt. daily for the first week, 12 pounds per cwt. the second week, and 14 pounds per cwt. the third and fourth weeks. One half of the calves were fed cold milk (about 50 degrees) as it would come from the cooler, and the others were fed milk at about body temperature. The milk seemed to be liked equally well, both groups gained at the same rate, no deaths occurred, and there was no scouring. Another group of calves less than two weeks old were also fed the cold milk with no apparent bad effects. In spite of these results it would seem advisable to feed warm milk during extremely cold weather or to young, weak, or sickly calves. Otherwise, badly-needed body heat will be used to warm the cold milk after it is swallowed.

The matter of feeding at regular intervals was tested in connection with feeding milk at varying temperatures, for it is sometimes believed that the temperature of milk fed to calves is not so important as feeding it at the same temperature and at the same time every day. Five calves between 4 and 14 days of age were fed with both the milk temperatures and feeding times varying constantly, while others were fed warm milk at regular times. Milk for the test calves ranged from 50 to 100 degrees, was fed at haphazard times, and several feedings were omitted completely. At the end of the test period, the mismanaged calves were just as healthy as the well-managed ones.

The matter of dilution was tested by diluting the milk at the rate of 1 to 3, or 25% water and 75% milk. This test was varied a little by giving half the calves warm milk, and giving the others cold milk. The dilution of warm milk resulted in much poorer gains than feeding undiluted milk, while gains were unaffected by diluting cold milk. The entire experiment was summarized as follows:

1. Warm milk (100 degrees) was as good or better than other temperatures of milk tested for feeding young calves.
2. Cold milk (50 degrees) was equal to warm milk for calves 14 to 42 days old.
3. Feeding cold milk or diluted cold milk had no apparent bad effects on the calves, so it might be fed during warm seasons if more convenient to use.
4. Feeding cold milk to younger calves merits more study, but it appears unwise to feed it to weak or sickly young calves, or to calves of any age during spells of extremely cold weather.
5. Feeding at regular intervals did not appear to be too im-

portant, and neither did feeding the milk at a constant temperature. Omitting feedings is not recommended, but otherwise
calves can be fed according to the convenience of the owner.
6. Dilution of warm milk reduced gains, so it cannot be recommended on the basis of this work.
7. Dilution of cold milk did not reduce gains, so it may be
practiced if desired.

How to Feed Milk Replacers to Calves

Feeding trials at the University of Illinois showed that dairy
calves receiving whole milk until they were at least two months old
outgained calves started on the recommended level of milk replacer
at five days of age. This isn't too surprising, for milk is a natural
food, and milk replacer shouldn't be expected to replace it entirely
for calf-raising.

In a series of tests, calves on milk replacers gained best when
fed whole milk for the first ten days, whole milk and replacer from
the 11th to 14th day, and milk replacer mixed one part to nine parts
of water from two to eight weeks of age.

Calves fed this ration gained 1.15 pounds a day compared with
1.26 pounds daily for calves on whole milk. Calves fed milk replacer
from five days to eight weeks gained less than a pound daily. Figuring whole milk at $3.00 per cwt., total feed costs ran $3.00 to
$4.00 less for calves fed replacer than for calves fed a total of 360
pounds of whole milk during the first eight weeks.

Probably most important of all, the tests demonstrated the importance of mixing replacer correctly. When workers tried mixing a
ration of one part milk replacer to six parts of water, calves
developed serious digestive troubles and gains dropped off.

How to Cull Cows

In the case of dairy cows, production records are usually considered first as a basis for culling. Extensive research has indicated
that no single body measurement or combination of measurements
is likely to be as dependable in predicting a heifer's production as
the production record of her dam, and the records of dams are not
very reliable for predicting the future performance of their daughters,
either. Accordingly, most authorities recommended that very little
culling be done on heifers before they have had a chance to show

what they are going to do in the milking line. On older animals, owners can start a culling program by asking these questions:

1. Have any of the first-calf heifers produced a third or more below the herd average? Such animals seldom warrant a second chance.
2. Have any of the second or third-calf heifers produced well below other heifers of the same age in the herd? They will probably continue to produce well below the average for animals of comparable age.
3. Have any of the mature cows produced less than 125 pounds of butterfat for the first four months of their lactation period? They will probably produce well under 300 pounds for the entire year. Do you want to keep that kind?
4. Are any of the animals going to be dry for more than five months? They will owe quite a feed bill by freshening time.
5. Are all of the cows pregnant that were supposed to be "settled"? A complete herd examination by a veterinarian may be in order to help decide which ones should be kept.
6. Are any of the cows nearing the end of their productive life? Such things as bad teeth and breeding troubles may indicate that certain older animals should be sold.

After these important questions have been answered, an owner can consider questions like the following:

7. Do any animals have undesirable habits, like fence-jumping, sucking themselves or other cows, kicking, stanchion-pulling, periodic "holding up" of milk, or extreme excitability?
8. Do any animals have undesirable physical characteristics, like crooked legs, sway backs, bad feet, weak pasterns, poor udder attachments, or pendulous udders? These may be inherited and continued in a herd for years by descendants.
9. Do any animals show signs of being "chronic bloaters" or frequent evidence of "crampiness" that may indicate the so-called "spastic syndrome"? These characteristics also have a good chance of being passed on to descendants.
10. Do any animals have regular attacks of milk fever, acetonemia, mastitis, kidney infection, or show frequent symptoms of "hardware trouble"?
11. Do any animals have "light" or completely dry quarters?
12. Do any animals leak milk, or are any of them "hard-milkers"?
13. Do any animals have udders which are lumpy with scar tissue which can be palpated with the fingers?

14. Do any animals have a history of retained after-birth, metritis, or other genital infection? Such animals often prove hard to get with calf again.

15. Do any animals have a history of being "shy breeders"? Unless her blood lines dictate otherwise, it is doubtful if it pays to keep a cow that has failed to conceive after five services, or is still "open" a year after her last calving. In addition to being an economic problem, such a cow has a good chance of transmitting her poor breeding qualities to her descendants.

When there is any uncertainty over which cows should be kept, it will probably be a good idea to rate all of the questionable animals on the entire table of points given, and then cull those with the lowest score.

In the case of beef cows, most of the questions asked about dairy animals should still be answered. Milk production can be quite an important factor to consider, even in beef cows. This is because the weaning weight of a beef calf is largely dependent on the amount of milk it has received. Accordingly, cows that wean light-weight calves are probably poor milkers, and might well be considered for removal from a herd. In addition, it will be a good idea to check back on the cows and see if any of them are potential carriers of undesirable inherited characteristics, like chronic bloating. The matter of dwarfism is especially important in beef herds, and any cow that has ever given birth to a dwarf should be culled automatically. Then, too, the matter of whether a beef cow is pregnant at culling time is extremely important, and so is the past record of breeding performance. As a matter of fact, beef heifers can actually be culled on this basis alone to make them different from dairy heifers that usually aren't considered for culling until after at least one lactation.

A beef heifer that doesn't calve as a two-year-old will probably miss dropping another calf in her lifetime. She may do even worse and never have a calf, or prove to be an alternate breeder that drops a calf only every second year. Calves from heifers can be used as a basis for culling, too. Work at the University of Arizona indicates that the first calf will be about 85 per cent accurate as a prediction of future calves. A light-weight first calf will be followed by other light-weights, and at the end of five years heifers dropping heavy calves will have produced about 250 pounds more of beef.

Size may be a factor in culling beef cows, too, for New Mexico work showed that large cows are better in several ways than small animals. Big Herefords stayed in the herd longer than little ones, had better calving records, and weaned more calves. Records showed that they averaged one and a half more calves than small cows during their stay in the herd.

After an owner has settled on the factors he wants to use as a basis for culling, he has to consider the best time for culling. There can be no hard and fast rule on this, especially for dairymen, but it will generally be best to cull in the late summer. There may be some price advantage in selling cull cows at this time before grass cattle get on the market in the fall. They will probably bring more in the spring, but the total maintenance cost can be greatly reduced by the elimination of winter feeding, and this will usually more than make up for a higher price in the spring.

Some beef raisers are participating in a performance testing program as a means of improving their herds, and in this program cows are culled strictly on the basis of their performance, and replacement heifers are selected out of the best producers in the herd. This is unquestionably the best method, but it may prove impractical for the average breeder. With this in mind, a simplified method of culling beef cows recommended by the North Carolina Beef Cattle Improvement Association is based on what kind of a calf is following a cow in July or August. It works as follows:

1. Separate the cows and calves overnight.
2. Examine both groups closely the next morning.
3. If the calves look better on the average than the cows, your bulls are helping.
4. If the cows look better, you should think about changing bulls.
5. Remove any cow that doesn't have a calf and put her in the cull pen.
6. Cull the calves on the basis of comparative size and grade, and turn culls back three or four at a time to find their dams.
7. When a cull calf is matched with its dam, put both in the cull pen.
8. Then go back to the calf pen and select the biggest and typiest heifers and mark them permanently as replacements for the cows being culled.
9. Sell all culls the day they are culled.

2.

FROM THE
VETERINARIAN'S STANDPOINT

The Different Kinds of Diseases

It's a common practice for people to think of diseases according to the body system they affect. Ailments are then listed as respiratory, digestive, genital, urinary, circulatory, muscular, osseous, cutaneous, or nervous troubles. A simpler classification is based on cause, and consists of ten divisions which look like this:

1. *Contagious.* Diseases transmitted directly from one animal to another. Bang's, tuberculosis, foot-and-mouth disease, and blackleg are examples.

2. *Infectious.* Diseases due to a specific organism, but not transmitted directly between animals. Lumpjaw, pyelonephritis, and lockjaw are examples. It is well to remember that all contagious diseases are also infectious, but none of the infectious diseases are usually considered as being contagious.

3. *Parasitic.* Diseases due to different kinds of parasites, such as mange, lungworm pneumonia, stomach worm disease, and lousiness.

4. *Deficiency.* Diseases due to different kinds of nutritional deficiencies. Goiter, rickets, salt sickness, and white muscle disease are examples.

5. *Metabolism.* Diseases due to some kind of an upset in metabolism that affects important body processes. Examples are milk fever, grass tetany, and acetonemia.

6. *Allergic.* Disorders due to an allergic reaction. Light sensitization, summer snuffles, hives, and serum shock are examples.

7. *Poisoning.* Disorders due to eating something that destroys tissues or interferes with normal body activities. Examples are sweet clover disease, lead, and prussic acid poisoning.

57

8. *Injuries.* Damage done by cuts, blows, falls, and other accidents, resulting in broken bones, wire cuts, and hematomas.

9. *Congenital.* Defects due to heredity or improper fetal development. Freemartins, blue baby calves, lethal factors, and monstrosities are examples.

10. *Miscellaneous.* Includes troubles that do not properly belong under any of the other headings, such as leukemia, tumors, eversion of the uterus, etc.

The Prevention of Disease

An extremely wise man once said that an ounce of prevention is worth a pound of cure, even if it doesn't get a man's name in the papers. With this being true, prevention shapes up as a real bargain, for it is the cheapest of all commodities on the farm, and certainly much lower-priced than drugs. In order to use preventive measures, causes must be recognized. As far as cattle are concerned, there are five big causes of disease which are listed in the order of their importance:

1. Exposure to infected animals.
2. Exposure to infected premises.
3. Lack of proper feed.
4. Lack of proper care.
5. Filthy housing and feeding conditions.

There is little question but that exposure to infected animals is the chief cause of disease in cattle. Thousands of beasts change hands daily and under modern conditions they may move hundreds of miles in a single day. Most of them are free of disease, but an occasional one is infected with something like Bang's disease. They may pass inspection even when tests are available, for they may be in the incubation or "coming down" stage and incapable of reacting. When tests aren't available the matter is made worse, for perfectly healthy-looking animals may be "carriers" of disease. An example is furnished by anaplasmosis, a disease that was pretty much confined to the southern states only a few years ago. Nowadays it is recognized as having spread over much of the United States through the movement of infected cattle. Whatever the actual disease, a single purchased animal can often be shown as the source of a bad outbreak. Infected animals are bad business for they make possible a doubling and redoubling of disease that can

cause disaster in a hurry. The original carrier infects one animal
and then there are two carriers. Each infects another and then there
are four. In short order there are eight, then sixteen, then thirty-
two, and so on. No wonder exposure to infected animals is the
biggest cause of disease!

Exposure to infected premises runs a close second in this respect. The selling off of "Bangers" and TB reactors and similar
carriers isn't enough to prevent contagious disease, for the animals
have probably left germs that will be able to infect healthy beasts
that may pick them up. Consequently, a campaign of prevention
calls for disinfection of buildings. Grounds may be infected, too,
but disinfection of the earth isn't too practical a measure. Instead,
manure piles may be moved out of barnyards and rubbish hauled
away so the sunshine has a chance to do a germ-killing job. In the
case of pastures, regular rotation is recommended, particularly for
the control of internal parasites like worms and flukes. If the pastures cannot be rotated, draining and fencing off of stagnant water
holes will help some.

In addition to an actual shortage of foodstuffs, the lack of
feed may mean a deficiency of certain essential minerals and vitamins. Such deficiencies are the sole cause of ailments like rickets,
goiter, "salt sickness," and different kinds of skin troubles. If they
don't actually cause disease, faulty rations may be responsible for
a "run down" condition that lowers the natural resistance of cattle
and so makes them more susceptible to troubles that would ordinarily be warded off.

The same thing is true in regard to lack of proper care, for
faulty management may also pave the way for disease. Pneumonia
often goes along with drafty quarters in a barn, just as shipping
fever may follow exposure to bad weather and exhaustion due to
various causes. Indigestion may result from irregular feeding, mastitis from insufficient bedding, constipation from lack of water, and
so on almost indefinitely.

Filthy housing and feeding conditions promote disease because
a great many kinds of harmful bacteria prefer to live in dark and
dirty surroundings. Calf diphtheria may result from eating out of
dirty feed boxes, and diarrhea from feeding milk out of filthy pails.
Foot rot and lockjaw germs like to be buried in manure. Ringworm
prefers to work on dirty animals kept in dark quarters, and the
same thing is true of lice and mange mites.

With the causes recognized, it's fairly easy to set up a practical
disease prevention program. In a condensed form it looks like this:

1. Avoid exposure to infected animals by:
   a) Buying cattle only from disease-free herds.
   b) Using available tests before buying even then.
   c) Isolating all purchased animals for at least a month after they are brought home.
   d) Refusing to take a chance on sick or suspicious animals that may be carrying dangerous germs.

2. Avoid exposure to infected premises by:
   a) Disinfecting buildings after an outbreak of disease.
   b) Moving manure and rubbish piles to give sunlight a chance to kill germs out-doors.
   c) Rotating pastures to break the life cycles of parasites.
   d) Eliminating wet places around tanks and in pastures.

3. Avoid feed deficiencies by:
   a) Furnishing balanced rations of good quality feeds.
   b) Supplying salt and minerals free-choice in separate boxes.
   c) Considering the extra requirements for growth, pregnancy, and milk production as well as those for maintenance alone.

4. Avoid trouble due to faulty care by:
   a) Eliminating drafts through broken windows, open hay chutes, etc.
   b) Providing shelter against blizzards and bad weather.
   c) Feeding regularly.
   d) Using plenty of bedding.
   e) Seeing that clean fresh water is available at all times.

5. Avoid filthy conditions by:
   a) Removing manure from barns every day.
   b) Installing plenty of windows and lights.
   c) Using clean instruments for dehorning, mastitis treatment, etc.
   d) Sterilizing calf pails after each feeding.
   e) Seeing that feed boxes are kept clean and free of spoiled feed.

When To Call a Veterinarian

It is neither practical nor necessary to call a veterinarian for every little thing that goes wrong with cattle. It is sometimes difficult to decide when help is needed, for animals that appear pretty sick may be fully recovered a short time later. On the other hand, immediate treatment may mean the difference between life and death for an ailing beast. There are exceptions to all rules, of course, but the following are examples of animals that warrant calling a veterinarian in most cases:

1. Those visibly sick and showing body temperatures of 103 and higher.
2. Those having "fits" or showing signs of having "gone crazy."
3. Those that try to freshen with calves in abnormal positions.
4. Those remaining "off feed" for more than 24 hours.
5. Those wobbly on their feet shortly before or after calving.
6. Those that "go down" and are unable to get up again.
7. Those showing signs of bad bloating.
8. Those with a persistent diarrhea.
9. Those losing weight while "eating their heads off."
10. Those showing evidence of having a contagious disease.
11. Those that die suddenly.

In the latter case a veterinarian cannot revive the dead, but he may be helpful in determining the cause of death. There are other times when a veterinarian should be called, but such instances are indicated under treatment of certain troubles. For example, "chronic bullers" or nymphomaniacs may require the attention of a veterinarian so that appropriate hormones can be injected directly into the blood stream. Cows that don't come in heat at all may merit examination by a veterinarian for the sake of discovering the cause. Aside from similar specialized services, the above list will serve as a satisfactory guide in regard to times when a veterinarian should be called for cattle.

The Importance of Diagnosis

A little browsing through this book will show that a great many diseases have one or more of the same symptoms. For example, a bad diarrhea may go along with completely unrelated troubles like poisoning, shipping fever, over-eating, Johne's disease, winter dysentery, stomach worm infestation, metritis, and assorted others. The same thing is true in regard to symptoms like coughing, constipation, loss of appetite, fever, paralysis, and decreased milk flow. As a matter of fact, we do not know of any disease that can be definitely identified by a single specific symptom.

Not so long ago a man asked us for something to "physic" a

cow that was "bound up" and decreasing in milk production. As matters turned out, the cow had acetonemia and. needed sugar instead of a laxative. Another owner killed a sick cow by drenching her with linseed oil. This was to be expected, for she had milk fever and so was unable to swallow. As a result the oil went into her lungs and caused gangrenous pneumonia. Similar instances of incorrect treatment might be given, for they're not at all unusual, and cost owners thousands of dollars every year.

All of which is a reminder that an accurate diagnosis is the first thing that's needed when cattle get sick. Without one, treatment is strictly a matter of guesswork, with remedies being tried blindly in the hope that something will eventually prove effective. Such a procedure is no better than gambling, with money being risked on drugs that may do no good at all. In addition, the life of an animal or the health of an entire herd may be at stake while time is being wasted. Anybody can treat a cow, but a man who is sure of the ailment is the only one who can treat her with the right kind of medicine. If you aren't sure, both you and your animals will be better off if you don't try to treat them. You wouldn't think of calling an M.D. who gave medicine to your family without first making a diagnosis of the ailment involved. Why do such a foolish thing as treating your valuable cattle before you know what ails them?

What Treatment To Use

Once a disease has been definitely diagnosed, an appropriate remedy must be selected. This is sometimes quite a problem, for several choices are often available. We are frequently asked to name the best remedy for certain ailments, but we always have to hedge a bit when answering such requests. This is because there isn't any "best" remedy for most diseases any more than there is a "best" brand of cigarettes or make of automobile or breed of cattle.

Foot rot may be used as an example. When caught early, chlorine, copper sulfate, coal tar disinfectants, butter of antimony, and other agents have been used with success and have their supporters. On the other hand, when infection is deep the germs may be out of reach of surface applications and require the use of something like sodium sulfapyradine solutions given directly into the blood stream.

The same thing is true of calf scours, for which many remedies have their adherents. Vinegar, alum, salol, bismuth, and various commercial preparations have all proven effective under certain conditions. However, calf scours has many different causes, so no one treatment can be expected to cure all cases. This statement is also true of mastitis, in spite of the highly colored claims made for different drugs and mixtures. Regardless of the disease involved, no single treatment will be 100 per cent effective, so there will always be times when accepted remedies won't effect cures.

A half dozen different veterinarians may have a half dozen different treatments for shipping fever that get results for them. Each of these veterinarians would naturally hesitate to change his treatment and gamble on a different one, even though it had been successful for another practitioner. Owners are likely to be the same way, and we don't blame them a bit.

Consequently, if you have a remedy that has worked well on your cattle, you should certainly continue to use it. However, warning should be made against depending on it too much, for it may eventually prove ineffective against a particularly stubborn case. When that time comes, something else should be tried.

If you don't already have an effective remedy, don't criticize your veterinarian because he can't furnish you with one. It may be that his "best" remedy just happens to be ineffective in your particular case in spite of the fact that it has always worked on similar cases for him before. There is also the chance that it is working, but that the animals are continually reinfecting themselves. Finally, it may be that there just isn't any successful treatment for the trouble.

A Home Veterinary Chest

We believe that a veterinary chest is desirable in every barn. It should be protected from dust and kept in an easily accessible place under lock and key. The lock will keep dangerous material away from children and also insure the availability of contents that might be needed in a hurry. Few drugs will be mentioned as needed, since the owner will probably have preferences of his own in regard to medicines. However, even with these left out, there are still quite a few items that are desirable in such a chest. The list includes:

1. Nose lead with rope.
2. Forty-foot lariat.
3. Six feet of ½″ rope.
4. Heavy scissors.
5. Long-handled hoof clippers.
6. Hoof knife.
7. Trocar and canula.

8. Metal dose syringe.
9. Odorless disinfectant.
10. Thermometer.
11. Obstetrical chains.
12. Hot water bottle with syringe attachment.
13. Bailling gun.
14. Drenching bottle.
15. Tincture of iodine.
16. Isopropyl alcohol.
17. Cotton.
18. Adhesive tape.
19. Gauze.
20. Mineral oil.

Symptoms of Sickness

The average cattleman spends most of his time around the herd and so comes to know his animals better than he knows most of his neighbors. As a result he quickly notices any changes like going "off feed" or a sudden drop in milk production or others such as coughing, watering of the eyes, trembling, and peculiar actions. Such things should prompt the checking of pulse, respiration, and temperature, since these body functions sometimes tell a great deal about an ailment and so help in making a diagnosis.

Almost any kind of infection or contagious disease can be expected to increase all three above normal. By way of contrast, disorders of metabolism like milk fever and acetonemia seldom cause any appreciable change. When infection is involved, the amount of deviation will often indicate the severity of an attack and the chances for recovery. The following chart shows the normal range of respiration, pulse, and temperature in healthy cattle:

Pulse	Respiration	Temperature
60-70	15-30	100.5-102.5

The above figures are based on averages and are given only as guides for cattlemen. The pulse is the same as heart beat and the range is for beats per minute. It can be determined by holding a watch and placing an ear against the lower chest just back of the left front leg so the heart beat can be heard. Calves and young animals have a faster pulse than mature stock. The rate is increased by such factors as excitement, hot weather, and exercise.

The respiration rate is that of breathing and the normal range is given in breaths per minute. It can be determined by observation, of course. An increased rate may be due to hot weather, advanced pregnancy, excitement, exercise, and recent feeding.

The temperature range is given in degrees Fahrenheit. It is determined by placing the bulb of a thermometer deep in the rectum and leaving it there about three minutes before a reading is taken.

The "Incubation" Period of Disease

The "incubation" period of disease has been greatly misunderstood. It is often pointed out that the term makes it sound like diseases are hatched like chickens. It may be that the matter isn't so much of a joke, at that.

In one case the germ of an egg is kept warm while a chick develops from it. In the other a germ of disease is nourished while infection develops from it. Emergence of a chick is the end result of the first "incubation" period, while symptoms of disease represent that of the second. Such a developmental period is required for every known disease, for immediate sickness never follows exposure as you might expect bleeding after cutting your finger. Everything considered, the variable time interval represents about the biggest difference between an incubation period for eggs and one for disease.

Chicken eggs require three weeks for hatching; no more, no less. The eggs of other birds have similarly definite incubation periods, but the situation is much different with diseases. They have no regular developmental period, and it may vary widely for the same disease on the same farm at the same time. For example, negative cows can become reactors to the blood test in as little as ten days after exposure to Bang's germs. At the other extreme, there are cases on record where it took several months for a reaction to appear after exposure to infection. To make the matter even more confusing, reactions have appeared at all times between those limits following exposure to the disease. The same sort of thing holds true for most of the other cattle diseases.

A variable incubation period is generally explained by differences in the amount of exposure. A small number of germs that enter the animal once will naturally take longer to multiply and cause symptoms of sickness than will repeated doses of larger numbers. Other factors also have to be considered, including care and feeding and inheritance that govern the natural resistance of animals to disease. In the case of Bang's, at least, the stage of pregnancy at which infection occurs seems capable of influencing the incubation stage of the disease.

The Care of Sick Animals

Regardless of the actual ailment, good nursing is as important as good doctoring, for the best of veterinarians can do little for animals that are neglected between calls. As soon as a cow is noticed as being sick, it's a good idea to get her into a well-bedded box stall that is free from drafts. We personally believe in blanketing sick animals, too, even when they're running abnormal body temperatures. This helps to conserve precious body heat in addition to serving as protection against chilling. In cold weather it will be advisable to warm the drinking water for the same reasons. The regular ration is best replaced by a light laxative diet of warm bran mash and soaked beet pulp combined with small amounts of first quality hay.

If the ailment appears serious, a veterinarian should be called immediately for the purpose of getting appropriate treatment started early. This increases the chances of recovery, since it means that the sick animal will have a little strength and resistance left to help out the medicines that are used.

Keep Things Clean

No matter how much he knows or can do, a man is still a poor veterinarian if he is dirty. This is because dirt means germs and germs mean infection, especially if they are introduced into wounds or delicate tissues. Nor do they always advertise their presence, for hands and instruments can be laden with germs even when they look clean. In order to prevent infection and spreading disease, the following "don'ts" are suggested in relation to veterinary activities:

1. Don't overlook wearing rubber footwear around barns.
2. Don't fail to disinfect them and change clothes after being around sick animals, particularly if there's a chance they have a contagious disease.
3. Don't deliver calves, clean cows, make rectal examinations, etc., without first trimming your fingernails short.
4. Don't do the same things until after you've scrubbed and disinfected your hands and arms.
5. Don't use dirty instruments for dehorning, castration, etc., but keep them clean and disinfect them between animals.
6. Don't fail to boil hypodermic needles, milk tubes, etc., after each use. Simply dropping them into alcohol isn't enough to sterilize them.
7. Don't use them even then without first disinfecting the skin or end of the teat to kill germs in the area.
8. Don't cut the skin for any purpose without first disinfecting around the line of incision.

9. Don't forget to disinfect nose leads, halters, blankets, etc., after they have been used on sick animals. Boil them or soak them for half an hour in an antiseptic solution.

10. Don't fail to scrub and clean up around the vulva before delivering calves, "cleaning" cows, etc.

The Control of Bleeding

It sometimes happens that animals cut themselves and bleed quite badly. Before trying to stop the bleeding, owners should recognize that blood can come from either veins or arteries. That

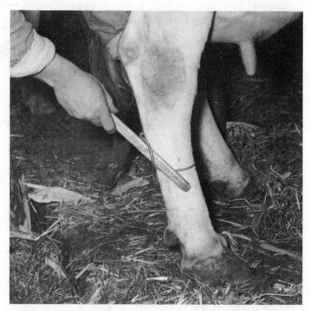

How a tourniquet is placed on a leg to stop bleeding.

from arteries comes in spurts corresponding to beats of the heart, while blood from veins is darker-colored and flows steadily. The control of bleeding after dehorning calls for a special technique that is described under that operation in the Practical Pointers section of this book.

In all other cases, bleeding from either arteries or veins is best stopped by locating the cut vessel and tying it off with a strong thread. A pair of forceps or even ordinary pliers can be used to close the cut end of a vessel in case of an emergency. If the cut is deep and the source of bleeding can't be readily located, a tourniquet can be used to control hemorrhage.

This is nothing more than a rope or cloth that is tightly tied or twisted around a leg to cut off the circulation of blood. If an artery is bleeding, the tourniquet is tied above the wound, for arterial blood comes directly from the heart. Bleeding from a vein calls for tying the tourniquet below a wound, since venous blood is returning to the heart. When a tourniquet is used it must be loosened for a few minutes every hour. Otherwise a complete lack of blood may cause gangrene in an area.

Minor bleeding can often be stopped by packing the wound with sterile cotton or gauze and then pressing it down firmly with

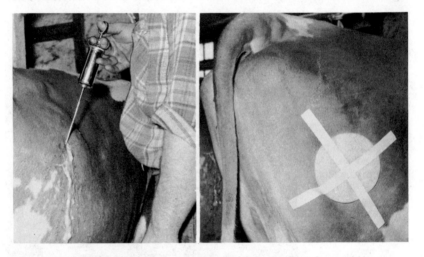

Left: Wounds being washed out with hydrogen of peroxide.
Right: Strainer pad taped in place as protective bandage for a wound.

the fingers. The use of flour, cobwebs, and similar material is not recommended for the control of bleeding since infection may easily result. Anything that isn't sterile may contain germs and be very dangerous for use in wounds.

The Treatment of Wounds

The first step in wound treatment is the control of bleeding just discussed. The second one is designed to prevent infection, and must be considered even when small cuts are involved. Germ-killing is best accomplished through first cleaning the wound with sterile dry cotton and then treating it with something like iodine or mercurochrome. Since water retards healing, its use is generally undesirable in wounds. Hydrogen of peroxide is very good for deep cuts, since its foaming action carries out particles of dirt that might otherwise be sealed in and cause pus formation at a later time. Drainage may be desired in deep wounds and this can be provided by packing the cut with sterile gauze and allowing an end to hang out to serve as a wick.

Several effective salves and ointments are available for promoting wound healing, but one of the very best is the penicillin ointment packaged in tubes for the treatment of mastitis. It is best squeezed out into wounds once a day. Scarlet balsam and thuja ointment are especially good for promoting healing of wounds located on joints or other places where constant movement keeps breaking them open. Whenever possible, it is generally advisable to bandage wounds lightly for protection against dirt that may cause infection.

The location of a wound will often determine whether or not it is to be closed by stitches or metal clips made especially for this purpose. Such treatment is not desirable when cuts are on the legs or in other areas where there is considerable strain on the skin, since tension will generally cause the sutures to tear out. The edges of minor wounds can sometimes be held together with bandages or adhesive tape. When bandages aren't too practical, an application of flexible collodion will serve to seal cuts against contamination. In hot weather it is desirable to swab the wounds with something that will repel flies. Iodoform powder and pine tar are old favorites for this purpose, while Smear 62 and the newer EQ335 are also effective against flies and will kill any maggots that may already be present in wounds.

This Business of Vaccination

Vaccination is a term that is commonly used rather loosely, for it correctly applies only to the injection of vaccine. Instead, it has come to be used for every kind of immunizing agent that is applied with a syringe. This has resulted in considerable confusion regarding the various products used for immunizing cattle against various diseases. Such confusion is regrettable, since there are striking differences in these products, and a lack of understanding may result in the wrong ones being used. In the hope of clearing up this matter a bit, a brief description is given for each of the four common immunizing agents:

Aggressin. Made from the fluid which collects under the skin following the injection of certain germs into animals. It is sterile and has been filtered through porcelain, so it contains no organisms, either living or dead. It was once used rather extensively against blackleg, shipping fever, and anthrax, but it has been largely replaced by other products at the present time. Immunity lasts for about a year, but takes a week or more to develop after the injection of aggressin.

Bacterin, also known as *Anaculture.* A weak salt solution containing killed organisms of the specific disease it is intended to be used against. Immunity lasts for at least a year, but also takes about ten days to develop following the use of bacterin.

Vaccine. A weak salt solution containing either living bacteria or live spores of certain diseases. Immunity is variable according to the vaccine used, but in all cases it takes about two weeks for development.

Serum, also known as *Antitoxin.* Made from the blood of immune animals. It is the liquid part of the blood which remains after the corpuscles have been removed. It gives protection within a few minutes after use, but the immunity lasts for only two or three weeks.

Logically enough, conditions should determine which product ought to be used. When disease hasn't appeared, aggressin, bacterin, or vaccine may be used, since there is time to wait while immunity develops. This slower-developing immunity has the advantage of lasting for quite a while. On the other hand, disease that is already present in a herd calls for the use of serum, since it gives immediate protection. Any of the other three agents represent a poor choice at such a time, since animals would probably be affected before resistance had time to develop.

Methods of Giving Medicine

There are five common methods of giving medicine to cattle. The best one will be largely dependent on the medicine, for some of the remedies can be given only in certain ways. Occasionally the time element also has to be considered in choosing a way to give medicine, for availability varies according to where drugs are placed. This will be mentioned in connection with each of the five methods listed below.

    1. INTRAVENOUSLY or directly into the blood stream through a vein. This is the fastest of all methods for getting results from medicine, since drugs don't have to be absorbed. Instead they are placed where they are immediately available. This fact makes the method especially desirable for use in emergencies like poisoning and attacks of milk

fever. The jugular vein of cattle is commonly used when medicines are given intravenously.

2. ORALLY or by way of the mouth. This is the oldest of all methods and calls for getting medicines into the stomach. Animals may be "drenched" or given liquids through a tube passed into the stomach. Powders may be mixed with feed or placed well back over the base of the tongue with a spoon or the hand. Pills and capsules may be given by hand or with a "balling gun." This is slower than intravenous medication, since drugs must be absorbed from the digestive tract before they get into the blood stream to act on other parts of the body.

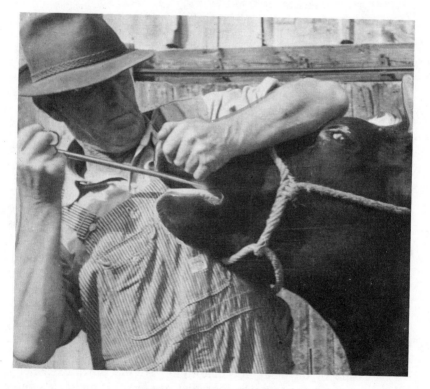

Giving pill with balling gun.

3. PER RECTUM or by introduction of liquids into the lower bowel. Only a few drugs are suitable for use in this manner, but it's usually easier to give medicines orally anyway.

It is slower-acting than when drugs are placed in the stomach. Absorption occurs in the same way, but the smaller area in the rectum naturally slows it down.

4. INTRAMUSCULARLY or into the muscle. Care must be used in selecting medicines, for some drugs will destroy flesh when given in this manner. Action is a little slower than when drugs are given orally, with absorption occurring through the capillaries and blood vessels abounding in muscle.

5. SUBCUTANEOUSLY or under the skin. Absorption is the same as when injections are made into muscles. However, the smaller number of blood vessels in this area slows the process down and makes drugs available slowly over a greater length of time.

Anesthesia

Animals are bigger and stronger than men, so anesthesia is frequently desirable for making them sleepy enough so they aren't quite so hard to handle. More often, though, anesthesia is desirable for eliminating needless pain and suffering of dumb beasts. There are six general classes:

1. TOPICAL, which consists of applying certain drugs to the eyes or mucous membranes described under the anatomy of the skin found in the section on Skin Troubles. Since absorption is rapid from such surfaces, they soon become incapable of feeling after such treatment. The outer skin is less sensitive, so topical anesthesia is rarely used on it. Two per cent solutions of butyn sulfate are suitable for this purpose, and newer compounds are also available.

2. INFILTRATION, or "local," which consists of injecting liquids under the skin and into flesh of areas to be treated. This is the type of anesthesia used by your dentist for extracting teeth.

3. NERVE BLOCKING, which consists of injecting liquids only into the main nerve supply to a certain area. It may be a single nerve like the cornualis that is blocked off on each side of the head for dehorning. At the other extreme, it may be the three or four that are blocked on each side of the backbone to cut off feeling in the flank areas when a calf is being delivered by caesarean section.

4. SPINAL or EPIDURAL, which consists of injecting liquids directly into the spinal cord to block off all nerves that

branch from it behind the point of injection. One or two per cent solutions of procaine hydrochloride are suitable for both this and the two preceding types of anesthesia.

5. FREEZING, which is the name often mistakenly applied to "local" or infiltration anesthesia. The real type of freezing calls for the use of ethyl chloride which is sprayed onto the skin. Rapid evaporation of this chemical causes fast cooling and actual freezing of tissues which makes them insensible to pain. It is suitable only for minor surgery, since frozen areas thaw out in a few seconds.

6. GENERAL, which consists of rendering animals completely unconscious. The inhalation of drugs like ether and chloroform is a possibility, but not very practical on cattle. Instead, it is easier to give drugs intravenously for general anesthesia. The best ones are carefully balanced solutions of chloral hydrate, magnesium sulfate, and sodium pentobarbital which come ready-mixed and available for immediate use.

Certain drugs may also be given orally to induce general anesthesia. Chloral hydrate is popular for this purpose, and is the "Mickey Finn" or knockout drops frequently mentioned in gangster stories. Dosage will depend on the animal. Practically all general anesthetics are highly poisonous and should be used only by individuals who have had experience in handling them. Otherwise the general anesthesia can change into a permanent variety.

Cattle Diseases Transmissible to Man

BANG'S DISEASE. When it attacks man this infection is known as undulant fever. Human beings usually acquire it from cattle by drinking raw milk from diseased animals. There are also some other ways in which infection can occur. Vaginal discharges may be flicked in the eye, or germs may be picked up through the handling of warm raw beef. It's also possible for germs to be picked up while delivering calves or "cleaning" infected cows that retain the afterbirth.

TUBERCULOSIS. Infection usually follows the drinking of raw milk from diseased cows, but it may also occur through the air, particularly in poorly ventilated barns where the air is foul and moist. Tuberculosis of the skin may result from handling diseased carcasses.

ANTHRAX is almost always acquired by human beings through the handling of infected meat or hides. Infection through milk is possible, but animals afflicted with anthrax probably would be too sick to be giving milk.

RABIES. Although exposure is usually through the bites of animals like dogs, cattle infect people too. It is not uncommon for affected animals to act like they were choking on something stuck in their throats. In making an examination of the mouth or while drenching sick animals, owners frequently get their hands well-smeared with dangerous saliva and the virus may get into the blood through cracks or cuts in the skin.

FOOT-AND-MOUTH DISEASE is rare in man, but still a possibility when infected animals are being handled. Infection may occur either through drinking milk or handling diseased tissues.

COWPOX usually affects the hands and arms of milkers. There seems to be two forms of this disease that closely resemble each other. The virus-caused type produces true cowpox, while the other type is believed due to bacteria and causes so-called "milker's nodules" on the hands of human beings.

MILK SICKNESS. Uncommon nowadays as the acreage of wild pastures decreases. It is poisoning caused by drinking the milk of cows that have eaten either white snakeroot or the rayless goldenrod. In various sections this ailment is also known as slows, puking fever, and alkali disease. It is historically important because it caused the death of Abraham Lincoln's mother.

LEPTOSPIROSIS. Probably generally spread through the breathing of urine mist in cow barns, but drinking of raw milk and the handling of raw beef are also possible methods of infection.

SARCOPTIC MANGE. Acquired by human beings through body contact with infected animals. Caused by mites that burrow under the outer layers of skin and aren't particular whether they live on man or beast.

RINGWORM. A disease caused by fungus. Man acquires the disease through body contact as in the case of mange.

LUMPJAW or ACTINOMYCOSIS. Another fungus disease which may attack man, although it seems doubtful that it ever spreads directly from cattle.

TOXOPLASMOSIS. A disease caused by a parasite which may invade practically any tissue or organ of the body.

Q FEVER. The means of infection isn't always known, but ticks found on cattle or dust from infected premises that is inhaled are usually blamed for the trouble.

SEPTIC SORE THROAT. Really a human disease. However, the causative germs may become localized in the udders of cows and be given off in the milk to infect man.

SCARLET FEVER. Another human disease that is spread by cows under the same conditions as given for septic sore throat.

DIPHTHERIA. Milk-borne epidemics of this disease have appeared, but infection has nearly always been traced back to a human carrier. In some instances udder sores were found to contain diphtheria bacteria contracted from infected milkers.

TYPHOID FEVER. This disease is often transmitted through milk, but the cow is never to blame, since she can drink germs without getting the disease. Contamination of milk always occurs through human handling.

TAPEWORMS. Human beings become infected with these parasites when they eat raw or improperly cooked beef that contains the larvae of *Taenia saginata*.

The "Carrier" Animal

Whenever and wherever disease control problems are discussed we're pretty sure to hear considerable about the so-called "carrier" animal. In the strictest sense of the word it can be one that is visibly

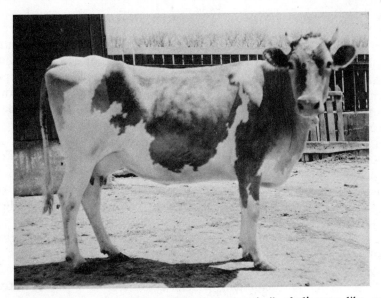

This apparently healthy animal might be a "carrier" of diseases like anaplasmosis, lepto, vibriosis, trichomoniasis, etc.

sick and showing symptoms of disease while giving off germs to infect clean animals. It can also be one that is in the "incubation stage" of some disease and carrying germs without being actually sick and capable of spreading infection. However, the carrier animal is generally thought of as being one that has completely recovered from an attack of disease but still carries and gives off germs that may infect clean cattle. The brute is then generally referred to as a "recovered carrier" capable of spreading infection wherever it goes.

A great many of our more serious cattle diseases are spread by these carrier animals. Bang's disease is an example of one, and tuberculosis represents another. Anaplasmosis, leptospirosis, trichomoniasis, vibriosis, and several other ailments are also spread by carrier animals. Fortunately there are tests of different kinds that will generally show up such dangerous critters. However, the apparent good health of animals may encourage buyers to neglect precautionary testing. Such neglect is often costly, for a single carrier animal can be the means of starting an outbreak of disease that will eventually bankrupt an owner. With this fact recognized, purchasers will do well to be careful about the kind of animals they bring home.

"Silo Filler's Disease," Nitrogen Dioxide Poisoning

For years we have realized that silos which have been empty all summer may be dangerous at filling time because of an accumulation of carbon dioxide. Danger isn't limited to empty pits, either, for accidents may occur after a break in filling or for a few days after silos are filled. This is because carbon dioxide is heavier than air, and may accumulate in low places or near the surface of silage so there isn't enough oxygen to support life. An old test for safety consists of lowering a lighted lantern into the silo. If it goes out, the silo is unsafe. However, in recent years we have become aware of a new danger that may be associated with newly-filled silos. It has been given the name of "silo-fillers' disease."

This trouble is due to accumulations of nitrogen dioxide given off by new silage during the first few days after filling. Nitrogen dioxide has been recognized as a hazard in certain industries for many years, especially when welding or the handling of nitrate films was involved, but it wasn't pin-pointed as a farm danger until 1956. This is a bit strange, for Wisconsin scientists noted

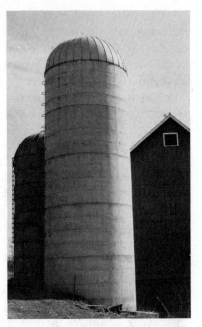

Your silo may be a death trap near filling time.

this gas in silos as far back as 1949. At that time they found that nitrogen dioxide collected at the bottom of the silo chute, and that it was present in 115 parts per million of air. It is generally considered dangerous at concentrations of only 15 to 25 parts per million.

Along in 1954 a strange sickness began affecting farmers in two or three drouth-stricken Missouri counties, and one known death resulted. However, this sickness attracted little more than local interest. Then in the fall of 1955 two Minnesota brothers died under mysterious conditions, and autopsies showed that they had inhaled nitrogen dioxide. Questioning brought out the fact that about a month earlier both brothers had tried to climb up the chute of a silo that had been filled with corn silage the day before. Strangling fumes had driven them down, coughing and gasping. This started doctors at the Minnesota Medical College looking for other cases, and they eventually proved that the gas had killed an additional farmer and had made three others seriously sick. This "silo fillers' disease" has probably existed ever since silos first came into use, but it is believed that many illnesses diagnosed as atypical forms of pneumonia in past years were really cases of nitrogen dioxide poisoning.

Chemists explain that nitrogen dioxide is produced by the reduction of nitrates to nitrites by bacteria working in the acid conditions that exist in silage. Nitrites are converted to nitrous acid, which breaks down to form nitric acid, and this in turn is changed to nitrogen dioxide when it comes in contact with air. The gas is evidently formed in greatest amounts from silage made of corn grown during an exceptionally dry summer. The danger of nitrogen dioxide is also increased when silage is made from immature plants or corn grown on fields that have received heavy applications of nitrogen fertilizer. Danger isn't limited to corn silage, either. In every test made on grass, oat, or corn silages at the University of Minnesota, variable amounts of gas were found. In Wisconsin, tests on three silos filled with corn and two silos filled with alfalfa, all showed a positive reaction to the presence of gas.

Immediately after the gas has been inhaled, victims may be aware of only a slight irritation of the nose and throat. A little later there may be shortness of breath, a choking sensation, and coughing which brings up a brown or bloody sputum. During the first week of illness there is a fever and a general weakness much like symptoms caused by various other lung troubles. It is unlikely that any doctor will be able to make a correct diagnosis unless he knows that the patient has been exposed to fumes from silage. The usual antibiotic treatments for lung infections have no effect on this particular trouble. Many patients will appear to be recovering during the second week, only to suffer a severe relapse about the beginning of the third week. Considering the serious nature of this trouble, we feel that most of our readers will be interested in knowing how to play safe by preventing "silo fillers' disease." Scientists associated with the USDA recommend the following procedures:

1. Remember that nitrogen dioxide is heavier than air, and that it settles on top of silage or at the bottom of the chute.
2. Look for yellow or brown fumes in or around a silo, and stay away if they are seen. Use a flashlight if the silo is dark.
3. Don't allow anyone to enter the silo unless the blower has first been run for 10 to 15 minutes, especially during the first 10 days after filling. If the blower has been taken away wait at least a week before going inside a filled silo.
4. Always leave the chute door open at the surface of the silage to prevent accumulation of the gas there.

5. Provide extra ventilation at the bottom of the chute when silos are attached to barns. Some owners have placed a large ventilating fan in this location and run it for several minutes before anyone enters the area.

6. If there is a separate silage room, it may be desirable to provide an outside door to let gas escape at the floor level.

7. Fence off the area around the base of the silo to keep children and animals away from this dangerous area from the beginning of silo-filling until 10 days after the job has been finished.

8. Since silo gases may be trapped indefinitely under a plastic cover, remove it carefully, regardless of whether it is used in regular or trench silos. Better yet, ventilate the area well for a couple of weeks before the silo is opened.

Three years of trials at the University of Minnesota (1958-60) have indicated that sodium bisulfite or sodium metabisulfite may be the means of preventing the formation of toxic gases in silos. This common grass silage preservative was added to corn, oats, and alfalfa silage at the rate of 8 to 10 pounds per ton of ensiled material with good results. Dr. Joseph Scaletti, in charge of the trials, stated that the addition of sodium bisulfite prevented the formation of toxic gas regardless of initial concentration of nitrates in the forage, maturity of the crop, the amount of nitrogen fertilizer that had been supplied to the growing crop, or the level of moisture in the ensiled material.

At first it was feared that the addition of sodium bisulfite might interfere with normal fermentation of silage so that forage containing large amounts of nitrates would be unchanged and able to cause nitrate poisoning of livestock receiving it. The trials showed it did not do this to any extent, although it delayed reduction of nitrates for about two days. However, by the fourth or fifth day following ensiling, the reduction of nitrates was equal to that in untreated silage, so no additional problem is anticipated along this particular line.

At this time scientists are still looking for a quick test that will show the presence of nitrogen gases. One that looks good at the University of Minnesota consists of a potassium iodide starch-treated paper that will turn blue if the gas is present. This test is similar to the litmus paper test for acidity. Danger is not increased by a high concentration of nitrate in plants, for fermentation of silage should reduce the nitrate completely within two weeks.

"Farmer's Lung"

A disease similar to what is commonly called "farmer's lung" was first reported from England in 1932, but it attracted little attention in this country until a couple of Wisconsin doctors summarized 39 cases in the summer of 1958. These cases were seen over an eight-year period in a dairy section, and several of them had been treated previously without the ailment being recognized for what it actually was. Authorities now believe that the ailment is much commoner than available figures indicate, for only the severest cases are likely to come to the attention of doctors, and it is impossible to estimate the number of farmers who may be in the early stages. If farm folks recognize the possibility of such trouble, they may give their doctors information that will help them to make a correct diagnosis.

This ailment is entirely different from "silo fillers' disease" which is caused by nitrogen dioxide given off by new silage, and is also called "farmer's lung" in some areas. It is caused by common mold dust, and attacks are brought on by working with hay, grain, fodder, and silage. There is evidently a difference in susceptibility, for the disease can strike any one of a number of persons who have lived and worked together on the same farm without affecting the others. Attacks are rare in the summer, and are much more likely during the winter when stored feeds are being handled in closed buildings.

The outstanding symptom of "farmer's lung" is a shortness of breath which may be suggestive of a heart condition. Other symptoms include coughing, headaches, shaking chills, loss of weight, blood-stained sputum, and a fever that may reach 106 degrees. In severe cases something like flu or pneumonia may be suspected. A characteristic that will often help to identify the trouble is the fact that shortness of breath may persist for several weeks when the patient is being treated for some kind of lung infection. This is not surprising, for treatment with drugs and antibiotics is of no value at all. Recovery from one attack is likely to be followed by another as soon as the patient is exposed to the causative dust again, and one of the Wisconsin farmers reported four attacks in five weeks. People who are sensitive to the dust may have recurrent attacks over a period of several years. Some degree of permanent lung injury may result from just a single attack, and repeated attacks may eventually damage the lungs so badly that labor of any kind is impossible, even in surroundings where there is no troublesome dust. Accordingly, an early diagnosis is important so that people can immediately get away from farm work that is dangerous for them. This represents the only practical solution. Research workers at the University of Wisconsin have developed diagnostic procedures for identifying "farmer's lung" during the early stages before it has had a chance to do much permanent damage to the lungs, and your doctor will doubtlessly be familiar with these procedures.

The only preventive measure recognized is the wearing of a respiratory mask like those used in industries where there is a heavy concentration of dangerous dust. No matter whether you've ever had symptoms of "farmer's lung" or not, it will still be a good idea for you to wear one of these masks any time that it is necessary for you to work in dusty places on the farm. The masks may be obtained through your doctor or local drug store, and may be the means of preventing serious trouble for you.

Warm that Water!

Although there are several cheaper fuels, a great many cattlemen use hay and grain to heat their animals during the winter. This happens when animals are furnished with ice-cold drinking water. The water has to be warmed to body temperature after being swallowed, and extra feed is used that might otherwise go for weight gains or milk production. In addition to causing such waste, the cold water can be to blame for indigestion that causes cattle to go off feed.

When cattle are being watered outside at streams or tanks, a spell of cold weather may induce an attack of indigestion in an entire herd of steers or dairy cows. Shivering animals will not drink as much as they will when they are warm, and often won't get enough for their actual needs. Owners may not realize how great these needs really are.

A good dairy cow will need somewhere between three to five gallons of water for each gallon of milk she produces daily, and steers will need at least a gallon daily for each hundred pounds of weight.

There are two good reasons why cattle are most likely to suffer from a lack of water during the winter. For one, they are able to get considerable water with their green feed during other seasons. For another, they won't be so cold during those other seasons that they have a natural tendency to drink less. This trouble can be greatly helped by warming the water in cold weather.

What you do about warming it will depend considerably on

your farm conditions. You can use various kinds of heaters that burn wood, coal, or oil, but electricity is more popular for warming the water. A cup can be obtained which contains a heating element around the riser pipe which brings the water up from below frost level. Such a cup will take care of about 50 cattle, and the operation cost will be considerably less than for a tank heater. A similar, but larger element can be obtained for tanks, or an entire insulated tank can be purchased. Having a thermostatic control pays for itself in fuel savings, since there are no benefits from heating water above ordinary well water temperature. A setting of around 40 degrees is about right. Owners must guard against the tank water level falling below the thermostat level, or a burned-out element will result.

Many owners make use of thermo tape and a thermostat, with the water pipe being wrapped with the tape to keep it from freezing. The water tank is then heated with a regular heater. Electricity can be saved by using an insulated tank and water pipe. A practical tank can be made by putting a 30-gallon barrel inside a 50-gallon barrel and insulating between the two, with a float being used to keep the water at the proper level.

As an extra improvement, it will pay you to build some kind of a windbreak around the tank to protect your animals while they are drinking. They will still be cold enough on some of those winter days, even when they have a chance to get out of the wind.

Watch that Summer Water!

During the summer months stagnant drinking water may cause trouble for stock through poisoning by green algae or "water bloom." Danger isn't limited to algae poisoning, either, for there are other possible sources of trouble. All kinds of disease germs may live in stagnant water, and epidemics of contagious diseases have often been traced back to such a source. Dead animals in tanks have caused deaths from botulism. Socalled "mouth-sores" have been blamed on dirty drinking water, while milk cows that stand bellydeep in filthy water have a good chance of developing mastitis. Water may also harbor the eggs and larvae of many internal parasites. Bloody scours and coccidiosis have been caused by contaminated water, and bad infestations with stomach worms and liver flukes have been traced back to this source.

Muddy ground around tanks and pond edges endanger cattle in another way. Deep tracks in mud eventually dry out into sharp-edged craters that are baked so hard they are able to cut the feet of animals. Besides causing lameness, these cuts may furnish a lodging place for mud-borne germs like those of foot rot and lockjaw.

Troubles that go along with mud and stagnant water are often collectively known as "stale pond" diseases. Most of these ailments can be cured, but owners lose money through decreased weight, less milk, and decreased resistance to other diseases. Accordingly, preventive measures are generally more practical than treatment after infection has occurred. A suitable summer program calls for:

1. Emptying and cleaning water tanks at least once a week.

2. Draining, fencing, or filling stagnant pools.

3. Equipping tanks with automatic valves to prevent over-running.

4. Concreting or providing drainage around spring-fed tanks to eliminate mudholes in such places.

5. Following measures recommended to prevent algae poisoning.

Getting Ready for the Show

In the late summer a great many cattle are readied for shows and fairs in various parts of the country. Every year some of the owners forget to do certain things, and such forgetfulness results in trouble of different kinds. We're not much concerned about such things as grooming and training and showmanship. Instead, we're interested in neglected details of management that often cause troubles for owners. Those are the things we'd like to consider here.

First, make sure that your health papers are complete and that you have all that are needed to meet show requirements. It sometimes takes longer than you expected to run tests, look up vacination slips, and get other papers together.

Second, make sure that your animals are protected against shipping fever. If you wait until the day before you start out, you can still use serum, but it's neither so effective or long-lasting as bacterin. However, the bacterin should be injected at least two weeks before animals go on the road in order to give them the desired protection. Depending somewhat on the shows you're making, it may also be desirable to vaccinate your stock against diseases like malignant edema, blackleg, and leptospirosis.

Feet must be trimmed, for no animal can move well with over-long toes or thick pads on the soles. Good foot trimming means close trimming, and since there is always some danger of tenderness afterward, the job shouldn't be put off until the day before showing.

Feeding is important, but the average owner is fully capable of doing it with a ration that will give best results. Consequently, we're more interested in methods of feeding than we are in the feed itself. Changes in rations are to be avoided whenever possible, since even a minor one like substituting "new" oats for those from last year may be enough to cause an attack of indigestion that soon takes the "bloom" off a show animal. When changes are unavoidable, they should be made gradually. Animals should be fed at regular intervals, too, since irregular feeding may lead to extreme hunger and result in overeating when feed is finally available. It's usually a good idea to take feed with you to the show. It may be either better or worse than what you can get on the grounds, but it will be what the cattle are used to and the plan will eliminate the danger of feed changes. It is also well to feed the animals at home out of the same boxes that will be used on the road.

Mentioning feed suggests that water changes often cause trouble at shows, too, for many cattle lose weight at a critical time simply because they don't drink enough water. Animals that get water from tanks or cups at home may refuse to drink from pails until they're forced to by extreme thirst. You can avoid part of this trouble by watering your animals only from pails for a week or so before they leave home, and then taking the same pails with you on the road. If animals don't mind the pails, they may object to water because it tastes and smells different than that at home. This happens quite often, for most of the water on fairgrounds is chlorinated. It isn't very practical to haul water with you, but you can mix a little molasses with the drinking water for a couple of weeks before you leave for the fair. You can do the same thing on the road, and the molasses will smother tastes and smells so the cattle won't be able to tell any difference in the water.

The above are a few of the things that an owner can do to avoid serious trouble later on when the chips are down in the show ring. Don't forget them in your preparations, for they're just as important as training and grooming the animals. Neglect of these details may not make cattle actually sick, but such carelessness can easily throw them out of condition just enough to make the difference between a prize winner and an also-ran.

About Undulant Fever

Once upon a time there was a man who didn't believe that people could get undulant fever by drinking raw milk from cows that were infected with Bang's disease.

"I'm perfectly healthy," he would boast. "Yet I've been drinking raw milk from Banger cows all my life. So have my brothers and sisters, and they're big and strong. My own kids were weaned on the stuff, and they're all right, too. Undulant fever from raw milk? Phooie!"

We hear stories like that quite often, and most of the time they're perfectly true. In fact, there are probably millions of people in the world who have drunk raw milk from Bang's-infected cows without getting undulant fever. There are at least three logical reasons why they have been able to do it.

First, all cows that have Bang's disease don't continually give off Bang's germs in their milk. It seems to be a case of "some always do, some seldom do, and some never do." So far as we know, there are no figures on the actual percentage of Banger cows that belong in each group. We only know that Bang's germs are often found in the milk given by diseased cows, and that those germs are capable of causing undulant fever in man. Plenty of experimental work and hospital cases have verified both facts.

Second, it is likely that many people are able to successfully resist the germs of Bang's disease. This is particularly true if the number of germs is small because the milk from infected cows has been greatly diluted with that from disease-free animals. Human resistance may be either natural or acquired through continued drinking of infected milk. Since the eating of even something like arsenic in gradually increasing amounts will eventually make people immune to it, you can see that there's nothing especially new about this acquired resistance angle.

Third, it may be that people have previously suffered an attack of sickness that was not recognized as undulant fever. In such a case, recovered individuals are likely to have a permanent immunity much like that following a bout with chickenpox.

Whatever the explanation is for the small number of people that acquire the infection in such a manner, it becomes increasingly clear that many cases of undulant fever are due to the drinking of infected raw milk. In addition, undulant fever may be due to Bang's disease germs that enter the body in other ways.

One of the commoner sources of human infection is represented by bovine uterine discharges. In the case of Bang's-infected females, it is pretty well known that the uterus is loaded with millions of germs during the period when the calf is developing. Some of these germs may escape before the calf's birth, a lot of them at calving time, and quite a few more for several weeks afterward. They are carried out with discharges and the germs may start infection in various ways.

We know one chap who was infected by a drop of contaminated material that was flicked into his eye by the tail of a recently-fresh cow. Then we frequently hear of undulant fever that followed bare-handed "cleaning" of a cow or helping a calf to be born. When cows are infected, a new-born calf and the afterbirth alike are swarming with germs, just the same as the uterus and the discharges from it. Then the dirty hands may carry the germs to the mouth or eyes. Cuts on the hands or even "hangnails" on the fingers will furnish a doorway for Bang's germs to enter the body. Such a doorway may not even be needed, for these particular germs are sometimes able to penetrate the unbroken skin.

All of the above still doesn't explain cases which often occur in people who drink no milk and keep no cows. Many of these cases can be traced back to swine, for these animals get Bang's disease, too. Anyway, sows are a distinct possibility, since the germs live in the uteri of these animals about the same as they do in cows. If owners don't help them at farrowing time, they have a chance of picking up the germs at butchering time.

The live germs of Bang's disease are often found in the warm blood and meat of newly-killed hogs, and infection is entirely possible from such a source. In fact, investigation has shown that large numbers of undulant fever cases can be traced back to the slaughtering of swine. The carcasses of cattle are not so likely to cause human infection through handling.

It is suggested that this difference may be due to the swine type of disease being more dangerous for man. Another possibility is that Bang's germs are found more often in swine blood than they are in cattle blood. Or it may be that both of the above factors are involved to some extent.

As a farmer you are probably more interested in avoiding undulant fever than you are in germ differences. The following procedures will help you in that respect.

1. Have all goats, swine, and cattle tested regularly to reveal the presence of Bang's disease on your farm.

2. Drink nothing but pasteurized or boiled milk unless it is known to come from Bang's-free animals.
3. Eat only butter, ice cream, and other dairy products made from the same kind of safe milk.
4. Thoroughly wash and disinfect hands after handling raw meat at butchering time.
5. Do the same thing after dehorning or castrating animals.
6. Grease hands and arms thoroughly with mineral oil or unsalted lard when assisting animals at parturition time, and wash thoroughly afterward.
7. Keep hands away from eyes, nose, and mouth when working with possibly Bang's-infected animals.

When Bang's Suspects Show Up

Suspects that show up when herds are blood tested for Bang's disease are of interest to practically everyone who raises cattle. Dairymen are likely to be most concerned over them, for the suspects can cause ring test reactions that then require blood testing of an entire herd. However, beef raisers and dairymen alike are apt to encounter suspects in routine herd testing or testing of individual animals for sale. When they show up, an owner usually wants to know why, especially if previous tests have been clean. We can't always give a definite answer, for there are several possibilities.

1. Animals may have recently been exposed to Bang's germs. These germs may have been brought in by purchased animals, or carried in on the feet of animals and human beings or been present in the semen of a bull that serviced a cow, either naturally or artificially. Exposed animals may then show up as suspects, even if they have resistance enough from vaccination to keep them from going on to become full-fledged reactors.

   Even the most highly resistant animals are pretty sure to show at least a slight temporary reaction following exposure to these germs. Depending somewhat on the number of germs that are swallowed, these suspects may or may not become worse until they finally end up as three-plus reactors to the blood test.

2. Animals may be official calfhood vaccinates that haven't completely cleared up after vaccination. These suspects are apt to be first-calf dairy heifers that were vaccinated when they were close to eight months old. Since beef

heifers mature a little more slowly, they aren't likely to remain as suspects for long periods afterward, even when they are close to eight months old when vaccinated.

3. Animals may have been vaccinated after they were eight months old, or even as adults, so they will react to the blood test in some degree for the rest of their lives. This is sometimes the case in herds that were once badly infected with Bang's and where all of the animals were vaccinated as adults in the hope of ending an abortion storm.

4. Animals may have once been reactors that have partially recovered so that they now show only a partial reaction to the blood test. These animals are likely to be valuable older animals that have been held over from the days when it was possible to retain reactors in a herd.

5. Animals may be bulls that were vaccinated, either through error by a veterinarian or because of an owner's belief that vaccination of bulls was helpful in protecting his herd against Bang's disease. Such vaccination has at least one disadvantage, for bulls are then likely to remain as reactors for life because the injected Strain 19 germs set up permanent living quarters in the testicles.

6. Animals may be females in an advanced stage of pregnancy. Although this point is hotly disputed, the fact remains that heavily pregnant cows sometimes produce certain hormones which may cause varying reactions to the blood test, even though they are completely free of Bang's disease.

7. Animals may have recently been turned to pasture or changed over onto a new type of green feed. The exact mechanics of this reaction aren't understood. It is generally believed that antibodies produced by intestinal irritation, or estrogens naturally present in the green forage are responsible in some way for changes in a blood test that would otherwise be completely negative. Such reactions disappear in a short time.

8. Animals may have recently suffered a severe attack of diarrhea due to something like winter dysentery. Again the exact cause is unknown, but it is theorized that antibodies produced by the infection resemble those of Bang's disease closely enough so that the blood test is slightly affected. This type of reaction soon disappears, too.

9. Animals may be calfhood vaccinates that have recently been vaccinated against shipping fever, malignant edema, or blackleg. Reactions to the Bang's test following such vaccination are explained by the fact that the injection of unrelated antigens may cause the formation of antibodies in the blood which are specific for antigens injected at an earlier date. Such an occurrence is often referred to as a " recall" phenomenon.

    With this possibility in mind, it is recommended that testing of official vaccinates be deferred for at least 30 days after they have been vaccinated with specific or mixed bacterins to protect them against other diseases.

10. Animals may have come in contact with swine that were infected with Bang's disease. Although cattle aren't susceptible to the swine type of Bang's disease, they may be sensitized by exposure to the swine type of germs so they will show up as suspects on the regular blood test. Accordingly, this possibility furnishes another reason why swine and cattle shouldn't be allowed to run together.

Why Test Cattle for Tuberculosis?

People often ask us why livestock authorities still insist on compulsory tuberculosis testing of cattle at five-year intervals. They point out that the disease is now eradicated in this country, and that the testing program might therefore be discontinued. Even if the disease did exist in a few isolated spots, they question that it would do any damage like it once did. Since tuberculosis germs are killed by pasteurization, and most cities and towns have laws forbidding the sale of raw milk, it wouldn't seem that tuberculous cattle would have much chance of infecting human beings. Well, questions about the need of continued tuberculosis testing of cattle always remind us of a case in our own experience.

It concerned a dairyman who had regularly tested his herd under the cooperative state-federal program for over 20 years. Like most of his neighbors, he had never lost a cow because of tuberculosis. Yet in the course of a routine physical checkup, doctors discovered he was afflicted with tuberculosis. Investigation showed that his wife and two children also had the disease, and it was decided that the cattle ought to be tested for tuberculosis, too. This seemed needless at first, since the whole herd had been negative to a test a little more than three years earlier. However, a test at this time showed all of the older cattle and most of the young stock as reactors, with several animals being so badly affected that they were "tanked" when slaughtered. The people might conceivably have been affected through drinking raw milk, or working around the infected cattle in a poorly ventilated barn where they had a chance to breathe in the germs. Living together in a single house, the family members could easily have infected each other after the disease was once started.

However, it was a bit hard to explain how infection might have started in the cattle, for no new and possible "carrier" animals had been purchased for years. This fact suggested that the human beings might have been infected first, since diseased people can give tuberculosis to cattle just as cattle can transmit the disease to human beings. So far as we know, the original source of trouble was never determined.

For our purpose it doesn't make any difference, since all we want to do is show that cattle unexpectedly contracted tuberculosis on a supposedly clean farm where such danger was never considered. The same sort of thing can happen in beef herds, although the disease does not have so good a chance of spreading as it does in dairy barns. People aren't the only ones in danger, either, for swine may easily be infected through drinking raw milk or following cattle in feed lots. Like human beings, these animals may then serve as spreaders to carry the disease wherever they go.

It is true that times have changed in the last 50 years, and there's certainly a lot less tuberculosis in cattle than there was in the days right after World War I. However, there is still some left, for every test picks off a few diseased animals. If those animals were left alone they would infect others to infect still others until eventually we would have a bad mess of tuberculosis in this country again. Even if we could remove every last infected cow brute with a single stroke, the remaining clean ones would still have a chance to come in contact with occasional human beings that were carriers of tuberculosis. Without regular testing these exposed animals would then have a chance to start another epidemic of bovine tuberculosis so the disease might get pretty bad again in the course of 15 or 20 years. Those are the reasons why we personally feel that it will always be desirable to test cattle for tuberculosis. As a matter of fact, maybe a test once every five years isn't often enough.

When TB Reactors Show Up

Every once in a while we run into reactors that remind us that tuberculosis of cattle isn't completely wiped out in the United States. There are several possible reasons why TB reactors or suspects may show up in a herd that was previously clean.

1. Purchased animals may have been infected when they were brought onto a farm to infect animals in the home herd.

2. Home animals may have come in contact with tubercular people who worked around them.

3. Cattle may have been exposed to swine or chickens that were allowed to run with them, especially in barns. Older chickens are quite likely to have the avian type of tuberculosis, and swine are highly susceptible to it so they are easily infected. Although cattle are completely immune to this type of the disease, it may still cause trouble, for exposure to either infected swine or poultry may sensitize them so they react to the test for bovine tuberculosis without being diseased at all. An examination after death at the packing plant will then result in a report of "no visible lesions" so that the owner will blame the veterinarian for doing a bad job of testing. Nothing can be done about such cases, for there's no practical way of telling what type of TB is causing a reaction, and animals have to be eliminated from the herd in order to be on the safe side.

4. Cattle may have been exposed to infection of the type referred to as "skin tuberculosis" on page 259 of this book. Reactions can't be safely blamed on skin infection, though, for the nodules are found in both tubercular and healthy animals, so reacting animals have to be removed from the herd.

5. A recent report has it that infestation with liver flukes may cause cattle to react to the tuberculin test. Although there is no definite proof of this, the fact remains that TB reactors have been slaughtered and no visible lesions found of anything but those caused by flukes. It is possible, of course, that these animals had been exposed to some type of bacteria found in the swampy areas usually associated with fluke infestation.

6. It has also been reported that cattle afflicted with lumpjaw or wooden tongue will sometimes react to the tuberculin test. The same thing is probably true of various other organisms that resemble those causing these two troubles.

With these possibilities in mind, owners will do well to hesitate a bit before condemning the TB test as inaccurate because it resulted in the elimination of cattle that showed no visible lesions when slaughtered. No test is 100 per cent accurate, and the tuberculin test is no exception. However, over the last 35 years it has been right a lot oftener than it's been wrong, so we are in favor of depending on it in spite of its limitations.

About Disinfectants

Although they depend on various principles for effectiveness, different kinds of chemical solutions are generally considered as the most practical germ-killers for farm use. The coal tar disinfectants act through coagulation and complicated chemical reactions. Chlorine combines with bacterial protoplasm to form entirely new compounds. Lye is effective because it has a caustic or corrosive action on most types of organic material. Although chemical disinfectants are like hot air and steam because they require direct contact with bacteria to kill them, such contact may not occur in a routine disinfection job. This is because there are a couple of factors that may prevent it.

Surface tension that we used to illustrate by floating a needle on water is probably the most important. Being present everywhere in nature, this acts as an elastic membrane which serves to protect bacterial cells. Accordingly, it is necessary to lower or destroy surface tension before a good job of disinfection can be done. The coal tar disinfectants may make the situation worse by coagulating organic material around organisms so they can't be touched by the solution. Even water has a fairly high surface tension which can diminish the effectiveness of a disinfectant solution. For this reason it is often advisable to combine disinfectant solutions with soap or some kind of a detergent which will act as a "wetting agent" by means of lowering the surface tension.

Then it must be remembered that the same disinfectant may vary in effectiveness according to the premises where it is used and the type of bacteria that is involved. For example, practically all disinfectants will work better on clean floors than on dirty ones. Lye can be taken as an illustration of how effectiveness depends on the particular type of bacteria involved. This chemical will destroy practically all other types of disease organisms, but it is completely ineffective against the germs of tuberculosis which are covered by a coating of wax. Regardless of the disinfectant used and where it is used, though, three factors will determine its effectiveness.

1. The dilution factor. As a general rule, the stronger a disinfectant solution is, the faster and more efficient its action will be.
2. The time allowed for action. Ordinary disinfectants don't act instantly, so time must be allowed for contact and destructive action.
3. The temperature of both the solution and the atmosphere must be considered, since most chemical actions are speeded up by raising the temperature.

When these factors are remembered, owners can often do a better job of disinfecting by making helpful changes in regular procedure. If the solution and weather is cold, the time of exposure and the strength of the solution can be increased. If there is little time available for disinfection, the solution can be applied hot and extra strong. If the solution is made up extra strong, it will also act quicker in cold weather.

The following recommendations from the USDA can be safely followed for these diseases:

1. Brucellosis (Bang's disease), shipping fever, tuberculosis. Use 1 cup of USDA-approved (stamped on container) cresylic disinfectant mixed with each 2 gallons of water to make a 4 per cent solution.
2. Anthrax and blackleg. Use five 13½ ounce cans of lye mixed with each 10 gallons of water to make a 5 per cent solution. For truckbeds, let the solution remain in the vehicle for 8 hours, then wash out with water before using again.
3. Vesicular exanthema. Use one 13½ ounce can of lye mixed with each five gallons of water to make a 2 per cent solution.

When Milk Doesn't "Stand Up"

The methylene blue or reductase test which is used in most milk plants is nothing more than a measure of the activity of bacteria which are present in the milk. Bacterial growth causes certain changes in the milk, with the extent and time required for those changes dependent on the number of bacteria present. The test makes use of this fact, with a specified amount of milk being mixed with a smaller amount of standard methylene blue solution to give the sample a uniform blue color. It is then placed in an incubator so bacterial growth is encouraged. Certain types of bacteria then reduce the blue color until the milk is white again, with the length of time required for reduction representing the interval that milk "stands up." A large number of certain bacteria will cause loss of color in an hour or so, while milk that is exceptionally clean will "stand up" practically all day.

It sometimes happens that bacteria which cause mastitis can also reduce the blue color so milk doesn't "stand up." However, *Streptococcus agalactiae* germs are the ones most often causing mastitis, and these organisms have practically no reducing power at all. The same thing is true of most staphylococci germs, which are usually ranked second as a cause of mastitis. The situation is much different if some of the coliform or corynebacterium species are involved, for these organisms are often high-speed reducers. As a general rule, though, most types of reducing bacteria get into milk after it is drawn from cows. There are several possible ways in which this can occur.

The commonest cause is dirty utensils, for milking equipment requires thorough scrubbing and disinfection twice a day. It isn't enough to draw cold water through a machine after milking and then throw the teat cups in a jar of sterilizing solution until they are needed again. Aside from actual dirt, there are other things that can cause trouble, for such things as dents, rust spots, and open seams in cans, pails, and tanks can encourage bacterial growth.

When the equipment is both clean and sound, bacteria may get into milk from the air if dairymen make a habit of pouring it into open pails in the barn. The chances of such contamination are increased if the barn is dusty or poorly ventilated.

Sometimes trouble is traced back to such things as filthy stables and muddy barnyards, especially when the udders aren't washed before milking. If the udders are dirty it won't do much good to use spotless equipment and carry the milk into the milkhouse before pouring it.

It may be that slow and improper cooling is the reason why milk doesn't "stand up," for bacteria grow pretty fast until it is cooled down to around 50 degrees Fahrenheit.

Finally, the methylene blue may be reduced by an enzyme instead of bacteria. These enzymes are frequently found in the milk of cows that have been milking for a long time. In such cases the milk may be clean and have an exceptionally low bacteria count, but still fail to stand up for more than an hour or two.

Listed according to their order of importance, the causes of milk failing to "stand up" look something like this:

1. Incomplete washing of milking equipment and parts.
2. Use of milker inflations that are old and cracked so that sterilization is practically impossible.
3. Improper sterilization of milking equipment and parts.
4. Exposure of milking equipment and parts to wind-blown dust between milkings.
5. Failure to wash udders before milking.
6. Slow cooling of milk.
7. Storage of milk at a temperature that is not low enough to stop bacterial growth.
8. Use of milking equipment that is pitted with rust, has open seams, or is dented.
9. Pouring milk in barns.
10. Allowing milk to stand in open containers.
11. Mastitis and "bad" milk.
12. Enzymes in the milk of cows that have been milking for long periods.

When the Bacteria Count Goes Up in Milk

Within the last few months we have had occasion to call at three different dairy farms where the owners were in danger of being "shut off" at the receiving plant because of a sudden increase in the bacteria count of their milk. In all three of these cases a dairy fieldman had visited the farm and after looking things over had advised the owner to call in a veterinarian because the trouble was due to mastitis. One owner had purchased a California Mastest kit for use in locating infected animals, and had already disposed of three cows at the time of our visit.

However, sampling of the cows indicated that something other than mastitis was to blame for the high bacteria count. On the first farm we found five affected quarters involving three cows in a herd of 34 milking animals, and in another nine affected quarters involving five cows in a herd of 42 milking animals. On the third there were seven affected quarters involving six cows in a herd of 27 milking animals. We considered this low level of infection as unlikely to be causing trouble, and were sure of it when holding out milk from these infected cows had no effect on the bacteria count.

At about the same time that we were making these calls we visited another farm where the owner was having mastitis trouble so bad that it was often necessary to use a dozen or more strainer pads for a single milking. We sampled this herd and discovered that about three-fourths of the cows and over half the quarters were infected with an especially bad type of mastitis. In spite of this, he had never had any complaints from the milk plant, and his bacteria count was under 25,000 day after day. He had called us of his own accord because he was worrying over his decreased milk production and not because he was in danger of being "shut off" at the receiving plant on account of a high bacteria count.

We have mentioned these cases only to show how a bacteria count may not be related to mastitis trouble at all. In the past fifteen years we have had this point brought to our attention many different times. Our personal experience is not unusual, either, for investigators at the University of Wisconsin have reported the same thing as true in many of the herds they have visited. One report in particular concerned a herd of 43 cows with 97 quarters that had been treated once or more times for mastitis. These figures represented 79% of the cows, and 57% of the total quarters, yet the official Board of Health bacteria count was 30,000 on the day milk samples were drawn by the University workers.

We have no desire to quarrel with dairy fieldmen on this matter, but we would like to point out that a great deal of investigational work indicates that causes other than mastitis are much more likely to be involved when the bacteria count of milk suddenly goes up. In the vast majority of cases it has been shown that the bacteria isolated were types not capable of causing mastitis, so that they must have reached the milk after it was drawn from the cows. Contamination of this kind can occur in several different ways.

In the first case we mentioned earlier, trouble was finally traced back to the dry storage of milking machine inflations between milkings, and it was promptly corrected by returning the inflations to lye storage during such periods. In the second case the owner was found to be using an ineffective sterilizer on his equipment. It was all right when he bought it, but it was a powder containing volatile ingredients that required storage in a closed container. Instead, he had left it in an open can, and as a result of continual exposure to the air, the powder had gradually been oxidized to the point where it had little more sterilizing power than cake flour. In our third case a window in the milk house had been opened to provide ventilation during a spell of hot weather. Unfortunately, the open window had also provided an entry for considerable dust from a nearby cornfield which had found its way into the bulk tank between milkings. There are some other causes of a high bacteria count in milk, but they can all be grouped in a listing like that represented by the first 10 items given as causes of milk failing to "stand up" under the reductase test. This list can be found on page 95.

In summarizing this subject, we might say that although it is possible for mastitis to cause a high bacteria count in milk, it is not very probable that this disease will do it. Therefore, it is not a very good policy to blame mastitis for a high bacteria count every time that some other cause can't be discovered right away. It may take a little extra time, but it's very likely that a painstaking investigation will show that the services of a veterinarian aren't needed at all for eliminating mastitis in a herd that suddenly becomes unable to produce low-bacteria milk.

Don't Produce Adulterated Milk

The matter of antibiotics in milk has received considerable publicity, for their presence constitutes adulteration under the Federal Food, Drug, and Cosmetic Act. Many articles have recently appeared in publications, and there is no doubt but what the crackdown against milk containing antibiotics is gaining momentum. Some dairies have permanently suspended producers when milk showed traces of antibiotics, temporarily refused the milk from others, and still other producers have been fortunate to get off with a warning from the dairy fieldman. Such action has resulted in a flood of questions from dairymen. We will list here some of the commonest of those questions, together with what we believe to be the correct answers.

Q. Granted that milk shouldn't be adulterated with anything, what other reason is there for all this fuss about antibiotics in milk? They sure aren't dirty, and small amounts shouldn't do any harm.

A. There are four good reasons:

1. Some people are allergic to certain antibiotics and become seriously sick, or may even die, when exposed to extremely small amounts of them. Dr. Donald Rosanove of the Mayo Clinic recently told the Minnesota State Veterinary Medical Society that 83 deaths were reported in 1958 from this cause, and others probably went unreported, since the symptoms are similar to a heart attack.*

* The Farmer, February 20, 1960, p. 8.

2. Other people may become desensitized to the germ-fighting powers of antibiotics through repeated exposure so that, when they are badly needed in times of illness, they may do them no good.

3. Antibiotics may inhibit bacterial growth so that small amounts of them interfere with the manufacture of certain cheeses.

4. A very small amount of antibiotic-carrying milk, once mixed with pure milk, can contaminate an entire tank car or truck.

Q. How do antibiotics get into milk?

A. Usually after they have been used to treat cows for mastitis, either through udder infusions, intramuscular injections, or introduction into the blood stream. They may also get into the milk after they have been used on animals to control other diseases, like foot rot and pneumonia. Feed containing antibiotics can cause adulteration of milk if it is not fed according to directions, and one dairyman of our acquaintance got into trouble by using antibiotics in his bulk tank to lower the bacteria count of his milk.

Q. What should be done with the milk from a quarter that has been treated with antibiotics to control mastitis?

A. It should be held out from the rest of the milk for at least 72 hours afterward. We know that claims are made for various antibiotics that milk needn't be held out so long, but we feel that the milk from treated cows should be considered as possibly adulterated for that long, anyway.

Q. When only one quarter of a cow is infused with antibiotics, what should be done with the milk from the other quarters?

A. The milk from all four quarters should be held out, even though there is no significant diffusion of antibiotics into the untreated quarters. We advise this because it is illegal to sell milk from unhealthy cows, and from a technical standpoint any cow that requires treatment for mastitis cannot be considered as healthy.

Q. What should be done with the milk from a cow that has been given an intramuscular injection of antibiotics?

A. This will depend on the kind used. Some penicillin compounds have been found in milk 10 days after such an injection, and consequently aren't recommended for use on lactating animals at all. If your veterinarian makes such an injection, ask him how long the milk should be discarded. If you make the injection yourself, look on the label of the product used for information in regard to the length of time milk should be held out.

Q. Can this discarded milk be fed to calves?

A. We don't favor the feeding of such milk to calves when the affected cow is seriously sick and requiring extensive medication. However, milk from the average cow that is mildly affected should be all right for calves, and might even prove beneficial. Many commercial calf feeds contain antibiotics which have been intentionally added for the control of infection.

Q. How are antibiotics detected in milk?

A. Usually at the receiving plant through inhibition tests involving the growth of certain types of bacteria. However, the Food and Drug Administration recently announced a new method of detecting penicillin which is sensitive and so fast that truck drivers can test milk from bulk tanks when it is picked up at farms.

Q. How long does it take to run tests at the plant?

A. The test generally used takes 2½ to 6 hours, but a supersensitive test takes 18 hours and is used when it becomes desirable to completely eliminate antibiotics in milk from a given area. This test is sensitive enough to detect a single 100,000 unit dose of penicillin that has been used in one quarter of a cow even after her milk has been diluted with that from over 160 other animals.

Q. Can a farmer check his own milk for antibiotics?

A. Not at this time, but it has been suggested that manufacturers mix dyes in the antibiotic ointments used against mastitis, so that milk would be colored as long as any antibiotic remained in the udder.

Q. Getting away from antibiotics, what should be done with the milk from cows that have been treated with sulfas and other drugs, either by udder infusion or other methods?

A. Although milk containing residues of these drugs probably won't constitute a human health hazard, they will be considered as adulterants if they affect the inhibition tests used on milk, so we recommend that it be discarded for 72 hours after treatment, too. Here again, the fact that treatment is needed signifies that this cow is unhealthy and one from which milk cannot be legally sold.

Q. What about milk from cows that have been fed "crumbles" and other feeds containing antibiotics?

A. Tests at the University of Rhode Island indicated that there was no contamination of milk from cows fed such feed at the recommended rate of 0.1 mg. per pound of body weight, but there was when cows were fed at the rate of 0.5 mg. per pound of body weight, so there seems no danger if the feeds are fed at recommended levels.

Recent legislation by the Food and Drug Administration requires label statements on drugs and antibiotics, telling owners the period of time required to discard milk after they are injected into lactating animals. An older law still requires similar labeling for udder-infusion of antibiotics and drugs.

As far as antibiotics and drugs are concerned, then, an owner can keep them out of milk simply by holding out milk from treated cows for the specified period. If he does this he will have to keep a pretty complete record of treatments. Some veterinarians have simplified this job for dairymen by pasting tags on the hips of treated cows, giving the date of treatment and date·on which milk can be sold again. Owners doing their own treating can do the same thing to help them remember.

However, antibiotics do not represent the only source of adulterants in milk, for pesticides of different kinds can get into it in at least five different ways:

1. Contamination of milking equipment, like tanks and pails.
2. Exposure of milk to sprays.
3. Exposure of cows to sprays.
4. Cows eating feeds contaminated with pesticides.
5. Cows drinking water contaminated with pesticides.

Pesticides pose a much more difficult problem than antibiotics and drugs, for contamination is sometimes hard to avoid. A farmer can spray a field for insects or weeds, or the state may spray an area for mosquitoes. A run-off after a rain may then form puddles or drain into a pond where cows drink, and a pesticide like DDT can lodge in the fat of cows and remain for long periods before traces no longer appear in the milk. Receiving plants can't run tests like they can for antibiotics, since pesticide tests are very expensive and practically impossible to run routinely in the plant. Accordingly, the responsibility for keeping pesticides out of milk becomes that of the dairyman. He can do this by observing these "don'ts," released by the Dairy Industry Committee:

1. Don't use anything but USDA approved sprays on walls, ceilings, and animals.

2. Don't use anything but USDA approved baits.
3. Don't contaminate milk or milking equipment when spraying in barns and milkhouses.
4. Don't contaminate feeds and drinking water when spraying in barns.
5. Don't use scatter baits or "barn sprays" inside milkhouses.
6. Don't spray animals in closed buildings.
7. Don't dust cows with methoxychlor or malathion powder within five hours of milking.
8. Don't feed fruit pomace and cannery wastes, unless you are sure they do not contain pesticide residues.
9. Don't fail to follow label directions when spraying cows, buildings, pastures, and crops, especially in regard to the time of spraying.
10. Don't allow cows to graze on fields that have been treated with DDT, toxaphene, chlordane, aldrin, dieldrin, heptachlor, or aramite.
11. Don't feed dairy cows plants that have been treated with any of the above. Treatment with phosdrin, dydox, endrin, methoxychlor, dibrom, malathion, and sevin will not keep forage from being fed, but it can be fed only after the period of time specified on the label.
12. Don't feed dairy cows ensilage made from plants that have been treated with any of the above, except under conditions noted.
13. Don't use pesticides that have been stored for long periods. Information on the label won't be up to date, and properties of the compound may have changed with time.

About Q Fever

A three-year (1958-1960) study at the University of Illinois, involving testing of over 8000 dairy animals, showed that 16% of the herds and 7% of the animals were positive. A recent investigation showed the presence of Q fever in nearly 23% of the 541 herds producing milk for the Milwaukee market. Testing in other states shows substantial evidence that Q fever infections are numerous through the Midwest. Human infection has been reported in Iowa, Wisconsin, Nebraska, and Ontario.

This disease is of little importance from a veterinary standpoint, for although affecting cattle, sheep, goats, and possibly other animals, it doesn't cause them to appear sick. Instead, it is considered as a serious occupational hazard for farmers and other people living near, handling, or having access to livestock.

It is caused by an organism of the rickettsiae group which has been given the name of *Coxiella burnetti,* and the disease is known as Q fever because it was first described in Queensland, Australia. Although the means of spread is not always known, it has been shown that ticks may act as carriers, and that the inhalation of rickettsiae-laden dust may also serve as a means of infection.

In the United States, *C. burnetti* has been found in both the lone star tick and the wood tick. Even if these ticks don't actually bite people, a possible method of human infection is the inhalation or wound contamination with the highly infective dried feces of the ticks. One authority believes that the great majority of people suffering from Q fever have been exposed to contaminated dust from dairy barns, or sheep and goat pens where diseased animals have been kept in the past. Most human outbreaks have occurred among people working with livestock in packing houses and stockyards, or in areas where indirect contact with animal products or dust is possible. Infected cows may give off rickettsiae with afterbirth, thus seeding the premises with millions of organisms. The rickettsiae are also found in milk, but they are destroyed by pasteurization. However, the drinking of raw milk might be a means of human infection.

In human beings, Q fever is characterized by sudden onset, high fever, headache, chills, weakness, and the development of an atypical pneumonia. In many respects the symptoms resemble a severe attack of influenza. An incubation period of about two weeks after exposure is followed by a period of fever that runs between 101 and 104 degrees. A dry cough develops on about the fifth day, with some pain in the chest. There are some variations in symptoms.

These variations are believed due to the fact that infection through the respiratory system results in an atypical pneumonia, while infection through the skin is characterized by fever, headache, and chills lasting one to three weeks. Involvement of the lungs can be demonstrated by X-ray examination, but the changes due to infection cannot be told from those caused by a virus pneumonia.

With proper care, there are few deaths from Q fever. However, an attack of pneumonia may cause a patient to require a much longer time than expected to regain normal health. In fact, it is fairly common for the recovery period to be quite long, even in the mildest of cases.

A definite diagnosis depends on isolation of rickettsiae from the blood or saliva, or through appropriate blood tests. Treatment with various antibiotics may aid in reducing the duration of fever and length of illness, but miraculous responses must not be expected from any of them.

No definite recommendations can be made in regard to preventive measures because there is a lack of knowledge in regard to how the disease is spread. However, it must be remembered that ticks are potentially dangerous and should be treated accordingly. Good ventilation and sanitary practices are desirable for reducing the dust hazard. Although Q fever may never be a disease of major importance in this country, cattle owners should recognize it as a danger, anyway. Up until the time investigational work was carried out, it wasn't considered as much of a problem in Wisconsin and Illinois, either. It may be more widespread in other states than anyone suspects, too.

Insecticides May Be Dangerous

We once visited a farm where several beef cattle had died shortly after being dipped to control mange mites. The owner couldn't believe that dipping was to blame, for he had followed directions to the letter in making up the solution. At about the same time we called at a dairy farm where three calves had died after being sprayed to control flies. The insecticides were to blame in both cases, but the contributing factors were different.

The beef cattle had been dipped in an emulsion that was not intended for use in a dipping vat, but was supposed to be used as a spray. This is an important point, for research has shown that some emulsions tend to form in large particles, either at the time of mixing or after standing. These particles of insecticide may then be deposited on the hair to give a strength many times that of the original emulsion. The formation of large particles is possible in practically all insecticide emulsions, but it is most dangerous in dipping operations. This is because a vat usually contains thousands of gallons, and each dipped animal is exposed to most of the contents. In contrast, when an animal is sprayed, it is seldom exposed to more than a gallon of emulsion. Knowing this, most manufacturers now produce insecticide concentrates with excellent emulsifying characteristics, and specify on containers whether or not they are to be used in dipping vats.

In the case of the dairy calves, the deaths were believed due to the type of sprayer used. The concentrate was mixed according to directions, and the particles in the emulsion were of a satisfactory small size. However, the concentrate had a tendency to settle out, and the hand sprayer used was not equipped with an agitator, of course. As a result, the last calves sprayed received an exceptionally strong dose of insecticide. It could have happened the other way around, too, for some concentrates have a tendency to "cream" or rise to the top of an emulsion, so that the first animals sprayed receive a dangerous dose of insecticide. In addition to the two illustrations we have given, there are some other ways in which insecticides can be dangerous for cattle, and for human beings as well.

One of the commoner ones is using emulsifiable concentrates that were manufactured for use on plants. The same active ingredient may be involved, but there is an important difference between plant and animal sprays. The plant-type emulsions are generally designed so that considerable insecticide is left sticking to the leaves, and we have already pointed out that this is an undesirable characteristic when emulsions are used on animals.

Another one is the use of insecticide on extremely young animals that are usually two to eight times more susceptible to poisoning than adult animals. The same danger, due to increased susceptibility, is present when young animals are given insecticides by mouth instead of being dipped or sprayed with them. This increased susceptibility is believed largely due to the relative ratios of body surface to body weight.

Another danger is represented by improper storage of insecticides in areas where they may be reached by cattle. Under the same heading can be included failure to dispose of empty containers and small amounts of left-over insecticides.

Another one consists of failure to read and follow directions in regard to mixing and application.

Finally, carelessness in handling can cause injury to human beings. It must be remembered that all of these insecticides are poisonous for people, and should be handled accordingly.

With the foregoing facts in mind, owners will do well to observe the following recommendations in regard to insecticides:

1. Make up emulsions in strength according to directions.
2. Determine if the concentrate is intended to make an emulsion to be used as a dip or spray, or both.

3. Determine if the concentrate is intended to make an emulsion to be used on plants or animals.
4. Use a sprayer equipped with an efficient agitator.
5. As an alternative, make up a small amount of emulsion and let it stand to see if the concentrate has a tendency to settle out or rise to the top.
6. Be careful about using insecticides on young calves.

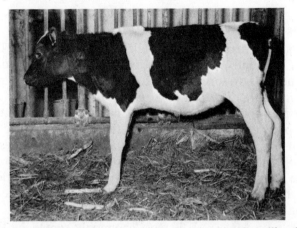

Be careful when using insecticides on young calves like this one.

7. Store all insecticides in a safe place, preferably under lock and key, in original, tightly-sealed containers.
8. Burn all combustible used containers, and keep out of smoke.
9. Puncture non-returnable containers, and handle returnable containers according to manufacturer's directions.
10. Be careful when handling insecticides. Wash before eating, after working with them, use appropriate protective clothing and respirators; remove clothing and wash thoroughly if insecticide is spilled on skin or clothing, change clothes daily.
11. Be sure not to contaminate feed and water when insecticides are being used.
12. Refrain from using insecticides in closed or poorly ventilated buildings.

3.

CONTAGIOUS DISEASES

Bang's Disease (Brucellosis)

CAUSE. Generally a germ called *Brucella abortus*. However, *Brucella suis* and *Brucella melitensis*, causing Bang's disease in swine and goats respectively, are also capable of causing this infection in cattle. The causative germs are occasionally found in the blood and various body organs for short periods of time, but usually persist permanently only in the udder, lymph glands, or pregnant uterus of the female and the testicles or accessory sex organs of the male. It is possible for steers to contract brucellosis, with the germs lodging in lymphoid tissue. There is little chance that such animals will transmit the infection as is the case of breeding stock.

MEANS OF SPREAD. It is most commonly spread by the movement of diseased animals. Infected females are believed to give off germs in vaginal discharges for about a month before and a month after calving. Calves from such animals are likely to be covered with germs, regardless of whether they are aborted or carried full term. Once dropped in barns or pastures the germs may be spread in many ways. Dogs may carry home infected material like parts of aborted calves. Germ-bearing litter may be dropped from stock trucks. Wild carrion-eaters like skunks, foxes, and crows may carry germs on their feet and pigeons or sparrows may do the same thing after visiting infected barn yards. Visiting neighbors, salesmen, stock dealers, and veterinarians are possible carriers, too. Chickens are frequent carriers, and so are rats that may actually become infected. Bang's germs may travel to clean farms through water in streams or drainage ditches. Home animals may bring back germs after being on exhibition or leased out for service. Regardless of how they are actually moved, the germs generally get into animals through being swallowed with food or water. However, Bang's disease may possibly be spread by the act of service, too. Bulls may become infected after breeding diseased cows that are discharging germs. Once infected, bulls may pass the disease on to cows that are bred to them either naturally or artificially, for germs are sometimes present in the semen.

SYMPTOMS. The commonest one is abortions that occur at about seven months, although they may happen at any time. There is nothing special about them to distinguish the abortions from those that may be caused by several other conditions. However, a large number of calves that are lost at about seven months in a herd is enough to cause suspicion of Bang's disease. As is usually the case with abortions due to any cause, they are likely to be accompanied with retained afterbirth. Breeding troubles are common in diseased herds, even when there are few abortions. Other symptoms include lowered milk production, poor body condition, and an evident lowered resistance to other diseases. Cows usually abort only once, and thereafter carry their calves full time. However, they generally remain as carriers and spreaders of germs that affect heifers as they come along and cause them to lose their first calves. A single abortion isn't an infallible rule, for some cows may abort twice or even oftener. In other cases there may be no abortions at all, with infected animals evidently having enough natural resistance to save their calves without having enough to keep them from becoming reactors and carriers. Swellings on the knees and hocks known as hygromas sometimes furnish evidence of Bang's infection, and so do rotten areas on the afterbirth where it has been fastened to "buttons" or cotyledons in the uterus. In common with a great many other troubles, calves from Bang's-infected dams may be born covered with a filthy yellow slime that tells of scouring before they were born. In males the testicles may become either shriveled or greatly swollen, while metritis and vaginal discharges are common symptoms of infection in females. An examination after death often shows nothing beyond swelling of the uterine "buttons" and the presence of a little pus in the organ.

DIAGNOSIS. Most practical through laboratory methods. Several tests depending on the presence of *Brucella* antibodies in the milk, blood, vaginal mucus, and semen have been used. The most common one is probably the standard plate test of blood. Although not 100 per cent infallible, neither is anything else that has been devised by man. After years of use it has demonstrated itself as being better than any other available procedure. It depends on the presence of so-called antibodies that appear in the blood stream after animals become infected with brucellosis. Blood serum is mixed with so-called antigen which is a suspension of stained dead *Brucella abortus* germs in a saline solution. Serum that contains the specific antibodies has the effect of clumping the dead germs and causing them to settle out. A large amount of infection means an increased clumping ability due to large numbers of antibodies. This faculty is used in running the blood test to indicate the severity of infection.

A calibrated pipette is used to measure out serum in the amounts of .04 cc., .02 cc., .01 cc., and .005 cc. A standardized drop of antigen is then added to the four serum amounts to give the familiar dilutions of 1:50, 1:100, 1:200, and 1:400 that are seen on the test cards. With smaller amounts of serum being used in each succeeding dilution, the test really measures the amount of antibodies that are present. The blood of a badly infected animal will probably contain enough antibodies to clump antigen even

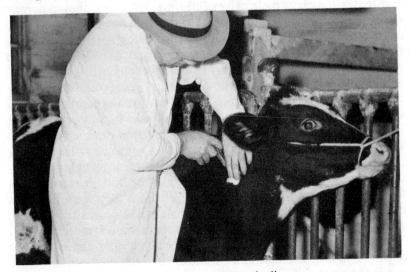

Vaccinating a calf for Bang's disease.

with the small amount of serum that is used in the 1:400 dilution as well as in the others. When clumping occurs in all four dilutions the animal is said to be a "four plus reactor." The status of all animals is determined by the extent to which clumping occurs in the various dilutions. It may be marked, barely noticeable, or entirely lacking in any of the dilutions to give readings of "plus," "incomplete," or "negative." Animals that show complete clumping in two or more of the dilutions are commonly called reactors. Those that show reactions of lesser extent are classed as suspects, while those showing no reactions at all are considered negative.

The plate test results are interpreted differently for officially vaccinated and nonvaccinated animals. Thus a vaccinate might still be classed as negative while showing an incomplete or complete reaction in the 1:50 dilution, while a nonvaccinate with the same reactions would be classed as a suspect.

A reactor cow must be considered as both a carrier and spreader, even though she doesn't abort her calves. Suspects aren't spreaders, but they may develop into reactors, so they have to be treated with caution. Any kind of a reaction to the blood test can generally be taken as meaning that involved animals are infected with Bang's disease to some extent. Reactors are likely to remain as such, although a small number of them will eventually throw off the disease and again become negative to the blood test. Suspects will do one of three things; go on to become reactors, remain as suspects, or clear up. In most cases they eventually become reactors.

A negative test shows that antibodies have not been formed in the blood, and this is generally taken to mean that infection is not present in an animal. However, animals that are in the "incubation" stage after exposure would not be shown up by the test because infection had not yet become strong enough to cause the formation of antibodies. Testing at a later time might easily show them to be suspects or even reactors. This possibility must always be considered when the blood test is run, for cows will sometimes even abort their calves before they show a reaction to the blood test.

Since nearly all infected cows shed *Brucella* antibodies in their milk, the milk ring test (MRT) is a practical means of detecting brucellosis in dairy herds. It serves as a screening device to identify possibly infected herds, and also as a practical way of repeatedly testing the same herds. A MRT report classifies a herd either as suspicious or negative, and suspicious herds are checked by blood testing each animal in them.

The test is run by adding 0.03 cc. of stained *Brucella* antigen to a well-mixed 1-cc. sample of milk. It is then oughly mixed and either incubated for an hour or · allowed to stand at room temperature for two hours. If the milk contains Brucella agglutinins, has enough butterfat, and possesses a cream-rising ability, the stained antigen clumps and is carried upward with the fat to form a deep-blue ring on top of the milk. If the specific agglutinins are not present, the antigen remains in suspension so that at the end of the incubation period there is a column of bluish milk capped by a white ring of unstained cream. Test results are usually reported in grades ranging from zero or negative up to four plus. When the ring of cream is white or practically white, the sample is given a negative rating. When the cream ring and milk below it are of about the same color, the sample is rated one plus or doubtful. When the cream ring is darkly stained and the milk is only slightly decolorized, the sample is rated two plus or weakly positive. When the cream ring is darkly stained and the milk is only partially decolorized, the sample is rated three plus or mildly positive. When the ring is darkly stained and is clearly separated from completely decolorized milk, the sample is rated four plus or strongly positive.

When the milk sample comes from more than 120 cows, it has been found necessary to modify the above procedure. This is done by using a 2- or 3-cc. sample of milk with 0.03 cc. of antigen. The exact procedure used will depend on the number of milking cows in a herd.

When most herds in an area are clean, the MRT supplies an inexpensive way of locating the few herds which should be blood tested. When the incidence of infection in an area is high, the ring test will probably not be justified, since most of the herds will have to be blood tested, anyway. Some states have started with blood testing and then adopted the MRT after the number of infected herds was greatly reduced.

The MRT has two principal disadvantages. First, a test that is sensitive enough to detect practically all infected herds will be sensitive enough to indicate some uninfected herds as being suspect. Such results are due to so-called "nonspecific" reactions which may be hard to explain. Second, logically enough, the MRT will not show up infected bulls, dry cows, or nonmilking heifers.

The market cattle testing (MCT) program is also used to detect infected herds and, like the MRT, represents a practical way of doing large-scale testing. Although of greatest value in beef herds or mixed beef and dairy herds, it is also useful in dairy herds being kept in areas where the MRT is not available. Its effectiveness is based on the fact that most owners regularly cull or sell surplus cattle from their herds.

Such animals are identified as to origin either at the farm, ranch, or stockyards by back tags applied by the owner, a veterinarian, or some other individual. A blood sample is collected from each animal at sales barns or slaughterhouses and sent to a laboratory for testing. If reactors are discovered, they are traced back to the herds of origin through the back tag numbers, and the entire home herd is then tested for brucellosis.

The recently developed card test appears to be a valuable addition to the older tests. The following advantages are claimed for it:

1. Simplicity.
2. Faster results.
3. Fewer retests required for elimination of brucellosis from a herd.
4. More accurate classification of problem cattle with a history of questionable plate or tube test results.

TREATMENT. None recognized at this time.

PREVENTION.

The best preventive program is composed of three parts. The most important one is concerned with sanitation, the next is calf-hood vaccination, and the third is regular testing, especially through MRT and MCT. Sanitary precautions are made up of ten major practices:

1. Avoiding the importation of infected animals by:
   a) Buying cattle only from certified Bang's-free herds.
   b) Testing all animals before buying them.
   c) Isolating them for 30 days after they are brought home.
   d) Retesting them at 30 day intervals until they freshen.
2. Blood testing the home herd regularly.
3. Eliminating reactors as soon as possible when they appear or isolating them for 30 days before and after freshening.
4. Isolating and retesting home animals that have been away.
5. Making people disinfect their shoes before walking in front of your cows.
6. Doing the same thing yourself when you've been on possibly infected premises.
7. Keeping chickens and dogs out of feed alleys.
8. Refusing natural service of bulls on outside cows.
9. Refusing to breed your cows either naturally or artificially to bulls not definitely known to be free of Bang's disease.
10. Eradicating rats on the farm.

Vaccination with Strain 19 is the second part. Research work and years of experience has led authorities to conclude that:

1. The best age for vaccination is between 4 and 8 months.
2. Revaccination does no good and may actually do harm.
3. Vaccination is best done with a 5 cc. dose given subcutaneously.

Calfhood vaccination has the strong points of:

1. Giving a resistance which protects most animals for at least two or three years, and probably for much longer periods.
2. Having a tendency to decrease the damage done by Bang's disease, even if vaccinates later become infected.
3. Being better than allowing heifers to become naturally infected through reacting animals.

It has the weak points of:

1. Not giving definite immunity, particularly in herds where a great many reactors are retained.
2. Creating reactions to the blood test that may persist for long periods of time to interfere with clean herd tests, certification, and the sale of animals.
3. Bringing up the problem of confusing test reactions due to vaccination with those due to natural infection. They can't be told apart at this time.

There appear to be at least five good reasons why bulls should not be calfhood-vaccinated against Bang's disease:

1. They can't possibly give birth to calves, so there is no object in trying to prevent abortions by bulls. If they don't abort, they won't be giving off infected discharges to contaminate feed and water.
2. Although bulls can swallow Bang's germs and become infected in the same way as cows, they ordinarily don't have such a good chance to pick up the germs with feed and water. Under dairy farm conditions bulls are generally kept by themselves, while cows run together so one infected animal has a chance to expose all the others. Germs may be carried on shoes to the feed alleys of cows, but people aren't likely to be walking around in a bull's manger. Under beef farm conditions bulls often run on pastures with cows, but they don't usually run with them all the time. Accordingly, most of the females have had their calves over a month before the bulls are turned in with them. Since diseased cows generally give off germs for only about a month before and after calving, they probably won't be acting as spreaders when they contact bulls. Any germs that are released will probably be killed by summer sunshine before they have a chance to infect the sires.

3. Since bulls aren't infected as often as cows, they aren't so likely to act as spreaders of Bang's disease through infected semen and breeding activities. If they are unlikely to be either infected or spreaders of the disease, there seems to be little object in vaccinating them against Bang's.

4. Bulls are likely to remain as permanent reactors to the blood test after vaccination, while heifers can be expected to become negative again within a few months. This difference is explained by physiology. Live germs introduced by vaccination can grow in females only in the pregnant uterus or the udder. Heifers between four and eight months old won't be pregnant, and they won't have much in the way of udders, so the germs soon leave their bodies. Bulls of any age have testicles which offer a permanent dwelling place for Strain 19 germs. They aren't eliminated from the body, and thus cause a continued reaction to the blood test. This failure to "clear up" may then interfere with sales and certification of a herd as Bang's-free.

5. In addition, harboring of germs in the testicles might possibly interfere with sperm production so bulls become poor breeders.

Although authorities recommend that calves be vaccinated between four and eight months of age, a little uncertainty still exists in regard to the best age for vaccination. This is due to the fact that vaccinated heifers are known to abort sometimes because of Bang's disease, while it's also known that others sometimes fail to "clear up" following vaccination and remain as reactors to the blood test for long periods afterward. Accordingly, owners often ask if these undesirable possibilities can't be avoided by vaccination at a certain age. The facts are a bit contradictory, since the correct vaccination age for preventing one trouble tends to encourage the other.

Young calves are naturally highly resistant to Bang's disease, and any germs that happen to be picked up are soon eliminated from their bodies. Vaccination, of course, consists of injecting a harmless variety of living Bang's germs. These harmless germs have to remain in the body for some time in order for resistance to be built up. Unfortunately, when they're injected into highly resistant animals, the germs have a good chance of being eliminated before much resistance is built up. These calves then aren't reactors to the blood test for very long after vaccination. On the other hand, these animals may have so little resistance that they become infected with Bang's disease so they abort in later life. This type of misfortune can be prevented by vaccinating the calves when they're a little older, but this practice has a disadvantage, too.

These older calves have much less natural resistance, so germs injected by vaccination don't leave the body so fast. Consequently, a strong resistance is generally established which is pretty sure to prevent later abortions. However, the long stay of the germs may cause animals to react to the blood test for long periods or be responsible for ring test reactions after they have freshened.

With the above in mind, owners have two choices in regard to the age for vaccination. They can vaccinate the animals at about four months and be reasonably sure that they'll soon "clear up" to the blood test without being equally sure that they won't abort later in life. Or, they can vaccinate heifers that are close to eight months old and be pretty sure that they won't abort, but without being equally sure that they won't remain as reactors to the test.

It is doubtful if adult vaccination is ever advisable except in cases where an abortion "storm" threatens in a herd. Even then it can't be completely depended upon to halt trouble, for resistance following vaccination takes time to build up, as previously mentioned. Aside from that, it also has certain disadvantages:

1. Reactions to the blood test may persist for life.
2. Abortions may be produced in occasional cows.
3. Persistent reactions may interfere with health regulations and the marketing of milk from vaccinated herds.
4. They may also interfere with sale of stock from such herds.
5. Raw milk from reacting animals, vaccinated or not, may contain germs that are dangerous to man.

Recognizing that the same plan may not be practical for all owners, the Bureau of Animal Industry has approved four different ones for the prevention and eventual eradication of Bang's disease.

Plan "A" calls for regular herd testing and prompt slaughtering of reactors to secure and maintain a certified Bang's-free herd. Calfhood vaccination may or may not be included and is at the option of the owner.

Plan "B" calls for regular testing, calfhood vaccination, and the temporary retention of reacting animals.

Plan "C" calls for calfhood vaccination without testing of the herd.

Plan "D" calls for adult vaccination and is little used.

The last three plans are intended for use by owners who are not immediately able to undertake test and slaughter under Plan "A." It is recommended that these plans be eventually discontinued in favor of the first one as soon as the number of reactors has been reduced to make the change possible.

Laws in the different states vary considerably, so before doing anything about a Bang's control program you'd better consult your county agent or local veterinarian. Lacking either one, you can still write the state livestock officials in your capital and get their advice. Depending on where you live, you may or may not be able to get your cattle tested and calves vaccinated free of charge under a combined state and government program. Since Bang's prevention and eradication is a big job, you will probably want all the help you can get on the matter. Once you have the facts, you can decide for yourself what course is best in your particular case.

Anaplasmosis

CAUSE. Two greatly similar parasites called *Anaplasmosis marginale* and *Anaplasmosis centrale*. Inside the body they are found only within the red blood cells. During spells of high fever they may infect 50 per cent of the total cells, and they can persist indefinitely in the blood of recovered cattle that then act as carriers. Sickness results from destruction of the red blood cells. The living place of the parasites outside of animals is unknown, but wild ruminants like elk and deer are known to be carriers of anaplasmosis and may be very important reservoirs of infection.

MEANS OF SPREAD. Generally believed to be principally spread by at least 19 different kinds of ticks that carry infected blood from animals. Mosquitoes and several varieties of blood-feeding insects, particularly horseflies, have also been proven as carriers. In addition, it is often spread by unclean instruments used for dehorning, castration, ear marking, and other operations, as well as equipment like pitchforks, nose leads, and hypodermic needles. As a matter of fact, anything that is capable of breaking the skin must be considered as a possible means of spreading anaplasmosis. Ticks which have fed on carrier deer have been shown as capable of spreading the disease to cattle.

Once pretty much confined to the warmer southern states, the movement of carrier animals has spread the disease to many of our northern states as well. These carriers are animals that have recovered from an attack and are permanently immune, but a large percentage of the them remain as carriers. When calves are born to carrier dams, they may be infected before birth.

SYMPTOMS. Infection due to *A. marginale* is the only type recognized in the U.S. and Canada today, and it is known as the "malignant" type of anaplasmosis. Common symptoms consist of animals suddenly going off feed in combination with complete stoppage of milk production and a fever of 104° F., or higher. Breathing is fast and the heartbeat may approach 100 per minute. The ears droop, constipation may be evident, and trembling may occur. Abortions are to be expected, probably because of the high fever and destruction of blood cells. Slobbering is also a frequent symptom. Urination may be frequent, but the urine is not bloody as in the case of pyelonephritis. A great many older animals can be expected to die within a day or two, with yellowing of the eyes and skin extremely noticeable shortly before death. Affected animals show a desire to eat dirt, probably an instinctive effort to replace essential minerals lost through the destruction of red blood cells. The disease is generally mild in calves up to a year old; severe, but seldom fatal in animals up to two years old; severe, and occasionally fatal in animals up to three years old; and exceptionally severe and often fatal in older animals.

Infection due to *A. centrale* was unknown outside of Africa up to a few years ago, and it is known as the "benign" type of anaplasmosis. In recent years it has been introduced into Australia and some of the Latin American countries as a possible means of protection against the severe form caused by *A. marginale*. Results of such work have been variable and not very satisfactory.

DIAGNOSIS. Made only in the laboratory through microscopic examination of the blood and fluorescent antibody testing. The detection of carrier animals presented a major problem for a long time, but the complement-fixation and capillary-tube agglutination tests are now used for this purpose. Because of the similarity of symptoms, anaplasmosis might be confused with such troubles as anthrax, blackleg, shipping fever, mineral deficiencies, and poisoning.

TREATMENT. Favorable reports have been made regarding the use of several drugs, including antimalarials, arsenicals, and dyes, but these reports are questionable because the results of treatment have been evaluated according to the number of treated cattle that recover. Conclusions formed on such a basis may not be very accurate because of the great variation in susceptibility of cattle that permits many recoveries without any treatment at all. None of these drugs has been demonstrated as having any effect on *A. marginale* or modifying the normal course of infection. None of them has eliminated carrier infection. Neomycin, erythromycin, tylosin, and Compound 10073 had no effect on the course of anaplasmosis in animals treated with these drugs.

At this time only chlortetracycline, tetracycline, and oxytetracycline have been effective in controlling the increase of *A. marginale* and changing the course of the disease. Recommended treatment consists of at least one injection of 3 to 5 milligrams of tetracycline per pound of body weight in combination with blood transfusion. Treatment is most effective when given early. The possibility of preventing carrier infection by feeding tetracylines has also been investigated and shown as promising.

Various dithiosemicarbazones have been reported as effective against *A. marginale* in tests made on calves. When given by mouth for three days at a daily dose of 100 mg. per kilogram of body weight, they compared favorably with oxytetracycline given intravenously for three days in daily doses of 10 mg. per kilogram of body weight. One of these, ethoxyethylglyglyoxal dithiosemicarbazone, was reported as being effective in adult cattle as well as calves.

Blood transfusions of one or two gallons are helpful in bad cases of anemia. A single one will usually be enough, but a second may be required a couple of days later. Although cattle may occasionally show allergic reactions and even die after such transfusions because of differences in blood types, this risk should not prohibit such treatment. There is really little to lose, for animals that need transfusions will probably die without them, anyway.

Along with medical treatment, animals should be isolated, given quiet, comfortable, shady quarters, be provided with plenty of good quality hay or pasture, and furnished with easily accessible, clean, fresh drinking water. Animals suffering from severe anemia should be handled as little as possible, since the destruction of red blood cells causes them to tire easily. When dangerously sick animals are on pasture or happen to be semi-wild range cattle, they are best treated where they are found, with shade, hay, and water being brought to them. Extremely excitable animals should be left completely alone, since efforts to treat or restrain them may cause determined resistance that results in heart failure and death. Occasional spraying with suitable repellents will make animals more comfortable at the same time that chances of infecting other cattle through tick and insect bites are being decreased. Other procedures that may be of value in the treatment of anaplasmosis include the intravenous injection of sugar solutions to provide strength and compensate for dehydration.

PREVENTION. Largely a matter of management designed to reduce the chances of infected blood being transferred to susceptible cattle from sick animals, wild animals, or apparently healthy carriers. Sanitary procedures should be followed when jobs like castration, dehorning, ear-tagging, blood testing, and vaccinating are being done. Instruments used for surgery of any kind should be rinsed free of blood and disinfected before reusing. When blood testing or vaccination is being done, needles should either be cleaned and disinfected before reusing or a sterilized different one should be used on each animal. Sick animals should be sprayed regularly in warm months to reduce the chances of clean animals being infected by ticks and bloodsucking insects. Susceptible cattle should be sprayed regularly during the warm months with approved pesticides or furnished with treadle sprayers or back rubbers that allow them to treat themselves. Experimental work has shown that the feeding of tetracyclines is an effective preventive measure.

Ordinary recovered cattle that remain as carriers are best sent to slaughter so they are removed as a source of infection. Valuable recovered carriers may be isolated, sprayed daily, and given feeds containing tetracyclines in the hope of making them non-carriers. Animals that die should be deeply buried, burned, or immediately removed from the premises.

A practical method of preventing anaplasmosis on a herd scale in areas where biting insects are the chief spreaders consists of establishing two herds. The herd is first blood tested and all reactors and carriers are removed to a location a mile or more away from the other animals. A distance like this is desirable to control spread by flying insects. In areas where wild animals exist as reservoirs of infection and ticks are important as potential spreaders, a program of isolation and testing will probably not be satisfactory. In such cases, a program of vaccination offers the best solution to the problem. Three different vaccines have been developed.

The first was a vaccine consisting of blood containing live *A. centrale,* which has been used in certain parts of Africa for over 50 years, and more recently in Australia and certain Latin American countries. Results have been variable and in general not very satisfactory. The use of this vaccine is not permitted in the U.S.

The second was a vaccine containing killed *Anaplasma* organisms. Experimental work has raised serious doubts about the immunity given by this product, so it cannot be recommended at this time.

The third was a so-called attenuated vaccine, consisting of a live *A. marginale* strain which was adapted to sheep. During repeated passages the strain became harmless for cattle while still giving immunity to vaccinated animals. Experimental work has demonstrated it as being highly effective against anaplasmosis. Today it looks like the best tool to use in controlling losses in areas where large numbers of cattle are already infected and non-infected cattle are always in danger of being exposed to anaplasmosis.

Rinderpest (Cattle Plague)

CAUSE. A virus which at various stages of the disease is present in all body tissues and discharges. It is widespread in the Eastern hemisphere, although Japan, the Philippines, Australia, and New Zealand are free of the disease. It is a serious problem in most of northern Africa, where large numbers of wild animals act as carriers and spreaders. It is not present at this time in Western Europe or the Western Hemisphere, although an outbreak occurred in Brazil in 1921. All ruminant animals are susceptible, but they vary in susceptibility according to species. For example, sheep and goats are so seldom affected that they are not vaccinated as a protective measure. Cattle and buffalo are the animals most commonly involved. Swine are susceptible, but vary in susceptibility according to geographical occurrence. It has been shown that swine are able to transmit the disease to either cattle or other swine.

The virus is readily killed by ordinary disinfectants, particularly lye solutions. It has been shown to be fairly delicate under wet or warm conditions, but will survive for several days in a dried condition, and for several years in a dried and frozen condition. Sulfas and antibiotics have no effect on the virus. It has been shown that the viruses of rinderpest, dog distemper, and measles are related in several respects. There are several different strains of rinderpest virus which vary in their virulence.

MEANS OF SPREAD. Usually through direct contact between infected and susceptible animals. Diseased animals may shed the virus from a day or two before showing fever, through the period when fever is shown, and for several days afterward. The delicate nature of the virus generally prevents indirect transmission through contaminated feed, water, and materials brought in by dogs, birds, and human beings. Mechanical transmission in blood by biting ticks or flies is a possibility.

SYMPTOMS. First, restlessness, constipation, and a fever of 104° F., or more. Discharges from the eyes and nostrils are seen in a day or two, animals go off feed, appear dull, are thirsty, and stop chewing their cuds. An examination of the mouth will show lesions on the lips, gums, and tongue, and a severe diarrhea is always shown. Coughing and difficult breathing are common symptoms, the coat becomes rough, and animals lose weight at a rapid rate so they become little more than walking skeletons in a very short time. Sores in the mouth cause profuse slobbering. From 25 per cent to practically all the animals in a herd may become affected, depending on the resistance of the cattle and the virulence of the virus strain that is involved. The death rate may also vary widely, but recovered animals are immune for life.

Opening a dead animal will generally show lesions in various parts of the mouth, pharynx, and upper part of the esophagus. The fourth or true stomach is apt to show bloody erosions, and this is also common in the large intestine.

DIAGNOSIS. Positive only in the laboratory through isolation of the virus or inoculation of test animals. Diagnosis by symptoms alone may be difficult because of the variation in virus strains and in resistance of cattle, and is further complicated by the similarity of symptoms to those of IBR and BVD. Accordingly, the appearance of suspected rinderpest in a region previously free of this disease should be checked out pretty thoroughly.

TREATMENT. None recommended, because quarantine and slaughter are believed to be the best course to follow when the disease appears in an area that was formerly free of rinderpest. This was demonstrated in the Brazil outbreak of 1921.

PREVENTION. This disease has never appeared in the United States, and in the event of an outbreak it is likely that it would be handled as foot and mouth disease has been controlled in the past. However, the use of vaccines may be desirable in countries where the slaughter of all exposed and possibly infected animals is impractical.

Some of these vaccines are made by passing the virus through animals other than cattle to change them so their virulence is reduced. The goat virus is too virulent for European cattle and, while the rabbit virus is suitable for use in European cattle it is too mild for use in zebu stock, and too virulent for breeds like African Ankoke, Sanga, and Ndama. No egg-adapted virus has been as stable at a satisfactory level of virulence as the goat- and rabbit-type vaccines. The tissue vaccine made by passage of the virus on calf kidney cells has several advantages, and is now the vaccine of choice for general use in Africa.

Vibriosis (Vibrionic Abortion)

CAUSE. A bacterium named *Vibrio fetus venerealis*. Organisms may be found in the digestive systems of aborted calves and in the reproductive tract, the afterbirth, and sometimes the liver of an infected cow. They may sometimes be found in the semen or reproductive organs of bulls.

A similar bacterium named *Vibrio fetus intestinalis* occurs naturally in the intestine of cattle, sheep, and swine. Although it sometimes enters the reproductive tract of sheep and cattle, and is the cause of epizootic abortion in sheep, it is relatively unimportant in bovine vibriosis, even though it is occasionally found in aborted calves.

MEANS OF SPREAD. Only through venereal means. Usually through natural service, with infected animals of both sexes being able to infect susceptible animals of the opposite sex. The disease can also be spread by artificial insemination with germ-bearing semen, but the infection is not transmitted from cow to cow through direct contact. It is generally considered that the spread of infection from bull to bull in artificial insemination studs is really venereal and results from contact with teaser animals, contaminated equipment, and clothing of handlers.

SYMPTOMS. The most important one was once believed to be abortions that might occur at any stage of pregnancy. However, the use of artificial insemination acted to control the disease in dairy herds, and today the outstanding symptom is breeding trouble, particularly in beef cattle of western range states. Abortions that occur at 60 to 90 days may easily escape notice, and signs of heat in supposedly pregnant animals may then be the first indication of infection in a herd. Sometimes a routine pregnancy examination of the herd will reveal an unusually large number of "open" cows that furnish evidence of a sterility problem. In addition, vaginal discharges, repeated breedings without conception, irregular heat cycles, and loss of weight in overworked bulls may be symptoms of this disease.

DIAGNOSIS. Definitely made only in the laboratory, although a tentative diagnosis can often be made on the basis of a history that indicates a herd-scale problem of breeding troubles. The causative organism may be found either in aborted calves, vaginal mucus samples from infected females, or semen samples from infected bulls. However, vibriosis is best diagnosed in bulls through the test-mating of virgin heifers. The heifers are then tested later by examining vaginal mucus. It will also be possible to make a diagnosis of vibriosis by using the vibriosis vaccine. This is best done by vaccinating and identifying part of the replacement heifers and breeding them naturally to the regular herd bulls. If vibriosis is present, the vaccinated heifers will have a high rate of conception and the unvaccinated heifers will have a much lower rate. If something else is causing breeding troubles, the conception rates of the two groups will be much the same. Blood tests have been found to be unreliable for the diagnosis of vibricosis. Under farm conditions it might be confused with troubles like leptospirosis, trichomoniasis, and problems due to poor management practices.

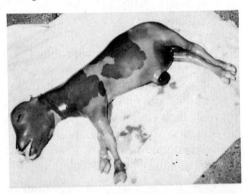

Calf aborted at five months because of vibriosis.

TREATMENT. Of doubtful value because reinfection occurs so easily. Intrauterine infusion with streptomycin has been recommended for cows, with 1 gram of streptomycin being given in two doses 48 hours apart in an aqueous vehicle. Experimental work has shown that a single subcutaneous injection of streptomycin (10 mg. per pound body weight) in combination with an application of 5 grams of a 50 per cent solution of streptomycin to the penis and prepuce would effect a permanent cure in bulls. However, these bulls became infected again when exposed to the disease later. Under ranch conditions the treatment of bulls would probably be of little value because they would become reinfected as soon as they bred a carrier cow.

PREVENTION. Begins with good management practices aimed at keeping the disease from getting started in a herd. This includes such things as maintaining a closed herd, keeping out wandering bulls, and refusing to use "loaner" bulls. When females are introduced, they should be:

1. Purchased only in herds that are known to be free of breeding troubles that might indicate the presence of vibriosis.
2. Isolated for at least 30 days after being brought home, and checked regularly for pregnancy until after they have calves.
3. Bred artificially to prevent possible infection of bulls.

The disease can be completely prevented in small herds by the exclusive use of artificial insemination with semen treated with antibiotics. A clean herd can be established by isolating virgin heifer and bull calves and eventually replacing an infected herd, but this will usually prove impractical.

Instead, a program of vaccination is recommended. All animals not vaccinated previously are injected with a single dose of vaccine a month or two before breeding and possible exposure. It will usually be more convenient to vaccinate older animals that are already protected by an earlier vaccination or infection sometime before they calve. It will be best to vaccinate all animals at once after the disease is diagnosed in a herd, since the older cows may not be protected by immunity following previous infection. Experimental work suggests that protection will be satisfactory if cows are vaccinated at weaning time, and vaccination of all females every year is recommended for best results. There is no data to show that vaccination of bulls would serve any useful purpose. The vaccine is killed, so there is no danger of producing the disease in vaccinates. Accordingly, many owners of noninfected herds surrounded by infected herds have vaccinated their animals as protection against accidental introduction of the disease.

Anthrax or Splenic Fever

CAUSE. A germ called *Bacillus anthracis*. The organisms are found throughout the blood and bodies of diseased animals.

MEANS OF SPREAD. Generally through the swallowing of germs or spores, although infection can also occur through cuts in the skin. Spores represent the dormant stage of the germs and are formed from organisms that are exposed to air through the escape of blood or body excretions from diseased animals. These spores may live in the soil for years and cause localities to be known as "anthrax districts." In past years tanneries have sometimes spread anthrax through the handling of infected hides. Germ-bearing liquid from the soaking vats was often dumped in streams to be carried to pastures. Germs and spores are also carried in grain or roughage grown on infected soil, and in some cases have been traced back to unsterilized bone meal and fertilizers of animal origin. When carcasses are left unburied, the disease may be widely spread by scavengers like crows, dogs, and wild animals. In one case an outbreak of anthrax was started by animals chewing on a piece of infected rope that had dropped off a rendering works truck. The swallowing of anthrax organisms is greatly encouraged by a combination of drouth and hot weather which leads to close grazing and the drinking of dirty water. Anthrax is also spread by mosquitoes and blood-sucking flies that successively feed on diseased and healthy animals. Spread may also be effected through the use of contaminated instruments used for dehorning, castration, and other types of surgery. Since vaccine has also been the cause of many outbreaks, some states have laws restricting the use of such products.

SYMPTOMS. Sudden death is the most striking one. Healthy-looking animals may simply drop dead or die within a few hours after slobbering, trembling, grinding their teeth and breathing fast. At other times they may live longer and show temperatures above 105 in connection with a pulse rate of nearly 100 and complete stoppage of milk production. Swellings may appear at the throat or in other regions of the body, and a bloody diarrhea is not unusual. Dark blood or bloody foam may escape from the mouth, nostrils, anus, and vulva. Dead bodies fail to stiffen in a normal manner, blood fails to clot, and decomposition sets in early. Opening a dead animal may show bloody areas of the skin and muscles, with bloody liquid in the body cavities. The spleen is commonly greatly enlarged, a fact which is responsible for the name "splenic fever." There are two good reasons why animals suspected of having anthrax should never be opened:

1. Blood and body fluids may be released to contaminate surroundings with spores.
2. Man is susceptible to this disease and is seriously endangered by handling infected material.

DIAGNOSIS. Definitely made only in the laboratory through culturing of organisms, guinea pig injection, and biochemical procedures. However, a tentative diagnosis may be made on the basis of history and symptoms shown by affected animals. When anthrax is suspected, it will be best to deliver specimens to the laboratory rather than mail them. Under field conditions anthrax might be mistaken for such troubles as lightning stroke, poisoning, blackleg, and other causes of sudden death. A veterinarian should be called promptly whenever anthrax is suspected, since an outbreak of this disease represents serious danger for human beings and animals alike in the entire surrounding area.

TREATMENT. Various antibiotics like penicillin and the tetracyclines have been used successfully in the treatment of animals affected with anthrax. However, if treatment is to be successful, these drugs must be given early in massive doses. Animals showing symptoms should be given aqueous penicillin intravenously in combination with procaine penicillin intramuscularly. Animals which react to vaccine should be treated with antibiotics.

PREVENTION. Vaccination is the most practical means in areas where anthrax is known to exist. This should be done every year a month or two in advance of the pasture season. When cattle are in badly contaminated areas, two doses of vaccine two to four weeks apart are recommended. A swelling may develop at the injection site in highly susceptible animals or older ones, and resistance in vaccinates may possibly be overcome by heavy exposure. When resistance breaks down, extra booster vaccinations may be advisable to prevent further losses. Different types of anthrax vaccines are available, and their selection should be left up to your local veterinarian or state officials who are familiar with the specific needs of an area. This is important in another way, too, for some of these vaccines contain living organisms, and their use is restricted by the laws of some states. Consequently, owners should check on this matter before undertaking to use them.

In case of an outbreak, sick animals should be isolated as much as possible, with healthy ones being moved to a different location and vaccinated for protection. Dead animals should be promptly burned or deeply buried in quicklime without cutting the skin. Body excretions of infected animals should be destroyed by burning. Premises should be thoroughly cleaned and disinfected after outbreaks, and a quarantine is desirable to prevent the moving of cattle, either living or dead.

Blackleg (Black Quarter)

CAUSE. A bacterium called *Clostridium chauvei*. Germs are distributed throughout the bodies of diseased animals.

MEANS OF SPREAD. Generally through the swallowing of germs, but also through contamination of skin wounds. The carcasses of dead animals represent the chief source of infection, for spores are formed both inside and outside the bodies. These spores will persist indefinitely in soil like those of anthrax, even when cattle are kept off pastures for years.

SYMPTOMS. Lameness is apt to be the first one noticed, but general sickness is soon shown by going off feed, trembling, fever of 105 and higher, fast pulse, and labored breathing. Along with other symptoms, swellings appear in various body muscles, chiefly in the hips, flanks, and shoulders. These swellings are small and painful at first, but soon become extensive and painless to the touch. Skin over the center of the swellings eventually becomes dry and paper-like. Gas in the tissues causes a peculiar crackling sound when the swellings are rubbed, and opening one of them usually reveals a dark, frothy liquid that has a peculiar sour smell. Muscles in the swollen areas are characterized by a metallic sheen that is easily seen. The disease is seldom seen in animals over two years old, but a milder form sometimes affects the older stock. Most of the young animals die within a day or two after symptoms appear, but those that recover at any age are immune to blackleg for life afterward. The formation of gas continues even after death and blackleg deaths are noted for excessive bloating that causes legs to stick straight out and forces bloody foam from the natural body openings. Blood clots in a normal manner and in this way is different from that of anthrax cases. Outbreaks are commonest when stock is on pasture, but may occur at any time of the year.

DIAGNOSIS. Definite only when *C. chauvei* germs can be found in tissues examined under the microscope. However, a highly fatal disease that affects young cattle and is distinguished by gassy swelling of muscles is always enough to warrant a tentative diagnosis of blackleg. Even then, the disease may be confused with others like anthrax, shipping fever, sweet clover poisoning, and malignant edema.

TREATMENT. Not very satisfactory unless the disease is caught in the early stages. Massive doses of crystalline penicillin in saline solution given intravenously are recommended to secure an immediate high blood level. This is to be followed by intramuscular injections of penicillin in oil in 3-million unit doses to prolong the action. Close inspection every day will be needed for detection of the disease in the early stages.

PREVENTION. Vaccination with bacterins has been proven as very effective for immunizing susceptible cattle. However, for seven to ten days after vaccination animals are more susceptible to infection, so losses may continue for at least ten days after vaccination. Since they contain no living germs, the bacterins cannot cause the disease.

Local conditions will determine the best time for vaccination, but in general, four months is considered the best age. However, if an area is badly infected, it will be advisable to vaccinate calves at about one month of age when immunity given by antibodies in the colostrum has been lost. Such animals should then be revaccinated at weaning time because the colostrum immunity may prevent proper action of the bacterin. If an outbreak occurs, it will be desirable to vaccinate all cattle less than two years old, with the exception of calves less than one month old. Since mixed infections are likely to occur, the use of a mixed bacterin gives extra insurance. Whenever possible, vaccinated animals should be separated from the herd and kept on dry feed for at least ten days following vaccination.

When animals die of blackleg, carcasses are best destroyed by burning. As an alternative, they should be buried deeply in quicklime. Such destruction is desirable because infection is distributed throughout the body at the time of death. Spores are highly resistant to heat and cold, and may persist in the soil for years. In addition, they can be carried by dogs, wild animals, birds, and floods to infect a large area if infected carcasses are not completely destroyed. Small patches of ground can be made fairly safe by burning a heavy layer of straw on them. It is believed that infected pastures may eventually become clean if a program of vaccination is followed every year to prevent the reintroduction of germs from carcasses.

True Cowpox

CAUSE. A virus closely related to that of smallpox in man. Present in infected tissues and harbored indefinitely in undisinfected stables. It is unknown where the virus exists between outbreaks and how it gets started in clean herds.

MEANS OF SPREAD. Often brought in with purchased animals and then spread from cow to cow on the hands of milkers or the inflations of machines. On some occasions outbreaks have been started by dairy helpers shortly after they were vaccinated for smallpox. Susceptible animals may also pick up the infection from contaminated stables where the virus seems able to live for long periods.

SYMPTOMS. The disease starts on the teats and udder as painful little red swellings that change into blister-like vesicles within a day or two. They are usually ruptured by the act of milking at this stage, but if undisturbed the vesicular fluid changes to pus before rupturing occurs naturally. In either case, scabs soon form over the ruptured vesicles. All stages of the disease may sometimes exist on the udder and teats of a single cow. Animals may "step" and kick at milking time because of the sore teats. Cowpox may persist in herds for months at a time, but recovered animals are usually permanently immune.

DIAGNOSIS. Based entirely on the appearance and location of the vesicles. It is practically impossible to tell it from false cowpox, although evident immunity after a single attack is sometimes helpful in this respect. The condition may also be confused with vesicular stomatitis, mud infection, suppurative dermatitis, and other causes of sore teats.

TREATMENT. It is doubtful if any drug does much good against true cowpox, but the teats can at least be softened a little and made less painful by certain agents. Zinc oxide, equal parts of glycerine and iodine, sulfathiazole ointment, and even plain vaseline or wool fat may prove helpful for this purpose.

PREVENTION. A thorough cleanup and disinfecting job is necessary in all barns where outbreaks of cowpox have appeared. Otherwise heifers and other susceptible animals may come down with the disease months after the last case has cleared up. In case of active infection, affected cows should be milked last and sanitary measures followed to prevent carrying the virus to clean cows. Scabs, cracks, and sores near the ends of the teats are particularly dangerous because they encourage invasion of teat canals by bacteria which may cause mastitis. Frankel in the Netherlands (*Tijdschrift Voor Diergeneeskunde*, January 1955) reports the development of a vaccine to protect cattle against cowpox.

False Cowpox (Pseudo-Cowpox)

CAUSE. A virus much like the one causing bovine papular stomatitis. It also appears to be the same one that causes so-called "milker's nodules" in man. This is the pox condition seen most often in cattle of the United States. Animals recovering from cowpox and human beings vaccinated against smallpox are susceptible to false cowpox infection, so it is evidently different from the viruses causing these diseases.

MEANS OF SPREAD. Evidently the same as for true cowpox.

SYMPTOMS. Almost exactly the same as for true cowpox, but different in that cows may be repeatedly infected after recovery from attacks.

DIAGNOSIS. Impossible to distinguish from true cowpox outside of the laboratory. However, the fact that lesions are usually smaller than those of true cowpox, and a history of repeated infection may help in making a tentative diagnosis.

TREATMENT. When applied after each milking sulfathiazole ointment is often very effective. Other remedies as mentioned under true cowpox may also do some good. In general, though, this is a highly discouraging condition to treat, for all kinds of different treatments can sometimes be used without noticeable improvement. Although it may occur under the best of conditions, such persistent trouble is often due to dirty barns and poor sanitary measures that permit continual reinfection.

PREVENTION. The same measures as given for true cowpox are recommended.

Foot-and-Mouth Disease (Aftosa, Aphthous Fever)

CAUSE. A virus that is found in blister-like vesicles that form in the mouth, between the toes, and on the tongue, lips, muzzle, udders, and teats of affected animals. It is also present in the milk and blood during periods when a fever exists. Authorities recognize at least seven types of this virus which are different enough so that immunity to one does not give immunity against the others.

MEANS OF SPREAD. Being one of the most contagious diseases known, it is easily spread by the movement of sick animals. It has recently been shown that the virus of foot and mouth disease may be present in the blood and urine for at least 246 days after recovery, so the possible existence of healthy-looking carriers must also be recognized. Garbage containing meat scraps and bones has often been involved as the cause of outbreaks, and when properly dried the virus may remain dangerous for years. This fact is important, for one United States outbreak was believed started by virus on straw which had been used to pack some imported flower bulbs. Since all cloven-footed animals are subject to this disease, swine, sheep, and goats must be considered as possible carriers as well as cattle. People like stockbuyers, salesmen and veterinarians may spread germs, while chickens, wild birds, automobiles, dogs, and other animals have also been mentioned as carriers. Reference to animals is a reminder that the common rat is susceptible to the disease, and so is recognized as extremely dangerous in diseased areas.

SYMPTOMS. Sore feet cause early lameness. Excessive slobbering, grinding of the teeth, and noisy smacking of the tongue are all typical and probably due to painful vesicles in the mouth. Infected animals can often be identified because of dirty noses, since soreness of the tongue prevents continual licking to remove mucus in a normal manner. The sore mouths also cause animals to refuse food and they lose weight rapidly because of this fact in combination with high fevers that dry them out. The sore feet cause animals to put in a great deal of their time lying down. Vesicles in different areas may be as large as two inches in diameter, and leave raw deep ulcers when they break open. These usually heal in a week or two but foot rot may follow infection in that area and bacteria of different kinds may invade teat lesions and cause severe cases of mastitis. Contrary to popular belief, the death rate is low and seldom exceeds more than one to three per cent in an outbreak, with the chief damage being done through loss of weight and decreased milk production. Recovered animals are subject to reinfection, for they are evidently immune for only about a year following an attack. Incubation period is one of the shortest, seldom more than four days and frequently less than 24 hours.

DIAGNOSIS. Definitely possible only in the laboratory or through the injection of experimental animals with fluid from the vesicles. Such injection is used to differentiate FMD from vesicular stomatitis in cattle. One animal is injected under the mucous membrane of the lips or tongue, while another is injected either intramuscularly or intravenously. If the infection is FMD, both animals will show symptoms within a short time, and if it is vesicular stomatitis, only the animal that was injected in the lips and tongue will show symptoms.

Under farm conditions FMD might be confused with bovine virus diarrhea, infectious bovine rhinotracheitis, rinderpest, malignant catarrhal fever, blue tongue, and various types of stomatitis other than the vesicular disease. Suspicious symptoms should always be immediately reported to state livestock authorities, or the federal veterinarian assigned to the state. Any delay may make a serious outbreak possible.

TREATMENT. None is recommended, since diseased and exposed animals have always been destroyed to eradicate the disease in the United States.

PREVENTION. In this country preventive measures have always consisted of rigid laws governing the movement of meat and animals in addition to the disposal of possibly infective material like garbage from ships. The use of vaccines is an alternative measure that may be desirable in areas where the slaughter of all exposed and possibly infected animals is impractical. Such products are used in European countries where national boundaries are close together and it is practically impossible to prevent constant reinfection from adjoining territories. More recently a program of repeated vaccination has evidently been successful in Mexico where it was used for the control of a foot-and-mouth disease outbreak.

Papular Stomatitis (Ulcerative Stomatitis, Muzzle Disease)

CAUSE. A virus that is believed to be distributed all over the world. The disease appears to be limited to cattle, although the virus may infect man and result in lesions similar to "milker's nodules" caused by the virus of "false cowpox." The disease was first reported in the United States in 1960.

MEANS OF SPREAD. Evidently through contact with virus present in discharges from the mouth and nostrils of affected animals.

SYMPTOMS. The disease is largely limited to calves, and is likely to be first shown by excessive slobbering and a crusty discharge from the nostrils. An examination will show that the lining of the mouth and nasal passages is inflamed and roughened by slightly raised papules. As time goes on, affected animals lose weight, become dull, and develop a dark, watery diarrhea. The papillary lesions increase in size and number while appearing on gums, muzzle, roof of the mouth, and under the tongue. Severe cases usually end in death. Opening a dead animal will show the typical lesions extending down the esophagus, and sometimes involving the first three divisions of the stomach.

DIAGNOSIS. Made definitely only in the laboratory through isolation of the causative virus. Under farm conditions it might be confused with troubles like diphtheria, wooden tongue, vesicular stomatitis, or BVD.

TREATMENT. None required for mild cases, since difficulty in eating will be the only symptom. Furnishing feed in liquid or gruel form will help through decreasing the amount of chewing that is required. The treatment of severe cases is likely to prove unsatisfactory, but sulfas and antibiotics may prove of value in controlling secondary bacterial invaders. Although an attack may last for some time, recovery is usually uneventful as the painful lesions heal.

PREVENTION. Largely a matter of sanitary measures consisting of immediate isolation of affected animals, and a complete cleanup and disinfection job on quarters after an outbreak has subsided.

Winter Dysentery

CAUSE. Once believed to be an organism called *Vibrio jejuni*. However, many authorities now suspect that the disease is caused by a virus, or possibly by two different infections existing at the same time. Its seasonal occurrence suggests that the stabling of animals is a predisposing factor. Climatic conditions and the type of ration may also be contributing factors. Since the disease never appears in a herd twice in the same year, it is likely that some degree of immunity develops following an outbreak.

SYMPTOMS. One or two cows suddenly show up as being affected with a watery brown diarrhea, and the trouble spreads rapidly in the herd. It is commonest in older animals, since calves and yearlings seem to have considerable resistance. Cows become "picky" about their feed, grow gaunt, and decrease by half or more in milk production. This decreased milk production represents the biggest loss from winter dysentery, since it seldom kills animals. The temperature, pulse, and respiration usually remain normal, and the disease is sometimes so mild that only a decreased milk production causes it to be noticed at all. At other times attacks are extremely severe, and the thin manure may be bloody or mixed with chunks of mucus. An outbreak commonly lasts for about a week, with scouring in animals usually ending on about the third day. The disease gets its name from the fact that it generally is seen during the winter or early spring months.

DIAGNOSIS. Based on typical symptoms and the affliction of older cattle during the winter season. The presence of blood in manure may cause it to be confused with coccidiosis and unusually severe attacks may be mistaken for shipping fever. It is often thought to be caused by spoiled feed or poisoning of some kind.

TREATMENT. The oldest is represented by intestinal antiseptics and astringents which are given by mouth, either alone or in combination. One of the best is a 50-50 mixture of pine oil and creolin which is given in 1- or 2-ounce doses and repeated every 12 hours as needed. Solutions of copper sulfate(5%) or chlorine (4%) are also suitable and are given in the same doses. An old favorite consists of 45 parts gum catechu; 45 parts sodium bicarbonate, and 10 parts of zinc phenolsulfate, given in doses of 1 to 3 ounces twice daily as needed.

Animals showing an extremely bad bloody diarrhea will probably be benefitted by additional medication. A half-and-half mixture of salol and bismuth subnitrate is useful both as an astringent and for giving a protective coating to the irritated walls of the digestive tract. It can be given at the rate of 2 to 12 ounces daily for a couple of days.

Various of the intestinal sulfas have been used with good effect in some cases, and several different commercial preparations are available in bolus form.

Greatly weakened or "downer" animals may require blood transfusions and salt solutions given intravenously to replace body fluids that have been lost through dehydration. Bran mashes and gruels made of concentrates with high food value are also recommended for such animals.

PREVENTION. Using care so that manure isn't carried into feed alleys. A shallow pan of disinfectant may be placed in a convenient place for dipping the feet, or rubber footwear may be removed before walking in front of the cows. Visitors, salesmen, stock buyers, etc., should be asked to stay out of feed alleys.

Shipping Fever Complex or Hemorrhagic Septicemia

CAUSE. Not definitely known, but generally believed to be a combination of stress factors like fatigue, hunger, anxiety, heat, cold, dust, fright, etc.; infection with one or more of several different viruses like those of IBR, parainfluenza, BVD-MD, PPLO, etc.; and infection with one or more species of bacteria like *Pasteurella, Streptococcus, Hemophilus, Pseudomonas,* etc. Shipment is not a requirement because a disease with similar symptoms often follows weaning of calves which never leave the ranch.

It appears likely that outbreaks are triggered by a virus, and that most of the symptoms shown are due to a bacterial infection.

The stress factors have the effect of lowering the body resistance to infection. However, other factors are evidently involved too, for newly purchased animals frequently start outbreaks in herds where there has been nothing to cause such decreased resistance. In such cases the importations seem to act as immune carriers of the disease.

MEANS OF SPREAD. Basically unknown, because attempts to transmit the disease experimentally have been generally unsuccessful. It appears that such knowledge must wait until the cause has been definitely identified.

SYMPTOMS. Primarily those of a respiratory disease, ranging all the way from an increased rate of breathing to severe pneumonia. A fever of 104° F. and higher is shown early. Affected animals appear dull, and often stand with their heads down and ears drooping. Feed is completely refused and weight is lost rapidly. Other symptoms include panting, coughing, grunting, thick nasal discharge, watering from the eyes, and slobbering. Either diarrhea or constipation may be shown. In some cases only one or two animals are affected, while in others practically the whole herd shows evidence of infection. Sudden deaths may occur of animals that had not previously been noted as appearing sick.

DIAGNOSIS. Usually based on a history of recent shipment, weaning, or exposure to other stress factors. Diagnosis may be difficult in herds where there have been no importations and the commoner stress factors do not exist. Under such conditions it may easily be confused with troubles like IBR, pneumonia, BVD-MD, etc.

TREATMENT. Usually effective if given early. Most veterinarians prefer injection of antibiotics like penicillin, streptomycin, and tetracyclines, either alone or in combination, but sulfas are often given as boluses or intravenously as solutions. When the number of sick animals in a herd is increasing, it will be advisable to treat the entire exposed group. Affected animals should be isolated immediately and individual treatment is recommended because administration of drugs in feed or water is usually not very satisfactory. This is because many of the sick cattle will not be eating or drinking.

Successful treatment depends on early detection of affected animals so they can be promptly isolated and treated. Animals showing even the slightest depression should be treated. Those responding promptly to treatment can be returned to the herd in a day or two. If treatment is delayed until pneumonia has developed, it is likely to be useless. The administration of serum appears to be of little value, and there is no good reason for using bacterin or aggressin when infection already exists in a herd. This is because the time required to develop resistance following vaccination may allow many animals to die. Temperatures can be taken twice daily during an outbreak, and any animals showing increases should be considered infected. They can often be isolated and treated before any noticeable signs of sickness are shown.

PREVENTION. Most practical through vaccination. Since viruses are widely distributed in cattle, most calves start out with considerable resistance acquired through the colostrum obtained from their dams. However, by weaning time most of this resistance has disappeared, and the animals are highly susceptible just at the time when they are likely to be exposed to the most stress factors. Logically, the vaccine is best used before the calves are exposed to the stress factors. This means vaccination at least two weeks before weaning and shipment to feed lots. The timing of vaccination will have to be approximated on a trial basis because existing antibodies from colostrum may interfere with action of the vaccine.

There are various types of vaccines, consisting of either killed or modified live viruses, singly or in combination with vaccines and bacterins against other diseases like IBR and BVD-MD. In the past, these have generally been injected intramuscularly, but it is possible that intranasal vaccination will prove more effective. Pasteurella bacterins have generally been ineffective, possibly because the available products were made up from different strains of bacteria than are involved now. Serum treatment may have failed because the serums were also prepared against the same strains of non-causative bacteria.

In controlled experiments no protection was secured from the use of penicillin and antipasteurella serum before shipment of cattle. Neither did the injection of antibiotics or the use of sulfas in the drinking water after arrival of the animals in feed lots serve to prevent the occurrence of shipping fever. Similarly, the use of vitamin A and large doses of penicillin and streptomycin were demonstrated as ineffective. It has been theorized that antibiotics given when animals arrive at feed lots are used too early, and thus have disappeared by the time that bacterial infection actually occurs.

Along with vaccination, certain management practices after calves arrive in feed lots will help to prevent outbreaks of shipping fever.

1. Put animals on good pasture for a week or so if it is available. Some operators have used rye and winter wheat for this purpose.
2. Feed a green-colored, good quality hay. Although different from the dry pastures most of these animals are used to, it may tempt them to start eating, and this is very important.
3. Feed small amounts of good quality silage for the same purpose, even though it will be a strange feed to most of the animals. Sprinkling a little grain or cottonseed cake over it may stimulate appetites.
4. Provide a constant supply of clean drinking water.
5. Watch the herd to make sure that greedy animals do not overeat.
6. Make sure that there is plenty of room at the feed bunks, and that they are low enough so that even small calves can eat easily.
7. Handle the animals as little as possible during the first few weeks, and postpone any activities like sorting, dipping, dehorning, worming, etc., until the calves are well started on feed.

Considerable publicity has been given to "preconditioned calves," but, although theoretically desirable, preconditioning may not always be practical. For one thing, owners are often reluctant to handle the calves for vaccination a few weeks before weaning. Then there is the problem of identifying and certifying the preconditioned animals. Feeding them hay and a light grain ration may be difficult under average ranch conditions. Finally, the rancher will have to be paid for the extra costs of preconditioning, and the buyer may be reluctant to pay this.

Johne's Disease or Paratuberculosis

CAUSE. A bacterium called *Mycobacterium paratuberculosis.* It lives in the intestines of infected animals, and greatly resembles the bacillus of tuberculosis, although it is somewhat smaller in size and much more resistant to destruction. Under favorable conditions it may exist in pastures for years, particularly those that are wet and marshy.

MEANS OF SPREAD. Probably entirely through infected animals, since the germs are believed given off only in the manure. They are then swallowed with contaminated food and water. It is believed that infection usually occurs early, often when calves are still with their dams. The incubation period is one of the longest known, sometimes lasting a year or longer.

SYMPTOMS. Although not always shown, the commonest one is a chronic diarrhea that usually returns if it is checked by dry feeds or medicine. Milk production decreases and weight is gradually lost, although the appetite usually remains good and the temperature shows no change in the early stages. The later course is variable, for symptoms sometimes disappear completely to recur after a few months or recovery may be permanent and complete without treatment of any kind. However, affected animals usually grow progressively thinner and weaker, and in the late stages are little more than rough-coated, sunken-eyed bags of bones that put in most of their time lying down. The disease is seldom seen in animals less than two years old, and symptoms often appear for the first time shortly after calving. High producing animals seem most susceptible, probably because heavy lactation tends to lower resistance to germs which ordinarily would do no harm. If a dead animal is opened, the small intestine often appears as alternate normal and enlarged sections, with the junction of the intestine and cecum or ileo-cecal valve often being markedly enlarged. Sometimes this particular area is swollen to twenty times its normal size. Like the expected diarrhea, enlargement of the intestine isn't always seen, and may be so slight as to escape notice. Johne's disease is much less contagious than tuberculosis, and usually causes loss of only one or two animals a year in diseased herds. There is probably no immunity, for animals that evidently recover generally continue to give off germs and are likely to come down with the disease again at any time.

DIAGNOSIS. Usually through the injection of johnin or avian tuberculin between layers of the skin. The presence of infection is indicated by a swelling at the point of injection as in the case of a test for tuberculosis. Both of these products can also be given intravenously, with a reaction being shown by shivering, scouring, and an increased temperature, while negative animals remain unaffected. Pieces from the lining of swollen intestines may also be examined under the microscope for *M. paratuberculosis*. From an owner's standpoint, a chronic diarrhea in combination with a steady loss of weight over a long period is strongly suggestive of Johne's disease. The symptoms are even more suspicious if they appear in high-producing heifers shortly after freshening.

Under field conditions Johne's disease might be confused with internal parasitism, chronic hardware trouble, liver abscesses, and malnutrition.

TREATMENT. None recommended, since symptoms are usually seen only in the terminal stages of infection. Although temporary improvement has been reported in some cases following the use of antibiotics and other agents, complete cures have not been effected. Instead, it is usually considered desirable to slaughter diseased animals so the source of infection can be removed from herds.

PREVENTION. Vaccines that have been tried are undesirable because they may cause vaccinated animals to react to the tuberculin test. Since the disease is usually spread by the movement of infected animals, cattle should be brought in only from herds known to be Johne's-free. Pasture rotation is desirable, and pools of stagnant water should be drained or fenced off. Outside feeding should be from racks or troughs, and never from the ground. Feed alleys and mangers in barns should be guarded against contamination with manure. Since infection apparently occurs early in life, this is another reason for early removal of calves from their dams. Once away from them, calves should be kept completely separated from older animals until they reach breeding age. Exposed older animals are apt to move out of the herd for some reason or other before the disease has a chance to develop to the stage where symptoms are shown. Animals that are purchased can be tested for the disease, and closely watched for a year or two afterward even if they show up as negative.

Mange (Scab, Scabies, Barn Itch)

CAUSE. Four different kinds of mites that burrow in or on the skin. They are called *Sarcoptes scabei bovis, Psoroptes communis bovis, Chorioptes bovis,* and *Demodex bovis* and cause sarcoptic mange (scabies), psoroptic mange (scab), chorioptic mange (symbiotic scab, tail mange), and demodectic mange, respectively. The sarcoptic and demodectic mites burrow into the skin, while the others bite and suck blood, but do not burrow. Eggs are laid and hatch out on the animals.

MEANS OF SPREAD. Unknown for demodectic mange, but others by direct contact of animals and migration of mites. The disease is carried through the summer on animals that harbor a few mites on the belly and other body areas where they are pretty much protected against sunlight.

SYMPTOMS. Itching is the most common except in the case of demodectic, which causes none at all. Areas first affected are commonly along the flanks, head, or neck, probably because of rubbing these parts against infected animals. Bulls may acquire the infection by serving cows, in which case the affected area is apt to be along the belly or inner surfaces of the legs. Hairless patches of skin sprinkled with small vesicles appear early, and a heavy dandruff is often seen. As infection becomes worse the skin grows wrinkled and greatly thickened and coated with an oozing eruption like a particularly filthy eczema. Eventually it takes on a leather-like appearance, with excessive rubbing leading to the formation of bloody scabs and crusts. Spread of the condition is largely governed by the body condition of animals, but it may extend over most of the body within two or three weeks. With the exception of demodectic mange which persists the year 'round, this disease is seen only during the colder months, since the mites are unable to withstand much sunshine. A lack of sunlight combined with a thicker, dirtier hair coat encourages breeding of the mites to cause the rapid development of symptoms. Severe infestation is often responsible for loss of weight, decreased milk production, breeding troubles, and often death. Demodectic mange is not generally serious, since the lesions are apt to be limited to nodules of varying size that discharge a creamy pus when they break or are opened. The greatest loss from demodectic mange results from damage to leather caused by lesions.

DIAGNOSIS. Definite only through microscopic examination of skin scrapings that discloses the causative mites or their eggs. The time of year when symptoms appear may help to indicate the nature of trouble, but even in winter time it may be confused with several other skin troubles. These include ringworm, light sensitization, stephanofilariasis, improper use of insecticides, lousiness, allergies, infections due to filth, and the newer X-disease.

All outbreaks of mange in cattle should be immediately reported to proper state or federal officials so that steps can be taken to prevent spread of the disease.

TREATMENT. Dips presently approved by the USDA for the treatment of cattle mange under supervision include:

1. Lime-sulfur dip made in the proportion of 21 pounds of unslaked lime (or 16 pounds of hydrated lime, not air-slaked lime), and 24 pounds of sulfur flour or flowers of sulfur to 100 gallons of water.

2. Commercial lime-sulfur preparations sold under various trade names.

3. Nicotine dip containing not less than 0.05% of 1% nicotine.

4. Commercial nicotine preparations sold under various trade names.

5. Dips made from approved toxaphene emulsions maintained at a concentration of 0.5%. Animals treated with such dips should not be slaughtered for food before the expiration of the waiting period prescribed by the Meat Inspection Act.

6. Various other dips approved by the USDA. Before a dip can be used the Division will decide whether its use will eradicate mange without injuring animals that are dipped in it. A list of these approved dips can be obtained from the USDA or inspectors of the Division. Some of the newer dips have the advantage of seldom requiring a second application, while the lime-sulfur dip, for example, must be applied several times at weekly intervals for a complete job. Regardless of what is used, the entire body must be treated or many of the mites will merely migrate to another area to start trouble there. No efficient treatment is known for demodectic mange, but it seldom does much damage anyway. The leathery condition of the skin may persist for weeks after the parasites have all been killed.

PREVENTION. Largely a matter of being careful about bringing infested animals into herds. It also pays to feed animals well, since those in good condition are less susceptible to mange than thin and poorly nourished ones. Buildings and equipment should be well

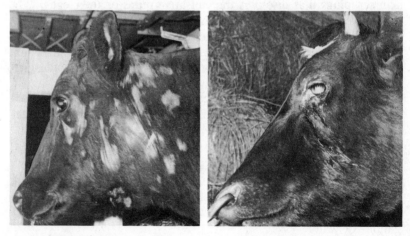

Sarcoptic mange of cow.   Pinkeye.

cleaned and thoroughly disinfected after an outbreak, for both mites and eggs can live for short periods after removal from animals. Consequently, they may be the cause of recurring attacks. Keeping animals clean and providing plenty of light in barns is also helpful in preventing mange, since the mites thrive in dark and dirty surroundings.

In case of an outbreak, infested animals should be completely isolated to prevent spread. Equipment like curry combs, clippers, etc. that is used on them should be sterilized in boiling water before being used on susceptible cattle. Even though demodectic mange does not spread readily from one animal to another, animals affected with it should also be isolated to be on the safe side.

Pinkeye (Infectious Keratitis)

CAUSE. Generally believed to be a germ called *Hemophilus bovis* which is found in discharges from the eyes and noses of infected animals.

MEANS OF SPREAD. Principally through the movement of carrier animals which have once had the disease, but show no symptoms of remaining infection. Once an outbreak has started, germs are rapidly spread by flies that alternately feed around the eyes of infected and healthy animals. The disease is believed to be carried through the winter in a chronic form by certain animals, and it seems to have no ability to spread before the arrival of flies. Such a theory is logical, for secretions from the eyes have been demonstrated as containing germs several months after apparent complete recovery.

SYMPTOMS. Watering of the eyes and swelling of the lids are particularly striking ones. Either or both eyes may be affected, with affected ones painful to the touch and usually kept closed to shut out irritating light. Discharges may cause matting of hair which may eventually come out to give the face a scalded appearance. The entire eyeball may become covered with a white film, and a raised yellow area may finally break open to leave a raw red ulcer. Infection may start here to affect the entire eyeball. Animals sometimes bellow and become violently delirious from pain. The most serious cases are apt to appear in range cattle that are exposed to dust and glaring sunlight, while mild attacks in dairy cows may show few symptoms other than a slight watering of the eyes. Most animals recover completely, although occasional ones are left partly blind. The average outbreak lasts about three weeks, with the biggest damage done by lost weight in beef herds, and milk production that may be cut in half for dairy herds. Young cattle are most seriously affected, for animals seem to retain considerable resistance after one attack, even though they aren't made completely immune. It does not seem so contagious as some of the other cattle diseases, for it is seldom that more than half a herd is affected in an outbreak. The incubation period is generally somewhere between two days and a week.

DIAGNOSIS. Usually based on the typical symptoms and evidence of being contagious. Sometimes confused with irritation due to dust and wind. Foreign bodies in the eye or injuries by weed stems, etc., may be thought to be pinkeye, but lack of spreading will generally serve to indicate the true nature of trouble.

TREATMENT. Good management is the most effective and practical. Affected animals are advisedly placed in dark quarters to avoid the irritation of flies and direct sunlight. Warm solutions of 4% boric acid or 1% argyrol may be used for washing out the eyes of gentle dairy cows twice daily. Mixed sulfa powders that are blown into the eyes with "puffer" tubes and various kinds of eye ointments may be useful in preventing the development of secondary infections, but it is doubtful if any kind of medicine has much effect on pinkeye itself. Treatment isn't recommended for beef animals, since the dust and wind and excitement involved probably does more damage than any good that can be expected from remedies.

PREVENTION. Largely a matter of avoiding the purchase of carriers. Since there is no test for pinkeye, this will probably be confined to purchasing animals only from herds where attacks of the disease haven't occurred. There are contradictory reports on the use of bacterins, vaccines, sterile milk solutions, etc., for preventing pinkeye, so the status of such products is not definitely known. In case of an outbreak, spread can be largely prevented by immediate isolation of affected animals. Healthy ones can then be checked daily for symptoms that merit their removal, too. The dark quarters mentioned under treatment are desirable for isolation, but if they aren't available the infected animals can be moved to a distant pasture as an alternative.

A dye that will persist for a couple of months or so has been used for painting on the skin around the eyes of white-faced animals to decrease the glare from sun rays, just as the cheekbones of baseball and football players are sometimes darkened with charcoal for the same reason. The formula for this dye is:

8 ounces of gum arabic powder
9 ounces of Nyanzol D lumps

16 ounces of hydrogen peroxide

The gum arabic is soaked for 24 hours in a pint of cold water. The Nyanzol D lumps are dissolved in 3 quarts of boiling water. The gum arabic is thinned with water to a pouring consistency, added to the hot dye solution, and enough water is added to make one gallon. When needed for use, this solution is warmed in water a pint at a time. The hydrogen peroxide is then added at the rate of 2 ounces per pint, and the dye is applied with a short-bristle brush. This dye can also be used for the prevention of cancer eye, and for everyday marking of cattle for reasons like culling and breeding.

Ringworm (Dermatomycosis)

CAUSE. In the U.S., usually a fungus called *Trichophyton album*. Another mold-like fungus called *Trichophyton mentagrophytes* has also been isolated from cattle in a small number of cases.

MEANS OF SPREAD. By direct contact with infected animals or contaminated surroundings and equipment. This last is important, for the disease may live for long periods in dark, filthy stables and can be carried on such things as curry combs and brushes. Spreading is helped by overcrowding in pens.

SYMPTOMS. Chiefly bald patches around the eyes and ears, although they may appear along the neck and on other areas of the body. These spots are covered with a dry gray crust and are evidently itchy, for animals sometimes rub and scratch them until

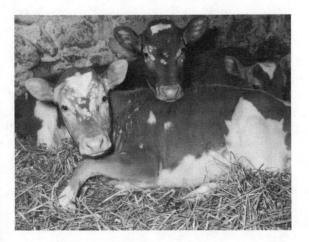

Calves with
ringworm.

bleeding occurs. Ringworm is commonest in young stock during the late winter, but may appear in animals of any age at any time of the year.

DIAGNOSIS. Definite by microscopic examination of skin scrapings and finding the threads or spores of the fungus. However, the typical gray hairless areas are usually enough to warrant a tentative diagnosis of ringworm. Under certain conditions it may be confused with other troubles listed under the diagnosis of mange.

TREATMENT. Begins with thorough scrubbing of lesions with mild soap and warm water. This removes scabs so remedies can come in direct contact with underlying fungus that would otherwise be pretty well protected. After that, treatment is apt to be a matter of choice, for ringworm is usually easy to kill. Both tincture of iodine and phemerol are old favorites and effective when applied daily a few times. So is the lime-sulfur dip used for mange, and in addition there are many satisfactory commercial products available under different trade names.

PREVENTION. Entirely a matter of management and sanitation. In case of an outbreak, infected animals should be isolated from other cattle while being treated and until the lesions have healed. Since the spores are capable of living a long time, pens occupied by infected animals should be cleaned up and disinfected before other animals are brought in. Equipment and objects likely to have been contaminated by the infected cattle should also be cleaned and disinfected. With the exception of lye, practically all of the recognized disinfectants are suitable for use. Barns and pens are best kept clean, dry, and well-lighted through the summer months to further decrease the chances of spores being carried over to cause outbreaks of ringworm during the following winter.

Leptospirosis (Lepto)

CAUSE. Several very similar organisms of the spirochete family. Although one called *Leptospira pomona* is most frequently involved, *L. canicola, L. hardjo,* and *L. grippotyphus* have been isolated from cattle and are all recognized as causative agents. At various stages of the disease the organisms can be found in the flesh, blood, milk, and urine of infected animals. The disease is most important in swine and cattle, but practically all domestic animals as well as chickens, are susceptible. In addition, many wild animals, including deer, foxes, skunks, raccoons, opossums, wildcats, bats, and rodents like rats and mice have been shown to be infected. *Leptospira pomona* received its name from the fact that it was first recognized in 1937 as the cause of illness affecting a dairy farmer living in Pomona, Australia.

MEANS OF SPREAD. Three facts indicate that swine act as a reservoir for leptospirosis:

1. It appears to be much more common in swine than cattle.

2. Large numbers of the organisms are excreted in the urine over long periods (usually considered to be 6 months), while carrier cattle give off much smaller numbers over a shorter period (usually considered to be 3 months).

3. The disease is easily spread from swine to swine and from swine to cattle.

An outbreak in a herd can usually be traced to either exposure of cattle to infected swine or to the importation of cattle that have had leptospirosis at some time and then remained as healthy-looking carriers. Outbreaks have been blamed on the contact of cattle with deer, but while it must be considered as a distinct possibility, the transmission of lepto by wild animals to cattle through contamination of forage or drinking water has not been definitely proven. Although man may become infected by animals, man rarely infects animals.

Direct transimssion through urine from infected cattle is believed to be common, and experimental work has shown that it is possible to infect susceptible animals by introducing leptospira into skin wounds, eyes, nostrils, or mucous membranes of the mouth. Infected urine that is voided on hard ground or concrete floors and walls might result in the splashing of tiny droplets into the eyes, nostrils, open mouths, or skin wounds of nearby cattle, and the switching of wet tails might have the same effect.

Indirect transmission is possible through contaminated drinking water, and ponds and lakes that cattle can wade into during the summer months should always be considered as possible sources of infection. Spread between neighboring farms might possibly occur through contamination of a common water supply with infected urine. In addition, grain or forage placed on the ground may also become contaminated with infected urine and spread the disease. It has also been suggested that the disease may be carried by bloodsuckers like flies, ticks, and mosquitoes. Whatever the method, infection must be transferred within a fairly short time, since leptospira soon die when they are separated from animals.

SYMPTOMS. In dairy cows the most important one is a completely limp udder that shows no evidence of infection at the same time that thick or bloody milk is being produced to cause suspicion of mastitis. There is evidently a mild and severe form of this disease, and both may be seen in the same herd at the same time.

In the severe form animals suddenly go off feed, breathe heavily, have a fast pulse, give bad milk, drop off to nothing in production, pass bloody or dark brown urine, run fevers anywhere between 103 and 107° F., and often die between two and ten days after first being noticed as sick. Abortions are common, particularly during the late stages of pregnancy. The skin often appears jaundiced, as do the eyes and lining of the mouth, and even the manure may be yellow. Animals sometimes show stiffness of the hind quarters and outstretched neck.

In the mild form dairy cows may show no symptoms other than a drop in milk production for a week or so, and the milk is more or less thick or blood-tinged during this time. There will probably be some abortions, and in beef herds this may be the only indication of trouble. The number of abortions varies widely, sometimes numbering only a few, but occasionally 25 to 50 per cent of the pregnant cows in a herd are affected. Cows, heifers, bulls, and steers of all breeds are susceptible, and have been involved at various times.

DIAGNOSIS. On the farm, through a blood test that is run much like the one used for detecting Bang's disease, but with a different kind of antigen. In the laboratory, through several kinds of other tests, or actual demonstration of the organisms after recovery from body fluids or tissue. The tests have the disadvantage of not showing up carrier animals, but it is hoped that a differential test will eventually be developed.

Guinea pigs and other animals are sometimes inoculated in the laboratory with suspected milk, blood, or urine to see if this will cause symptoms of the disease. It is well to note that inoculations may fail to produce infection if the test materials are not taken from animals carrying a fever, or the milk is not bloody, thick, or otherwise abnormal. On the other hand, animals may fail to show reactions to the blood test during the early stages of an attack, but the same animals will usually react to the test after apparent recovery. In its two forms the disease might be confused with such troubles as shipping fever, anaplasmosis, pyelonephritis, mastitis, liver abscess, and hardware trouble.

TREATMENT. None completely satisfactory in cases of the

severe type, but injections of antibiotics may help when infection is caught early. Streptomycin and dihydrostreptomycin have been shown to be effective in the treatment of calves. When dihydro-streptomycin was given to carrier animals intramuscularly at the rate of 5 mg. per pound every 12 hours for three days, carrier animals did not shed leptospires during the observation period. However, most authorities believe that outbreaks are best controlled by a program of vaccination to produce immune animals. All animals over two weeks old are vaccinated, and then revaccinated in about six months. Purchased animals are to be vaccinated at once, and then isolated for three weeks before being turned in with the home herd.

PREVENTION: On clean farms by:

1. Blood testing all animals for lepto before bringing them home.
2. Isolating animals that pass the test for 90 days, and then retesting them before releasing them into the home herd.
3. Keeping swine, cattle, sheep, horses, and goats completely separated to prevent spread between species.
4. Insisting that semen for artificial insemination comes from sires that are negative to regular tests for lepto. As an alternative, it is likely that the antibiotics generally used for the preparation of semen for insemination would probably destroy the organisms and thus make it safe for use.
5. Refusing to use bulls that have been "changed around" in a community, regardless of a clean blood test.
6. Having show cattle vaccinated against lepto a few weeks before they go to exhibits.
7. Having suspicious animals blood-tested for lepto, preferably after apparent recovery.

Vaccination with an approved vaccine is a valuable preventive measure in herds where the disease is just getting started or is likely to start because of outbreaks on nearby farms. When the type of *Leptospira* causing an outbreak is unknown, it is recommended that a vaccine effective against *L. pomona* be used because it is usually to blame. When laboratory reports show that a type other than *L. pomona* is involved, a vaccine for that particular type should be used. The development of a multivalent vaccine that would be effective against several types of *Leptospira* has been stated as desirable by the U.S. Livestock Sanitary Association. The vaccines presently available will not cause lepto or produce reactions to the blood test, but will give considerable resistance to the disease within two or three weeks after vaccination. Vaccination at least every year is desirable to maintain a satisfactory degree of immunity in a herd.

Other control measures recommended for infected herds include:

1. Isolating sick and suspicious animals.
2. Destroying milk from infected cows.
3. Burning or deeply burying materials like infected carcasses, bedding, afterbirth, and aborted calves.
4. Bringing in replacement animals not earlier than three months after the last case on a farm.
5. Following an intensive rodent control program.
6. Fencing off ponds and other open watering places.
7. Avoiding feeding off the ground.
8. Mixing chlortetracycline in the feed at recommended levels.

Trichomoniasis

CAUSE. A single-celled parasite called *Trichomonas fetus*. It is commonly found in the reproductive organs of both bulls and cows as well as in or on calves that are born to infected females.

MEANS OF SPREAD. Almost entirely by sexual intercourse, although cases have been reported in virgin heifers. Since the organisms are frequently found in the semen, infection is possible through either artificial or natural service.

SYMPTOMS. Breeding troubles of various kinds are the commonest. Cows may fail to "settle" after repeated breedings or come back in heat weeks after they were thought to be safely with calf. There are generally a few cows that will settle in diseased herds. Abortions may occur at any time, but are commonest during the first ninety days of pregnancy when they can easily be missed. Whitish discharges from the vagina are common, particularly a few days after breeding, and vaginitis is often a symptom of trichomoniasis rather than a disease by itself.

DIAGNOSIS. Definite only through demonstration of the parasites by means of microscopic examination. Vaginal swabs, vaginal washings, sheath swabs, sheath washings, vaginal discharges, or fluids from an aborted calf may be used for such examination. A single trichomonad is proof of infection, but failure to find one is not proof of freedom from the disease. This is because there may be few of the parasites, and they may be hard to find in an average sample. Various kinds of tests based on blood have been shown as unreliable for diagnosing trichomoniasis. A mucus test has been demonstrated as of value when a large number of cows in a herd was infected, but not accurate enough to identify individual animals that were infected. A herd history of breeding troubles and vaginal discharges may cause trichomoniasis to be suspected, but the same symptoms are also those of diseases like vibriosis, leptospirosis, and IBR abortions.

When a bull is suspected of being infected, but the organism cannot be demonstrated, the animal may be mated to several virgin heifers. Vaginal samples can then be taken from these animals ten days to three weeks after service. Sometimes the appearance of heat in infected females will be accompanied by the expulsion of uterine material containing trichomonads.

TREATMENT. Fortunately, complete sexual rest for three or four months will give most cows enough immunity so they will thereafter conceive without too much trouble. If pyometra develops, it should be treated as conditions warrant. Three injections of 50 mg. of diethylstilbestrol given a week apart may be enough, or it may be combined with infusion of the uterus with mild antiseptic solutions. Since many of these recovered cows will remain as carriers capable of infecting any bull that serves them, breeding is preferably done by artificial insemination.

Sexual rest does bulls no good, and for a long time they were considered as incurable if they contracted trichomoniasis. Today a German-made product known as Bovoflavine ointment is recognized as an established treatment for trichomoniasis in bulls, or a 0.5% acriflavine ointment can be used instead. However, treatment and follow-up testing will prove both expensive and time-consuming, so it has been suggested that treatment should not be started unless the bull is worth at least three times his market value. Treatments are repeated at about two-week intervals, and testing for evidence of persistent infection can start a week after the last treatment. At least six negative tests at weekly intervals has been recommended before the bull is used for breeding. It will then be best to use him on two virgin heifers, which are sampled 10 to 18 days later for examination. If *T. fetus* is found in any of the samples, a second series of treatment is started. This type of treatment can be expected to be effective in about nine cases out of ten.

Many other treatments have been used, including chloramine

silver nitrate, and iodides, but Bovoflavine has proven the most satisfactory. On the basis of reports, it appears that dimetridazole and metronidazole may be effective treatments for trichomoniasis in bulls. Unfortunately, at this time neither drug has received governmental clearance for use in cattle. In recent years it was reported that Berenil (a trade name) was an effective treatment for bulls with trichomoniasis. Seventeen bulls were treated by infusing the sheath with 100 cc. of 1% solution and massaging it for 15 minutes. The treatment was repeated daily for five days. Four bulls required two courses of treatment and only one bull remained infected.

PREVENTION. Entirely a matter of avoiding the purchase of infected stock and refusing natural service to outside cows. Caution must also be used in regard to either natural or artificial services for cows in the home herd. Although only a small percentage of cows are infected by semen because it carries only a few trichomonads, it has been shown that *T. fetus* can survive the processing and freezing of semen, so there is always a possibility that infection can occur even when artificial insemination is used. A cow infected through artificial insemination could then infect the rest of the herd if she was later bred naturally to the home bull. It has been reported that metronidazole can be added to semen in a concentration that will kill *T. fetus* without affecting spermatozoa. If this fact can be confirmed, it might help considerably in lessening the danger of infection from artificial insemination.

Imported cows should have a record of regular calvings, and bulls considered for purchase should show a satisfactory conception rate. There is no simple test for trichomoniasis, but the herd of origin should show evidence of freedom from suspicious breeding troubles. An outbreak of trichomoniasis could be detected early enough to prevent serious trouble by keeping complete breeding records and calling in a veterinarian to make a diagnosis in case of more than an ordinary amount of breeding trouble in a herd.

In case of an outbreak, the most practical procedure usually calls for giving all cows a period of 90 days sexual rest, and then breeding them artificially to a virgin bull.

A less satisfactory plan calls for the natural use of two bulls in a herd. One is used on all cows that have been previously bred, but only after they have been rested for 90 days. The other bull is a virgin, and is used exclusively on virgin heifers the first year.

The second year he is again used on virgin heifers and those that were bred to him the previous year, while the first bull is still used exclusively on the potentially infected older cows. This plan is continued until the herd is completely made up of clean animals, after which a single bull can again be used on all females.

In range country it may be impractical to do much more than try to control spread of the disease by regular testing of bulls and not turning them in with cows until most of the females have had a 90-day rest. Although it is possible for a cow to remain as a spreader and carrier of trichomoniasis after the 90-day rest period, such cases are rare, and a program of this kind is highly effective. There is no satisfactory vaccine for trichomoniasis at this time.

Tuberculosis

CAUSE. Usually an organism called *Mycobacterium bovis* which may be found almost anywhere in the body of an infected animal. Infrequently, cases have been reported from infection with *Mycobacterium tuberculosis,* the type of germ causing human tuberculosis. *Mycobacterium avium,* the type of germ that causes tuberculosis in chickens, sometimes attacks cattle, but does not affect the health of the animals in any way. However, the infection may cause reactions to the test for Johne's disease, and probably occasional ones to the test for bovine tuberculosis. Germs are given off in large numbers through the saliva, manure, and milk of infected animals.

MEANS OF SPREAD. Chiefly through the swallowing of germs with food and water, but also through the breathing of contaminated air in closed and poorly ventilated barns. Common sources of spread are represented by contaminated water holes, mangers, feed bunks, troughs, and tanks. Danger of infection is greatly reduced in drinking places where there is running water, since germs are then carried away about as fast as they are dropped. Feeding cattle from a single grain bunk or watering from a common tank is dangerous business, for a single animal can infect a whole herd in a short time under such conditions. Cattle have also been known to contract the human type of tuberculosis from infected people who were careless about spitting in the animals' mangers. Dry pastures are not likely to support *M. bovis* for very long, since the germs are quickly destroyed by direct sunlight. This is not true of wet pastures, because germs have been known to exist for almost two years in a moist outdoor environment.

SYMPTOMS. There are no definite ones, since animals may be infected with tuberculosis while appearing to be perfectly healthy. In well-advanced cases the disease is apt to cause gradual wasting away and decreased milk production. Coughing is sometimes a symptom and so is labored breathing. Listening to the lungs may or may not reveal abnormal breathing sounds. Diarrhea is a fairly common symptom and swollen lymph glands may press on the esophagus to cut off the normal escape of gas from the stomach and so cause bloat. Involvement of the udder may cause swellings of quarters that resemble those of chronic mastitis.

DIAGNOSIS. Generally through the intradermal injection of a little tuberculin on the under side of the tail near its base. These injection sites are then "read" three days later and any that show signs of swelling are considered as possible reactions indicating infected animals. In addition, a subcutaneous injection of tuberculin is sometimes made in the neck area (cervical test) when a diseased herd is being retested. Infected animals are sometimes picked up on postmortem examination in slaughterhouses, and a tentative diagnosis is confirmed by laboratory procedures on suspected tissues. Contrary to an old belief, tuberculin cannot start tuberculosis in animals. This is because it contains no germs, either living or dead.

TREATMENT. None recognized in the U.S., where a policy of test and slaughter has been followed since 1917. However, the so-called "anti-tuberculosis drug," isonicotinic acid hydrazine (INH) is known, and as early as 1957 favorable results were reported from intramuscular injection of 5 milligrams of INH per kilogram of body weight for 40 days. The drug can be given in feed or water, and has its greatest value in countries where there is a great deal of tuberculosis.

PREVENTION. Primarily a matter of regular testing and prompt elimination of reactors. Yearly testing is advised, since the once-in-five-years checkup by state and federal agencies may permit widespread infection of herds before the disease is discovered. Protection against the introduction of disease into a herd can be secured by making sure that all purchased animals are negative to a recent tuberculin test, and that they originate from a tuberculosis-free herd.

In case of an outbreak, all premises must be thoroughly cleaned up and disinfected before susceptible animals are brought in. It is interesting to note that lye is not a suitable disinfectant for tuberculosis, since the germs are protected by a waxy capsule.

Consequently, coal tar disinfectants or the newer quaternary ammonium products are required by law for use against this disease.

Various types of vaccines have been produced for cattle, but none has been demonstrated of value. As an added disadvantage, use of the vaccines causes sensitivity to tuberculin and thus interferes with test results. In countries where tuberculosis is a serious problem, the antituberculosis drug, INH, might be used as a preventive agent on exposed young animals.

Contagious Pleuropneumonia

CAUSE. A germ of the pleuropneumonia(PPLO) group called *Mycoplasma mycoides*. It causes natural disease only in cattle and other ruminants like buffalo, reindeer, bison, and yak, and at present is largely confined to Africa, Asia, Australia, and the Iberian peninsula. The disease has not appeared in the United States since 1892, but in these days of jet travel, outbreaks are always a possibility.

MEANS OF SPREAD. Believed only through the breathing of air infected with the lung secretions of diseased animals, since there is no proof at this time that the disease can be transmitted through the eating or drinking of contaminated material. Spread requires direct contact between diseased and susceptible animals, and the organism is given off for long periods by chronically affected animals and apparently healthy recovered carriers.

SYMPTOMS. Usually the first sign is occasional coughing which steadily becomes worse and is most noticeable in the morning while the animals are exercising or exposed to cold. The temperature may rise to 105° F. or higher, but in most cases symptoms develop slowly and there is little rise in temperature. Milk production drops off, animals go off feed, and breathing becomes faster and evidently more painful. A nasal discharge is often apparent.

In most outbreaks symptoms persist for about a month, but in acute cases animals may die within a few days. In an average herd about 40 per cent of the animals will die, another 40 per cent will either recover or become chronically affected, and the remainder will appear to be immune.

Opening a dead animal will show areas of various sizes in the lungs to be solidified and gray to brownish-red in color. The membrane over such areas is dull or reddened and may be covered with a fibrinous deposit. In most cases there will be a considerable amount of a yellowish fluid in the region around the lungs. Parts of the lungs may rot and become encapsulated.

DIAGNOSIS. Definite only through laboratory tests. However, a tentative diagnosis can sometimes be made on the basis of known exposure to diseased animals, knowledge that the disease exists in the area, the characteristic development of symptoms, slow spread of the disease in a herd, and postmortem examination that shows the typical lung lesions and yellow fluid in the pleural cavity. Under field conditions it might be confused with shipping fever and practically any of the other contagious respiratory diseases.

TREATMENT. None recommended in the United States, for diseased and exposed animals are supposed to be destroyed if the disease ever appears again in this country. Sulfas and organic arsenicals have been used in other countries with fair results in reducing the death rate. Penicillin and streptomycin are reported as of little value, but oxytetracycline and chloramphenicol have given encouraging results.

PREVENTION. If it appears in a new area, all animals in the vicinity should be quarantined and examined regularly for at least a year to detect symptoms of pleuropneumonia. In old areas of infection, diseased and carrier animals should be isolated to protect susceptible cattle. Disinfection is considered unnecessary because *M. mycoides* is quickly destroyed in natural surroundings and the disease is considered to be spread only through the inhalation of infected air.

Vaccination has been used in areas where contagious pleuropneumonia is a problem, but results have caused doubt as to the value of many of them. A live vaccine produced on chicken eggs has been widely used and appears to be quite effective against the disease. However, authorities agree that vaccines are needed to use on cattle with different degrees of resistance, and which happen to be exposed to different strains of the causative organism.

Granular Vaginitis (Granular Veneral Disease)

CAUSE. Unknown, although generally believed to be of an infectious nature. Many agents have been blamed, including various types of viruses, bacteria, and even protozoa. A recent report indicates that an organism named *Mycoplasma bovigenitalium* may be the cause. This disease is also known as nodular vaginitis and nodular venereal disease.

MEANS OF SPREAD. Essentially unknown, although claims have been made of the disease following exposure to various organisms and discharges from affected cattle. It is easily spread by the breeding act, but has been found in virgin heifers and animals that were bred artificially. Calves have been suspected of becoming infected through drinking milk from diseased cows. Once started in a herd, animals of both sexes may be affected.

SYMPTOMS. The commonest one is the appearance of whitish granules on the lining of the vulva. In severe cases these may merge so they cover practically the entire vulvar lining. They are seldom found in the vagina proper, but are generally confined to a small area around the vulvar opening. Accordingly, the disease is really a vulvitis instead of a vaginitis. In advanced cases there may be swelling and inflammation of the vulva in combination with grayish discharges that leave dark crusts on the vulvar tufts of hair. Badly infected animals appear uneasy and show pain when urinating. The same type of granulation develops on the penis and in the sheath of infected bulls. However, the worst part of the infection has a tendency to be localized at the end of the penis, and swelling and soreness may be severe enough so that bulls refuse service.

The average course of the disease is about two months. However, it is believed that recovered animals may carry a mild form of the disease indefinitely, and possibly act as carriers to infect younger animals. Although once believed to be an important cause of breeding troubles in cattle, the disease is now considered as having little or nothing to do with sterility problems.

DIAGNOSIS. Tentatively made on the basis of the typical granules which are confined to the lining of the vulva. It might be confused with a true vaginitis due to such causes as trichomoniasis, IPV, and infections caused by various types of yeasts and molds.

TREATMENT. The most effective is 60 days of sexual rest for either bulls or females. Many different compounds, including sulfas and antibiotics, have been used for direct application; various types of douches like Lysol solution, and powders like silver picrate have also been recommended. However, none of these remedies have altered the course of the disease to any appreciable extent, so treatment may be a waste of time and money. Affected cows may be bred artificially without making the condition worse.

PREVENTION. Difficult to prescribe, since the true cause is

unknown. Diseased animals should not be bred to clean ones, of course, and a program of artificial insemination will certainly decrease the chances of infection appearing in a herd. It has been suggested that improved methods of raising calves might help to prevent many cases of this disease.

Infectious Pustular Vaginitis (IPV, Coital Vesicular Exanthema)

CAUSE. The same virus that is responsible for IBR (rhinotracheitis). It was first known in Central Europe as coital vesicular exanthema and a similar condition was reported in the U.S. during the 1920's where it became known as vesicular venereal disease. It was finally shown that the so-called "vesicles" were actually pustules, so the disease was renamed "infectious pustular vaginitis." Later work showed that it was the same disease that was originally reported from Europe as "coital vesicular exanthema," and was caused by the same virus.

MEANS OF SPREAD. Principally through the breeding act, although infection may be carried on curry combs, brushes, blankets, bedding, etc., and it has been suggested that transfer may also occur through tail switching of vaginal discharges. Most outbreaks can be traced back to a single bull or cow. This is not surprising, for investigation has shown that cows sometimes shed the virus for a year or more following apparent recovery from the disease. In addition, bulls have been known to harbor the virus for as long as 23 days after infection has occurred. To make matters worse, one attack gives only a short immunity, and animals may become infected over and over so that the disease is never completely eradicated in a herd.

SYMPTOMS. Common early ones are arching of the back, frequent urination, straining, and stamping of the feet. Itching of the vulva is evident, and the organ soon becomes swollen with the appearance of creamy discharges. The lining of the vagina usually becomes thickly sprinkled with pustules that sometimes merge to form sheets of a yellowish material. These structures eventually slough to leave raw ulcers of various sizes, with the lesions sometimes appearing on the outside of the vulva as well as inside it. The ulcers finally heal, with a typical case taking about two weeks to run its course. Similar lesions appear on the penis and lining of the sheath of an infected bull, with severe bleeding sometimes following attempted service. Lesions in bulls may result in adhesions of the penis to the sheath walls, and narrowing of the preputial opening to prevent extrusion of the penis. A vaginal discharge may persist in females for several weeks. Appetite and milk production is usually only slightly affected, and the disease does not appear to cause breeding troubles. However, the lining of the uterus may become inflamed through secondary bacterial infection.

DIAGNOSIS. Vaginitis in combination with the typical pustules in the lining of the vulva, particularly in recently bred cows, is enough for a tentative diagnosis of IPV. However, a definite diagnosis is possible only through laboratory procedures to isolate the causative virus or demonstrate inclusion bodies in the vulvar lining.

TREATMENT. Valuable only to prevent bacterial secondary infection, and should be confined to the use of nonirritating agents, since the genital mucous membranes are extremely sensitive. Solutions of mild antiseptics like 2% chlorine can be recommended, and the same is true of various eye ointments like sulfathiazole and 10% argyrol. The douching of the prepuce of infected bulls with oily solutions may serve to prevent adhesions of the penis.

PREVENTION. No definite recommendations can be given in regard to preventing the introduction of this disease into a herd. In case of an outbreak, breeding operations should be suspended while disease exists in a herd. Infected animals of both sexes should be isolated, and given sexual rest for at least a month after apparent recovery. Bedding used by such animals is best burned and their quarters should be thoroughly cleaned and disinfected before they are used by other animals. Blankets, brushes, etc., can be sterilized by boiling them for a few minutes. Immunity can be given by vaccinating with IBR vaccine, but it lasts for only a few months as in the case of the naturally occurring disease. The use of artificial insemination will help to decrease the chances of spread in a herd.

Catarrhal Bovine Vaginitis

CAUSE. An enterovirus which may be of different serologic types. This is particularly likely to be present in the feces of young animals.

MEANS OF SPREAD. Usually through the breeding act, but may also occur in virgin heifers. In such cases it is believed that infection occurs through fecal contamination of the vaginal lining. Since the resulting vaginal discharge may contain a high concentration of the virus, spread might then occur through this discharge.

SYMPTOMS. The most striking one consists of a jelly-like, yellow discharge from the vulva, which may be abundant enough to soil the tail and rump. An examination will sometimes reveal a considerable amount of this discharge on the vaginal floor. Although once believed to cause breeding troubles, it is now considered as having little to do with infertility problems. As a matter of fact, diseased cows have been known to conceive. Other parts of the reproductive system are not usually affected. Bulls are unaffected, even in herds containing infected females.

DIAGNOSIS. Definite only in the laboratory through isolation of the causative virus from the vaginal discharge. It can be distinguished from IPV through the absence of vulvar pustules, and from granular vaginitis by the fact that inflammation is not confined to the vulvar region. It might be confused with the vaginitis that accompanies other diseases like vibriosis and trichomoniasis.

TREATMENT. Recommended only in cases of infection due to secondary bacterial invasion, as treatment of the viral infection is ineffective.

PREVENTION. Most practical through the use of artificial insemination. Inasmuch as animals may be repeatedly infected, it appears that an attack either does not give immunity or that any immunity gained does not last long. Consequently, no attempts have been made to develop a vaccine against this disease.

Warts

CAUSE. A virus that is present in the warts.

MEANS OF SPREAD. Not always known, but suspected to be by direct contact or rubbing against infected animals. The virus is often carried on dehorners, tattoo forceps, bleeding needles, nose leads, and similar instruments.

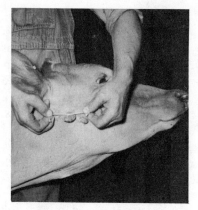

Tying off wart for removal.

SYMPTOMS. In young animals cauliflower-like masses of warts which appear gradually at first and then grow rapidly. The heads and sides of the neck are areas most often affected, with the disease being commonest during the late winter months when beasts are often overcrowded in pens. Warts on older animals usually appear on the udder and teats.

DIAGNOSIS. Usually not difficult, although a single wart on the shoulders might be mistaken for a melanoma.

TREATMENT. Warts in young animals will sometimes disappear if they are soaked daily with castor oil for a week or so. Wart vaccine injected subcutaneously at ten day intervals is often effective. Another method of removal is represented by surgery. Sometimes the removal of a few larger warts is followed by the disappearance of the remainder within a short time. A practical way of removing the warts is furnished by tying strings or twisting rubber bands around the bases of warts. Leaving them in place cuts off the blood supply and results in the warts dropping off in about a week without leaving a wound of any kind. Warts on teats are best clipped off with scissors while the cow is dry. Bleeding can be controlled by touching the wound with silver nitrate.

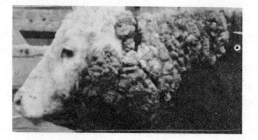

The head and sides of the neck are the areas most often affected by warts.

PREVENTION. No definite ones can be given. Warty animals should be separated from others until recovery is complete. In areas where warts occur regularly it may be desirable to vaccinate with wart vaccine without waiting for animals to become affected.

Bovine Virus Diarrhea or Mucosal Disease

CAUSE. A virus that is present in the manure, blood, and tissues of infected animals at various stages of the disease. It was first reported in New York in 1946 by Dr. Peter Olafson of Cornell University. Ten years later a similar disease was reported from Indiana in beef and dairy cattle. At about the same time a more severe form was reported from Iowa and adjoining states. At that time it was called "mucosal disease." It is now believed that all three of the outbreaks described were caused by a single type of virus. Investigation has revealed evidence of infection in cattle all over the world, and a survey of 38 of our states showed that it had existed at some time in all of them.

MEANS OF SPREAD. Not definitely known, but evidently chiefly through virus-bearing manure that is carried in various ways and swallowed with feed and water by healthy animals. Recovered animals may act as carriers, and deer and antelope may also serve as spreaders. Presence of the virus in the blood during periods of high fever suggests that blood-sucking insects might also possibly act as spreaders of the disease.

SYMPTOMS. Somewhat variable, since three forms of the disease—mild, acute, and chronic—are recognized. Early signs are usually dullness, coughing, rapid breathing, slobbering, and fevers ranging between 103° and 108° F. Animals lose weight rapidly, and milk production drops off to nothing. A watery, grayish, bad-smelling diarrhea appears. This diarrhea is the most characteristic sign of this disease, and may persist for three or four weeks, or continue off and on for months.

A little later on the muzzle dries and peels off, with considerable sloughing occurring in the acute type of the disease. A grayish discharge from the nostrils is common, and extreme loss of weight may cause the eyes to sink almost out of sight in the sockets. Severe ulceration may occur in the mouth, the eyes often water and are frequently covered with a bluish-white film.

Lameness often occurs, particularly in the chronic type, with the feet becoming badly swollen around the tops of the hoofs. This symptom may be seen early in an acute attack, with as many as a third of a feeder cattle herd being affected, and may be the first indication of infection in a lot. Many of the affected animals develop wrinkled, distorted, overlong hoofs. In both acute and chronic lameness, cattle often walk with their front feet well ahead of the body and spread apart while their hind feet are brought well up under the body so that the back is arched. Since their feet are obviously painful, affected animals lie down much of the time. Some of them will have a normal appetitie in spite of being rough-coated and in poor condition.

Calves are particularly susceptible to the acute form, and the death rate among them is higher than for older cattle in such an outbreak. In adult dairy cattle the disease may range from very mild to very severe, and frequently it causes abortions. There is also apt to be considerable variation in the number of animals affected in different outbreaks. However, the death losses are usually low, with about 10 per cent of the affected animals dying on an average. In addition to actual weight loss, deaths, and abortions that may occur weeks after recovery, feed lot operators also lose through reduced daily gains, poor feed conversion ratios, and an increased cost of weight gains.

If a dead animal is opened, the most noticeable lesions will be extensive ulcerations in the mouth. These will probably be found all the way down the esophagus, and inflammation and evidence of bleeding will probably be found all through the stomach and intestines. Watery swelling and extensive ulceration along with a fibrous membrane can also be expected throughout the digestive tract. Lymph glands along the tract may be watery and enlarged.

DIAGNOSIS. Largely a matter of eliminating other diseases with similar symptoms, although when present, the ulcers in the mouth are apt to prove helpful in identifying virus diarrhea. This disease may easily be confused with others like winter dysentery, shipping fever, malignant head catarrh, red nose, infestation with internal parasites, and poisoning.

Definite diagnosis can be made only in a laboratory through isolation of the virus and various blood studies. Such a diagnosis may be of little value in an outbreak because an outbreak may be over before one can be secured. In such an event the diagnosis would serve only as a warning and a basis for a control program.

TREATMENT. None recognized at this time other than that of a supportive nature. This includes blood transfusions for seriously weakened animals, the use of sulfas and antibiotics to control secondary bacterial invaders, and the oral administration of various diarrhea remedies. In addition, in case of an outbreak, it may help to decrease the amount of concentrates in a ration.

PREVENTION. Most practical through vaccination. The vaccine for BVD-MD has been combined with those for infectious bovine rhinotracheitis and parainfluenza, and such vaccination is both effective and economical. Because of possible interference with vaccine when calves have received antibodies with the colostrum from immune dams, there is no practical way of telling exactly when to vaccinate all the calves in any one herd. Accordingly, the best way to be sure of a high degree of protection is to vaccinate several times.

For the greatest degree of protection, it is recommended that calves be vaccinated at six to ten weeks of age, and again two or three weeks before weaning. In herds where there is little danger of this disease and calves are pretty well isolated, vaccination at, or shortly before, weaning time may give sufficient protection. However, it is advisable to give a booster shot a few months later, because the length of immunity following vaccination is not definitely known.

The vaccination of feeder calves after they arrive at the feed lot has some merit, but it is not without danger. Such animals may already be half-sick because of various stress factors, and in addition may have been exposed to the disease during shipment. Vaccines should be used to prevent disease, and not for treatment. Experience has demonstrated that severe outbreaks may result when animals are vaccinated while coming down with some kind of disease. Problems can be expected as long as cattle are vaccinated shortly after shipment. A better plan calls for isolating such cattle in a multi-lot operation and allowing them several days to recuperate and adjust to the new ration before being vaccinated. An even better plan consists of vaccinating the animals a couple of weeks or so before they ever leave home. The BVD-MD vaccines are both safe and effective when used on healthy cattle, but they aren't foolproof.

With this in mind, the following recommendations are made:

1. Isolate all new additions to the herd for an observation period of 30 days.
2. If such animals are known to be susceptible to BVD-MD, vaccinate them before allowing them to mingle with the home herd, because some of the natives may be carriers of the disease.
3. Do not vaccinate pregnant females since abortions may result.
4. Vaccinate nonpregnant cows three to four weeks before they are bred.
5. Vaccinate cattle which are going to shows, fairs, sales, feed lots, etc., at least three to four weeks before they are moved.

Infectious Bovine Rhinotracheitis (IBR), (Red Nose)

CAUSE. A virus which may produce symptoms of several other troubles in addition to those involving the respiratory system. The respiratory type of IBR was believed first seen in Colorado feed lots in 1950, and shortly afterward in California dairy herds. The first published report of an outbreak appeared in 1954. At this time the disease is known to have appeared in at least 16 of the western and midwestern states. It is also known as upper respiratory disease and necrotic rhinotracheitis, while the genital form is referred to in the United States as infectious pustular vulvovaginitis (IVP).

MEANS OF SPREAD. Not definitely known, but evidently through contact. However, in feed lots it may occur in pens that are surrounded by pens of unaffected animals, and cattle may share a common water tank, with animals in one pen remaining healthy while those in another come down with the disease. Evidence indicates that recovered animals may remain as carriers for several months. The close confinement of feeder cattle and large dairy herds seems to provide favorable conditions for the rapid spread of IBR.

SYMPTOMS. Rather confusing, for five different forms of IBR infection are recognized, and these may occur either alone or in various combinations. These forms are:

Respiratory: Cattle first appear dull, go off feed, and show a nasal discharge that is often tinged with blood. Animals develop a cough, run fevers of 104° to 107° F. or higher, pant, foam at the mouth, and water from the eyes. Dairy cattle drop abruptly in milk production. Diarrhea is not a constant symptom, but it may appear.

Affected animals often stand with their heads down and mouths open, breathing noisily and with difficulty. Many will have bad-smelling breath. The noisy breathing and bad breath account for the names "wheezers" and "stinkers" sometimes given to diseased cattle by cowboys. Some animals will become lame, and practically all of them will lose weight rapidly. Opening a dead animal will show lesions in the nostrils, larynx, and trachea, and sometimes involvement of the lungs. The muzzle and lining of the nostrils will be badly inflamed to explain the descriptive name "red nose." Animals under two years old seem to be more susceptible than older cattle. When young calves are affected, the disease is often more serious and causes more deaths.

Cattle may all sicken at once so an outbreak is over in a week or two, or they may become infected a few at a time so that an epidemic lasts for several weeks. Similarly, although most affected animals will recover from IBR in two to nine days, complications like pneumonia, diphtheria, lameness, and abortions may prolong trouble for a much longer time. Regardless of the number affected, there will probably be only a few deaths, and most of these will be due to secondary bacterial invaders that have caused pneumonia. Dairy cattle may develop acetonemia, probably because of failure to eat. Although the death rate is low, lost weight in feeder cattle and lowered milk production by dairy cows may represent quite a loss for an owner.

Genital: Begins with reddening of the vaginal lining. Pustules soon form in this area, and these give a granular appearance to the lining of the vagina and vulva. A grayish discharge develops, and sometimes a sort of diphtheritic membrane forms on the lining. When this membrane sloughs or is rubbed off, a bleeding raw surface is left. Depending on the involvement of secondary bacterial invaders, this form of IBR runs its course in three to eight weeks.

When the male is affected, the lining of the sheath and end of the penis becomes inflamed, with later pustule formation that gives a granular appearance to the affected tissues as it does to the vaginal lining of the female. Swelling of the penis and prepuce may occur so that the penis protrudes and cannot be retracted.

Eye: Inflammation of the various eye parts results in considerable swelling, and a grayish membrane develops over the eyelid lining to give it a granular appearance. This may cover only a part or the entire lining. The watering of affected eyes causes soiling of the facial hair below them. A nasal discharge also occurs which is watery at first and then becomes thick and gray. The eye itself may become slightly and partly clouded, and the entire eyeball may turn white if secondary infection occurs to cause keratitis.

Abortion: Appears to be increasing in recent years, but this may be due to the fact that IBR is being considered as a cause more often than in the past. It often happens that there has been an outbreak of an undiagnosed respiratory trouble, or exposure of the herd to IBR a few weeks before abortions occur. There can be no doubt that the disease is capable of causing abortions.

The causative virus was first isolated from aborted calves in 1964, and the recovered virus was then used to cause abortion in susceptible heifers. Later investigators have also reported the use of IBR virus to cause abortions in heifers.

Encephalitic (Nervous System): Researchers first reported that IBR virus caused a disease of the brain (meningoencephalitis) in Australian cattle, and shortly afterward similar results were reported in the U.S. It is currently believed that this type of IBR is comparatively rare.

It is usually seen in calves less than six months old, and starts with dullness and evidence of muscular incoordination like staggering. This is soon followed by frantic movements, convulsions, frothing at the mouth, and finally by paralysis. The course of the disease is short and usually ends in death.

DIAGNOSIS. Usually made definitely only in a laboratory, especially when the respiratory, abortion, and encephalitic forms are involved. However, IBR should be considered as a cause whenever any sudden onset of upper respiratory disease occurs in cattle. Fibrinous exudates in the trachea and nasal passages of a dead animal are strongly suggestive of IBR.

The eye form can usually be diagnosed in the .field by the granular appearance, the grayish membrane over the eyelid linings, the swelling, and the thick gray discharges from the eyes and nostrils. Evidence of eye inflammation during an attack of upper respiratory infection will support the diagnosis. It might be confused with an outbreak of pinkeye.

Neither should there be any great difficulty in making a tentative diagnosis of the genital form in a herd. The typical symptoms on a large scale would make it difficult to confuse with any other disease.

TREATMENT. No specific treatment is recognized for IBR itself, but secondary bacterial invaders that cause most of the deaths can be largely controlled by the use of sulfas, antibiotics, and various other agents. The injection of solutions containing enzymes directly into the windpipe will sometimes help to remove accumulations of phlegm and exudates from the breathing passages to lessen danger of suffocation.

PREVENTION. Most practical through vaccination. A satisfactory program will be dependent on the type of operation being carried on.

Breeding herd, either beef or dairy:

1. See that all herd additions are vaccinated at least two weeks before being brought home.

2. Insist that animals claimed to be vaccinated are accompanied by a certificate of vaccination.
3. Vaccinate all females three to four weeks before breeding.
4. Do this every year so that the "booster" shots will give good protection to calves at birth through the colostrum they drink.
5. Vaccinate all calves at five to seven months of age.
6. Do not vaccinate pregnant females.

Feeder calf operation:
1. Vaccinate all calves about three weeks before weaning or sale.
2. Vaccinate all calves at an earlier age if there is any danger of immediate exposure.
3. Revaccinate all early-vaccinated calves at about weaning time.
4. Do not combine IBR vaccine with other vaccines unless there is label approval by the vaccine manufacturer.
5. Give all buyers a certificate of vaccination with vaccinated animals.

Feed lot operation:
1. Vaccinate all calves two or three weeks before being shipped, if at all possible.
2. Otherwise, vaccinate all calves as soon as they are well on feed after arrival.
3. Do not vaccinate them as soon as they arrive at the feed lot.
4. If recommended by the vaccine manufacturer, vaccinate the calves for BVD—MD and parainfluenza at the same time as for IBR.
5. Inspect vaccinates daily for 30 days and immediately isolate for treatment any that show signs of sickness.

Texas Fever (Cattle Tick Fever, Piroplasmosis, Babesiasis)

CAUSE. A protozoan parasite, *Babesia bigemina*, which invades and destroys red blood cells. The disease is believed to have been introduced into the Western Hemisphere with cattle brought to Mexico during the Spanish colonization. In the early days this disease was associated with Texas cattle so much that it came to be known as Texas fever. Up until 1956 the only known tick-infested area in the U.S. was a narrow strip in eight counties of

Texas along the lower Rio Grande river. Reinfestation repeatedly occurs here through stray and smuggled cattle from Mexico, so this zone is kept under quarantine as a protective measure. However, an outbreak was reported from Florida in the spring of 1957.

MEANS OF SPREAD. These parasites usually require a tick for transmission. The ability to transmit is limited to a few species, primarily those of the genus *Boophilus,* in which the parasite is carried through the eggs to the next generation of ticks. In the United States *Boophilus annulatus* (southern cattle tick) was the chief transmitting tick, with *Boophilus australis* being involved in a small area of Florida. The ability of *B. australis* to live on deer has delayed completion of tick eradication in some of the swampy Florida sections. Other ticks act as vectors in various parts of the world.

After feeding on infected cattle, the female ticks drop to the ground, lay eggs, and die. The eggs hatch in anywhere from 18 days in the spring to six months in the late fall or winter. These larval or seed ticks then attach themselves to cattle and may transmit *B. bigemina* on their first feeding. After mating, the engorged females then drop to the ground to lay eggs of their own. The disease may appear in 10 days after infected seed ticks have fed on healthy cattle. It is also possible for infection to occur through castration and dehorning when instruments are not disinfected between animals. Recovered animals are immune for life, but they remain as carriers, and such cattle may act as a reservoir of infection.

SYMPTOMS. Somewhat dependent on the age of animals, season of the year, and amount of exposure. The severe form occurs in hot weather and begins with a fever of 104 to 107 degrees. Animals appear droopy, go off feed, and pant for breath. They are usually constipated at first, but may develop a diarrhea later. The eyes may be yellowed, and the blood is light-colored. The urine is likely to be bloody, with the color varying from light red to almost black, depending on the destruction of the blood cells. The mild or chronic form occurs in partly immune southern cattle or susceptible cattle that are infected in the late fall. There is usually no bloody urine in this form because of the slight damage to blood cells. Animals appear pale, stunted, thin, and in a weakened condition. Fevers may last for several weeks, but there are few deaths.

Opening a dead animal will show a spleen enlarged from two to four times its natural size, and the liver will also be greatly enlarged. The liver is likely to have a yellow color and often has a mottled appearance. The kidneys are generally swollen and dark, while the urinary bladder may contain bloody urine. No characteristic lesions will be found in other parts of the body.

Mature susceptible animals suffer most during hot weather, and about 90 per cent of those that sicken will die. The course of the disease is usually mild in animals under nine months of age, and very few of these will die. About one-fourth of the affected yearlings can be expected to die, and about half of the animals between a year and a half and two years will die if they contract the disease.

DIAGNOSIS. Positive only through microscopic examination of the blood that shows *B. bigemina* in the red cells. However, a tentative diagnosis can often be made on the basis of typical symptoms appearing in tick-infested cattle, and a knowledge that Texas fever exists in the area. Such a diagnosis can be supported if the same symptoms are produced when a susceptible animal is inoculated with a small amount of blood from a suspected animal. Under field conditions this disease may be confused with pneumonia, anthrax, leptospirosis, bacillary hemoglobinuria, pyelonephritis, anaplasmosis, trace element deficiencies, and infestation with internal parasites.

TREATMENT. Not practical in the U.S. where tick control is enforced. In other parts of the world remedies have included trypan blue, trypaflavine, and acaprin. Although effective, these drugs do not keep recovered animals from acting as carriers of the disease. Trypan blue has the disadvantage of staining the tissues bluish-green for several weeks. Trypaflavine is equally effective, but causes a temporary yellowish discoloration of tissues. It is given intravenously in 0.1 percent solution at the rate of 0.5 gram for young cattle and 1.0 gram for mature animals. Acaprin is as effective as the other two, and is favored because it causes no staining of tissues. It is injected subcutaneously or intramuscularly as a 5 percent solution in doses of 2 cc. per 100 kilograms of body weight.

Good nursing is an important part of treatment, with the affected animal being made as comfortable as possible in a shaded area and sprayed to remove ticks. Blood transfusions may be indicated for seriously weakened animals, and the same thing is true of dextrose solutions given intravenously. Good feed and fresh water should be easily available, and animals must be handled carefully to prevent excitement and over-exertion which might cause death.

PREVENTION. As practiced in the U.S., through the destruction of ticks in either one of these two ways:

1. Pasture rotation which calls for removing all animals from infested pastures for 8 to 10 months. Under such conditions the ticks then starve to death for lack of a suitable host.

2. Allowing animals to remain on infested pastures and treating them every two weeks with an approved dip of standard strength. The following are approved at this time by the USDA for the dipping of dairy cattle:
Pyrethrins plus Synergist—0.1% pyrethrin plus 1.0% synergist.
Rotenone—A 5% dust at the rate of 12 oz. per gallon of water.

The above may be used on beef cattle as well, and in addition solutions of lindane, malathion, ronnel (Korlan), toxaphene, Co-Ral, and Delnav may be used on beef animals. Otherwise these chemicals appear OK for use on dairy cattle, too.

A list of dips permitted for use in the official dipping of cattle for fever ticks may be obtained from the Chief, Animal Disease Eradication Branch, Washington 25, D. C.

Dipping cattle prevents the engorged female ticks from dropping to the ground alive, and laying eggs to reinfest pastures. Larval ticks that are already on the ground will be killed by later dippings if they manage to get on cattle, and they will starve to death if they do not. The time needed to insure eradication of ticks through dipping varies somewhat with the time of year when dipping is started. However, dipping at 2-week intervals for 8 to 12 months has given satisfactory results.

Young cattle can be immunized, either by inoculation with 1 to 3 cc. of infected blood or by the application of a few ticks carrying *B. bigemina*. Both methods produce a mild form of Texas fever, and are best used during the late fall or winter. In foreign countries, vaccination against this disease is often combined with vaccination against anaplasmosis. Vaccination against Texas fever is not recommended for animals over a year old, and even then the method is not without a small amount of danger.

Salmonellosis

CAUSE. Any one of several different types of *Salmonella* bacteria. *Salmonella bredeny* was identified as the cause of a California outbreak, while *S. typhimurium* was involved oftenest in Wisconsin cases. Parasitism, poor rations, weaning, shipment, other stresses, and practically anything likely to cause loss of condition can act as a contributing factor. Although once believed to be a rare disease in the United States, it has been diagnosed with increased frequency here in recent years. Florida authorities recognize it as a widespread disease in that state.

MEANS OF SPREAD. Chiefly through germs in manure from infected cattle that are carried in various ways and swallowed with contaminated feed and water by healthy animals. Recovered cattle may act as carriers, and rats, other wild animals, birds, poultry, and reptiles are also believed to be possible carriers.

SYMPTOMS. Dullness and refusal of feed are usually noticed first. Within a short time adult animals are affected with a dark, bad-smelling diarrhea, and carry a body temperature that ranges between 103 and 107 degrees. In later stages blood and mucus will be found in the manure, as well as occasional tube-like pieces of fibrinous material. Pregnant cows may abort. Symptoms in young calves are much the same, but the manure is often a yellow-green color. Hair coats become rough, and dehydration may make skeletons out of animals in a short time. Calves may die suddenly with no previous symptoms of illness. Opening a dead animal will usually show extensive hemorrhage and lesions throughout the digestive tract. Ulcers and large amounts of fibrinous material are likely to be found in the stomach and small intestine, while lungs generally show evidence of pneumonia. Young cattle are usually affected more severely than older animals.

DIAGNOSIS. Definite only in the laboratory through isolation of *Salmonella* organisms from manure or tissues of affected animals. However, a tentative diagnosis can often be made on the basis of typical symptoms, and the finding of much blood and fibrin in the digestive tract of a dead animal. Under farm conditions the disease may be confused with other troubles like winter dysentery, coccidiosis, virus diarrhea, enterotoxemia, poisoning, and infestation with internal parasites.

TREATMENT. None recognized as entirely satisfactory, although some of the broad spectrum antibiotics will frequently affect a temporary reduction in the body temperature of affected animals. Blood transfusions may help seriously weakened calves, while oral dosing with sulfas and chloramphenicol, and injection of immune serum has been reported of value. According to sensitivity tests, *S. newport* was susceptible to nitrofurazone and a mixture of neomycin and polymyxin, and similar findings were confirmed in regard to *S. typhimurium*. As a general rule, the chances of recovery are very poor for young calves, and fair for adult animals.

PREVENTION. Largely a matter of management concerned with general hygiene, aimed at eliminating contact with carrier animals and decreasing the chances of infected material being swallowed with feed and water. Vaccination of dams and calves with *Salmonella* bacterins may help, and the practice is followed in South Africa and Europe. The early separation of calves and raising of young stock in isolation are considered excellent practical measures. Animals should be handled so stress factors are reduced as much as possible, particularly those involving parasitism, diseases, and poor rations.

Toxoplasmosis

CAUSE. A protozoan-like parasite, *Toxoplasma gondii*, which may invade the cells of practically any part or organ of the body. Although the organism has been known since 1909, it was not recognized in cattle until 1953. All species of birds and animals may be affected, with cross-infection possible between different species. Even human beings can contract the disease from animals.

MEANS OF SPREAD. Not definitely known, for transmission has been proven only on a congenital basis with dams bearing infected young. However, it has been shown as capable of spreading readily among animals kept in close contact. Accordingly, spread is possible through contamination of feed and water with manure, urine, saliva, and nasal discharges, as well as inhalation of air containing *T. gondii*. Blood-suckers, like ticks and lice, are also possible spreaders.

Part of the life cycle is comparatively simple. After invading a host cell, the parasite reproduces to create hundreds of new organisms. Each parent cell develops smaller cells within itself which eventually fill the front portion of the cell and then break out, destroying the original cell. During multiplication, this aggregation of parasites is covered by a membrane and is called a "pseudocyst," which may represent the infectious stage that is transmitted to other animals. Spread of infection in the host's body is effected by the unencysted free parasites, possibly through the blood, for they can be found in it during certain periods of the infection. The parasites have also been demonstrated in the milk and meat of cattle.

Since practically any bird or animal is capable of transmitting the disease, no definite species has been named as the principal reservoir of infection. At various times dogs and rabbits have been considered, as well as sparrows and pigeons.

SYMPTOMS. Largely dependent on the type of tissues affected and the age of animals. Invasion of the lungs may cause panting, coughing, sneezing, frothing at the mouth, and a nasal discharge. Invasion of the brain and spinal cord will cause symptoms like tremors, shaking the head, grinding the teeth, staggering, and prostration with paddling movements of the legs. Invasion of the digestive tract may cause diarrhea, and invasion of the reproductive tract may cause abortions. Body temperatures may reach 106 degrees, but many animals will show normal or even subnormal temperatures. As a matter of fact, attacks of this disease are sometimes so mild that no symptoms are shown. Young animals will usually die within two to six days, but older animals will sometimes recover. Such animals are likely to remain as spreaders.

DIAGNOSIS. Definite only in a laboratory through isolation of *T. gondii* from the tissues or body fluids of suspected animals. Under farm conditions it might be confused with other troubles, like diseases of the mucosal disease complex, leptospirosis, listerellosis, shipping fever, or poisoning.

TREATMENT. Not too satisfactory, but extensive tests have shown that sulfamethazine, sulfamerazine, sulfadiazine, and sulfapyrazine have some value against *T. gondii,* while pyrimethamine has also been demonstrated as being fairly active against this organism. Combinations of the above drugs appear to give the best results. Most young animals can be expected to die, regardless of what is done for them.

PREVENTION. Since the complete life cycle of *T. gondii* is unknown, and the means of transmission is also unknown, no recommendations can be made at this time other than those dealing with general sanitary measures.

4.

DIGESTIVE TROUBLES

The lips must be considered as the beginning of the digestive system, with the mouth, cheeks, and teeth also being included. The tongue is particularly important because it is so widely used for bringing food to the mouth. Its fore part is rough to the touch because of points that project backward and help in grasping roughage, while the back part is conspicuous because of a raised prominence. Just beyond it is the pharynx which is used for both swallowing and breathing. When food is being swallowed the soft palate raises to keep material out of the nose, while the epiglottis folds back to keep food or water from going into the lungs. At all other times the soft palate lies flat to close off the back part of the mouth, and the pharynx is used entirely for breathing.

The salivary glands must be mentioned since they provide the large quantities of saliva that are needed for the digestion of dry feed. There are three of these, all paired so there is one on each side of the head. The parotid lies pretty much back of the lower jaw with a portion extending up under the ear. Its duct passes along the edge of the cheek muscle, crosses about the middle of the lower jaw bone, ascends on the other side and finally empties into the mouth at a point opposite the fifth upper cheek tooth. Blocking of this duct causes trouble mentioned elsewhere in this section. The parotid partly covers the larger mandibular gland which lies close to the lower jaw, and the sublingual glands are located beneath the tongue.

The esophagus is about three feet long in adult animals and connects the pharynx and stomach. The cow has a single stomach that is divided into four parts, so she is commonly believed to have four stomachs. All food that is swallowed for the first time goes into the rumen or paunch which takes up most of the abdominal space on the left side. Digestion in this stomach is pretty much by bacterial action, and "cuds" are raised from it for further chewing. The second stomach is called the reticulum or honeycomb and gets its name from a lining which actually does resemble the structure of a honeycomb. Depressions of this nature favor the holding of nails, wires, etc. so most cases of hardware trouble originate here. When "cuds" are swallowed after rechewing they usually pass directly into the second stomach. The third stomach is called the omasum or manyplies and gets its name from a lining which resembles the leaves of a book. It is here that fatal impaction often occurs with fine material like chaff. The fourth or true stomach is known as the abomasum and is the only one of the four that contains digestive glands. It connects with the small intestine through a valve known as the pylorus. A raised part on this valve known as the Torus pyloricus is often involved as the cause of chronic bloating in young calves.

The small intestine is generally considered as being made up of three parts although there is little difference between them. In the order of appearance they are called the duodenum, jejunum, and ileum. The bile duct opens into the duodenum, which is a reminder that the liver and gall bladder are also parts of the digestive system. The liver gives off the hepatic duct and the gall bladder gives off the cystic duct, and these join to form the bile duct. The pancreas is also part of the digestive system and gives off a duct which empties into the duodenum about a foot behind the bile duct.

The ileum joins the cecum, which is considered as the beginning of the large intestine. It is at this junction or the ileo-cecal valve that the most pronounced lesions of Johne's disease are often found. The large intestine or colon represents the terminal part of the digestive system. The last foot or so of it is called the rectum and the actual opening to the outside is the anus.

Choke

CAUSE. Usually apples, ears of corn, potatoes, and similar objects that have been swallowed whole. Greedy animals may choke after bolting dry feed, and it is frequently caused by foreign bodies like wire or pieces of tin. Strong drugs like chloral may burn the tissues to cause swelling that is to blame for choking.

SYMPTOMS. Bloating and slobbering are usually the first ones. The head may be lowered and the neck stretched out while grunting, coughing, open mouth breathing, gasping, chewing movements, and attempts at vomiting are also common. Animals seldom try to eat or drink, and crazy actions may appear in the late stages.

DIAGNOSIS. Made through seeing or feeling the obstruction, which is possible only when it is in the upper part of the throat.

When located further down the use of a stomach tube may be the only way of discovering the true nature of trouble. Choke may be confused with bronchitis, bloat from feeds, rabies, wooden tongue, and paralysis of the pharynx.

TREATMENT. First of all a matter of removing the obstruction so gas can escape from the stomach in a normal manner and lessen danger from bloating. When the esophagus is completely blocked it may be necessary to "tap" animals so they will live until the object can be removed. When located in the upper part of the throat it is best to bring foreign bodies back out through the mouth. Sometimes this can be done by simply reaching in and pulling them out with the fingers. At other times it is desirable for two men to work together. One stands on each side of the animal and places a hand below the obstruction, then both press upward with the thumbs. When raised far enough, one man can hold the object in place with both hands while the other man reaches into the mouth and removes it. A piece of baling wire bent double can often be effectively used for extracting slippery objects like apples or potatoes. The loop is slipped over and behind them and then pulled forward. A large clevis can be inserted flat and then turned up crosswise to hold the mouth open if desired while objects are being removed.

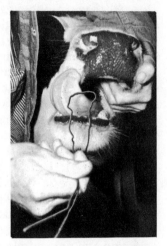

Using a loop of baling wire may be the easiest way of getting an apple or potato out of the mouth of a choking cow.

When located in the lower part of the esophagus, objects are usually best pushed on into the stomach. A five foot length of half-inch rubber hose with one end tied shut can be used as a "pusher," but it should be well lubricated with mineral oil or mild soap before use. Since unskilled use of such objects may cause serious damage to the throat, they are recommended only as emergency instruments. Arecoline given daily under the skin in 1 grain doses sometimes helps by increasing secretions that soften dry masses of feed and lubricate the esophagus to make swallowing easier.

PREVENTION. Largely a matter of careful feeding. Ear corn, beets, potatoes, and similar feeds should be chopped into small pieces. Turning cattle into root fields and apple orchards is a practice to be avoided, particularly in wet weather. The gulping of feed by greedy animals can be stopped by putting a few large rocks in the grain box so that only small amounts can be secured at a time.

Bad Teeth

CAUSE. Injuries that have chipped, cracked, or even split teeth. Sometimes irregular growth and uneven wearing that have permitted certain teeth to become overlong so they cut the cheeks or tongue.

SYMPTOMS. Slobbering is the commonest one, and cautious chewing is another. Mouthfuls of feed may be spit out if a tooth is hurt while chewing is being done. Water may be lapped or sipped in small amounts at a time if it hurts when teeth are contacted. Sometimes teeth are so sensitive that eating is practically impossible and in such cases the animals are reduced to little more than skin and bones through slow starvation. Secondary infections may occur in cuts on the tongue and in various places.

DIAGNOSIS. Made through examination of the mouth and the finding of abnormal teeth.

TREATMENT. Usually a matter of dressing down or "floating" teeth with a special long-handled file to remove rough edges or over-long points. Teeth that are split or otherwise badly damaged are best extracted. At this point it is well to remind owners that the front teeth of cattle are generally loose as a perfectly natural condition and are entirely serviceable even when they can be easily moved from side to side a bit.

Occlusion of the Parotid Duct

CAUSE. Usually a bit of roughage like a timothy head which enters the duct through the mouth opening and blocks it so saliva is backed up. In some cases a stone that has formed through deposits of calcium from the saliva acts as an obstruction.

SYMPTOMS. Swelling of the jaw on one side in the region of the parotid duct. Sometimes the seepage of saliva through the walls of the duct will cause the entire jaw to swell up within a short time. Considerable slobbering may accompany the swelling.

DIAGNOSIS. Generally based on the location and sudden appearance of swelling. Sometimes the obstruction can be felt in the duct close to the point where it crosses over the lower jawbone. May be confused with wooden tongue, lumpjaw, abscesses, bruises and hematomas.

TREATMENT. Surgical removal of the occluding object is the most practical. The incision in the duct must be closed with stitches to prevent a permanent fistula at that point.

Indigestion

CAUSE. (1) Overfeeding is the commonest one, particularly in the case of high-producing cows. (2) Lack of water is also common, especially in winter when drinking cups aren't available in barns. Water in tanks may be so cold that animals will drink but little when they have the chance. (3) Irregular feeding encourages overeating, since animals often become extremely hungry between meals. (4) Overripe roughages that are dry and fibrous like timothy hay and corn stalks. (5) Damaged feeds like heated grain, frozen silage, moldy hay, etc. (6) Indigestible substances like afterbirth, mudded hay, and dirty chaff. (7) Overeating when cattle break into corn fields, grain bins, apple orchards, etc. (8) Sudden changes of feed like old to newly threshed grain, clover to alfalfa hay, etc. (9) Sudden increase of feed for fresh cows.

SYMPTOMS. Dependent on cause. Cows generally appear suddenly sick, go off feed, stop cud chewing, decrease in milk production, and show evidence of constipation with few bowel movements. The pulse rate is apt to be increased, especially if fermentable feeds like apples or green corn have been eaten. The temperature is usually up a little, but in bad cases it may be normal or even below normal. There is often moaning, kicking at the belly, and grinding of the teeth. Chills may be evident and ears, horns, and teats feel cold with the muzzle appearing dry instead of moist. Lack of movement in the rumen may be detected by listening in the left flank, although sounds of rolling gas are common. Animals frequently become paralyzed and go down in a stupor like cows with milk fever, particularly when trouble has been caused by grain or green feeds like corn. Abortions may occur and bloating is generally present in some degree although it is frequently absent in cases due to dry feeds.

DIAGNOSIS. Usually based on a history that indicates overfeeding, overeating, or other common causes of indigestion. Symptoms aren't too dependable since they are the same as for hardware trouble, acetonemia, torsion of the uterus, poisoning, and any other number of ailments. Improvement is usually rapid following treatment when indigestion is causing trouble, and the failure of remedies is apt to be an indication of some other ailment.

TREATMENT. The most important part of any treatment is the

withholding of feed for a few days, although laxative feeds like bran mash may be given sparingly. Returning to normal rations should be done gradually. When bloating is present it should be promptly treated as described under that ailment for the relieving of that condition comes ahead of everything else. When cases are uncomplicated by bloat, the use of a laxative is indicated. Depending on size of the animal, a pound or two of Epsom salts may be dissolved in warm water and given as a drench or a quart or two of mineral oil may be substituted for the salts. Drenching must be done carefully and is described in the Practical Pointers section of this book.

An alternative method consists of giving medicines through a stomach tube, in which case two to five gallons of fairly warm water can be pumped in along with the laxatives already listed to encourage bowel movements. An ounce of turpentine and an ounce of spirits of ammonia can be added to the water and will probably prove helpful, too. After getting the medicine into the animal, the rumen can be stimulated into action by massaging the left flank with the fists in a movement from below upward. Such treatment can be continued for twenty minutes or so and results are usually shown by belching and movements of the rumen within a few minutes after massaging is started. Animals that have gone down and are half unconscious can sometimes be helped by the intravenous injection of 250-500 cc. calcium gluconate or 50 cc. of 30% sodium thiosulfate in combination with 500 cc. or more of a 50% glucose solution. Since loss of consciousness is usually due to absorption of poisons from feeds like green corn, 8-16 ounces of magnesium oxide given as a drench or by stomach tube is recommended as additional treatment. In severe cases a rumenotomy operation for removal of stomach contents through the flank may represent the only chance of saving animals. Such a step provides for getting fermenting material out where it can't do any more harm, anyway. Cows that act dull and fail to eat well after an attack of indigestion can sometimes be helped by giving them a grain of strychnine daily for a few days, but prolonged use of the drug is dangerous.

PREVENTION. Entirely a matter of avoiding the causes listed.

Bloat

CAUSE. Fundamentally a failure of gas to escape from the stomach through normal and regular belching. In the case of pasture bloat this is generally due to a lack of stiff stems and irritating material that ordinarily tickle the stomach wall and induce belching through reflex action. This point contradicts the old belief that bloating is due to excessive gas formation by certain green plants. As a matter of fact, a ration of alfalfa hay and grain really forms more gas in the stomach than does green alfalfa alone. However, bloating sometimes occurs on dry feeds when the rumen is paralyzed for some reason or other and becomes incapable of responding to irritating stimulation. Pasture bloat at times is also evidently caused by differences in the sugar content of certain plants. Rapid fermentation of large amounts of sugar in combination with a natural type of plant soap may result in the formation of countless bubbles and the appearance of so-called "frothy bloat" which is hard to relieve in the usual manner.

Bloating is frequently caused by different kinds of infections that enlarge lymph glands in certain locations and results in pressure on the esophagus that retards the normal escape of gas. Obstruction through choke causes bloat in a similar manner. Animals that lie on their backs or stretch out flat on their sides for long periods are apt to bloat for another reason. In such positions the liquid that is normally in the bottom of the rumen is shifted to the top and closes off the opening of the esophagus with a sort of water seal that prevents the escape of gas.

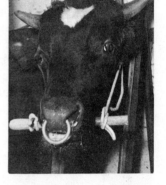

Tying a stick in a bloated animal's mouth will often help to relieve bloat by causing constant chewing movements.

SYMPTOMS. Mainly a swelling of the left flank which may become extensive and cause the entire body to expand like a balloon. In extreme cases animals froth at the mouth, fight for breath, and go down in convulsions. Death can result in a few minutes at times, with death being due to the absorption of poisonous gases like methane and carbon dioxide by the blood.

TREATMENT. The immediate services of a veterinarian are desirable. While he is coming, here are some things you can do yourself that may easily save the life of your bloated animal.

1. Tie a stick or large rope crosswise in the mouth. An eight-inch piece of an old pitchfork handle, with a small rope fastened to each end, makes a good bit for this purpose.

After drawing it well back in the corners of the mouth, the ropes are slipped up close to the teeth, the free ends are carried back and tied tightly together behind the ears. This "gag" will encourage chewing and movements of the tongue to induce belching.

2. Drench bloated animals with a mixture made of a half-pint each of warm milk and kerosene (or turpentine), and repeat treatment every half hour as needed.

3. Drench bloated animals with a mixture made by adding water to one of the concentrated aryls or silicone preparations made up especially for bloat treatment and available through your veterinarian. You may want to stock up with a few bottles of these compounds for emergency use.

4. Drench bloated animals with a mixture made by adding water to one of the ordinary household detergents containing aryl alkyl sulfonates. In an emergency the detergent can be be given dry, a handful at a time, and placed well back in the mouth so it has to be swallowed.

5. Keep animals on their feet and walking about, preferably uphill. This is because the gas has a natural tendency to rise, and keeping the head high helps it to escape.

6. Knead the left flank vigorously with the fists to force gas out of the rumen.

7. Pass a stomach tube through a mouth speculum, down the throat, and into the stomach to provide an outlet for the gas. If you don't have a stomach tube, you can substitute a five-foot length of ordinary garden hose. The mouth can be held open by a clevis placed cross-wise between the back teeth, and the hose passed through it so it isn't chewed up.

8. In extreme emergencies animals may be "tapped" as described in the Practical Pointers section of this book. When "tapping" is done with a knife, the resultant wound may take weeks to heal, since the escaping gas can be expected to carry stomach contents with it to cause extensive infection.

9. Whatever treatment you use, be sure to keep cattle away from water for at least three hours after the bloat has been relieved. Otherwise a recurrence of trouble can be expected.

PREVENTION. By:

1. Seeding pastures so they are half grass and half legumes and furnish forage capable of causing normal belching. It is generally hard to get a fifty-fifty balance the first year

because grass grows slower than legumes. However, A. R. Schmid of the University of Minnesota says that orchard grass may fit into such a scheme because it develops rapidly and gives legumes considerable competition the first year.

2. Keeping good quality hay in portable racks on pastures where cattle are grazing. The dry feed encourages belching.

3. Leaving old stack "butts" in pastures to provide dry roughage for the same purpose.

4. Making sure that water is available in the pasture, piping it there if necessary. This keeps cattle from drinking too much at any one time. Too much water in the rumen prevents normal escape of gas.

5. Waiting until legumes are in full bloom before pasturing them. The plants will then have stems stiff enough to irritate the stomach and cause belching.

6. Avoiding turning in on wet plants the first day. More water means more fermentation and more gas formation.

7. Being sure that cattle aren't extremely hungry when turned to pasture. Fill 'em up with hay or silage first.

8. Changing gradually from barn feeding. Allow on pasture for increasing periods of time each day until they're on it all day.

9. Keeping animals on pasture night and day after the change has once been completed, and giving them no chance to empty out between fills.

10. Keeping salt and minerals in separate boxes so the cattle can help themselves at all times and prevent bloat through the promotion of better digestion.

11. Dumping 50 to 100 pounds of calcium carbonate (feeding lime) in water tanks during the summer months. The value of this practice is disputed, but if it doesn't do any good, it at least will do no harm.

12. Mixing penicillin with salt or feed. Successful control of bloat by this method was first reported by B. F. Barrentine of Mississippi State College. It was found that a 100 mg. dose of procaine penicillin or a 63.4 mg. dose of potassium penicillin per head daily was effective in preventing bloat in yearling steers. Bloating was not prevented on the day of treatment, but was prevented the next day. Later tests showed that the penicillin was effective for only about 17 days, and bloating would then occur again, even though cattle were still receiving it. Additional study at the Mississippi Station

indicates that the effectiveness of penicillin can be extended by mixing other antibiotics with it. A combination of antibiotics gave adequate protection for 36 days. Doses of 100 mg. procaine penicillin and 63.4 mg. potassium penicillin are equal to 100,000 units of penicillin. Stock salt mixed with penicillin is available, but a surer way of getting the penicillin into animals is represented by mixtures which are sprinkled on the grain at feeding time. They are especially convenient for use on dairy cows. A teaspoonful of the mixture usually contains 75-100 mg. of the penicillin, and it is merely added to each animal's grain allowance every morning or night.

13. Spraying green forage with some kind of oil to increase the surface tension of rumen contents. Dairymen in New Zealand control frothy bloat by spraying their pastures with enough oil so that cows eat two ounces while grazing. Research workers at Iowa State College found that bloat was reduced by spraying enough soy bean oil or lard derivative oil over green-chopped alfalfa so that each animal got four ounces per day. In another Iowa State College experiment, giving each animal a pint of oil in the late afternoon completely prevented bloat during evening grazing, even though cows were turned on alfalfa during a severe bloat period in September. Based on work to date, peanut or mineral oil sprayed on dangerous forage at the rate of three ounces daily per animal appears to be a very effective way of controlling bloat.

14. Eliminating ladino, red clover, and alfalfa from the pasture program. Birdsfoot trefoil, a plant which has never been known to cause bloat, may be substituted for them, but it produces less feed than a grass-legume combination.

15. Clipping pastures regularly. Otherwise, grass becomes overripe and is left alone while legumes are constantly kept closely grazed and in their most dangerous stage of growth.

16. Strip-grazing pastures to keep certain areas from being grazed too closely. After a rain these areas are likely to come up with a dangerous new growth which is eaten first, of course.

Why All Bloat Cases Can't Be Treated the Same Way

Bloat in cattle may occur for the following reasons:

1. The ration may not contain stiff plant stems and sharp-

pointed leaves that ordinarily irritate the stomach and cause belching. Many beef raisers have discovered that bloat cases can be increased merely by cutting down the amount of hay fed.

2. Green plants may be eaten that have a natural tendency to cause "frothy bloat." There is a good chance that this type of bloat is commoner now than it was 20 years ago because of the development of new plants and improved strains of older ones. For example, alfalfa that is more resistant to winter-killing may also contain more sugars and saponins.

3. Indigestion. Usually caused by over-feeding or eating spoiled feeds like moldy silage, but anything that causes indigestion also has a tendency to stop normal digestive movements. When this happens, stomach gas accumulates to cause bloating.

4. Poisoning by either plants or chemicals. Regardless of the poison involved, bloating is actually due to the partial or complete paralysis of the digestive system as in the case of indigestion.

5. Diseases of some kind. They may be either non-contagious, like milk fever and lockjaw, or contagious, like rabies and shipping fever. Here again, bloating is due to paralysis of throat muscles and parts of the digestive system.

6. Hardware trouble. Objects that pierce the rumen may paralyze it so that gas accumulates there.

7. Ulcers of the rumen or abomasum. They may have the effect of paralyzing the stomach.

8. Stomach worms. Bloating is then primarily due to irritation of the fold at the junction of the stomach and small intestine. This results in swelling of the fold which then blocks the intestinal opening and prevents normal emptying of the stomach.

9. Foreign materials. These include such things as balls of plant fiber, after-birth, grain sacks, paper, and accumulations of hair which may interfere with normal digestive processes.

10. Deposits of fat or enlarged lymph glands. Pressure by them on various parts of the digestive tract can easily prevent the normal escape of gas from the stomach.

11. Choking. Something like a potato or an ear of corn or an apple may lodge in the esophagus so that belching is impossible, and in such an event gas naturally will accumulate in the rumen, even though normal breathing is possible.

12. The position of the body. When animals are stretched out flat or with their backs downhill, the liquid that is normally in the bottom of the rumen is moved to the top and closes off the lower opening of the esophagus like a water seal to prevent the escape of gas.

With so many different causes, it is easy to understand why all bloat cases can't be treated the same way. Animals that are lying down will often remedy themselves if they are raised so liquid no longer seals off the lower end of the esophagus. Bloat due to gas resulting from indigestion or grain can be corrected by passing a stomach tube, or "tapping" the upper left flank. Animals will often improve rapidly if a stick is tied cross-wise in the mouth so they chew constantly and keep the mouth open so gas can escape. When bloat is secondary to things like poisoning or diseases, the primary cause will have to be corrected to prevent a recurrence of trouble.

Treatment isn't so simple when so-called "frothy" bloat is involved, and this constitutes well over half the bloat cases which occur annually in the United States. This type of bloat follows the eating of lush green forage that contains dangerous sugars and saponins. Passing a stomach tube or "tapping" an affected animal won't relieve this type of bloat, for the froth just can't get out fast enough through a small opening.

"Frothy" bloat first requires treatment with something that will increase the surface tension of the rumen liquid so the bubbles are broken down and the gas is freed. The bloat can then be treated with regular methods. Grandpa probably didn't know why, but his old remedies, like kerosene and turpentine and mineral oil were effective because they increased the surface tension and broke up the froth in the rumen of bloated animals. As a matter of fact, our newer aryls and silicones are no better than the bloat remedies used by Grandfather. After the small bubbles have been broken up, animals will often start belching and releasing the gas normally within a short time. In cases of extreme emergency, when there isn't time for breaking up the froth, it may be necessary to slash open the left flank so the froth has a chance to get out in a hurry.

Hardware Trouble or Traumatic Gastritis

CAUSE. Cows seldom chew their food very thoroughly the first time, and so are likely to swallow a great many nails, staples, pieces of wire, etc., that they accidentally get in their mouths. Such objects are likely to be caught and held in the reticulum, which lies against both the diaphragm and the liver. If pointed in the proper direction, they are apt to be forced through the stomach wall by digestive movements, pressure in the latter stages of pregnancy or straining at the time a calf is born. If the diaphragm is punctured as well as the stomach, the heart or lungs may then be injured as well. When the injury is a little further back, the liver may be pierced instead of the diaphragm. Sometimes objects are short like tacks and incapable of doing much more than piercing the stomach wall. Regardless of any additional damage that may be done, piercing of the stomach alone is usually enough to cause infection and evidence of sickness.

SYMPTOMS. Dependent on the size of the object and the organs it pierces. Generally much the same as described for indigestion. A peculiar stiffness and reluctance to move are characteristic, and a cow that will jump a ditch or gutter probably doesn't have hard-

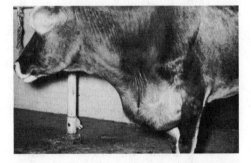

Swollen brisket and distended jugular vein due to hardware trouble. (Picture, courtesy Dr. W. J. Gibbons, A.P.I., Auburn, Ala.)

ware trouble. Arching of the back, tucking up of the belly, and trembling of muscles back of the front legs are all common symptoms of hardware trouble. Affected animals often spend a great deal of time lying down, with pain evidently being eased a little in this position. Pain may be shown when the floor of the chest cavity is bumped or the backbone is pinched back of the shoulders. Reaction to the latter occurs because natural bowing of the back away from pinching causes increased pressure on the stomach area where it has been pierced. When the heart is involved it is often possible to hear splashing or tinkling sounds when the organ beats. Bloody urine may result from heart injury, too. In the latter stages of such cases there may be swelling of the brisket and distension of the jugular veins. This trouble is far commonest in advanced pregnancy and at calving time. Attacks are of indefinite duration, for small objects may be sealed off and recovery complete in a few days while larger ones may cause severe internal injuries and death within the same length of time. Repeated attacks may occur because of short nails or wires that keep breaking loose and causing new injuries. At other times infection may spread abscesses through various parts of the body and cause a wasting illness that lasts for months.

DIAGNOSIS. Often difficult because the symptoms so closely resemble those of indigestion. However, a history of over-eating or access to spoiled feed will often help to indicate indigestion. Another diagnostic aid lies in the fact that bloating usually appears early in cases of indigestion while it appears late in hardware trouble if it appears at all. Then, too, indigestion usually responds rather promptly to treatment while hardware trouble does not. In recent years modified mine detectors have been used quite successfully by some men in the diagnosis of hardware trouble. These instruments aren't altogether dependable, for most older cattle carry pieces of assorted hardware in their stomachs which lay there and cause no trouble whatever but are shown up by the detectors whether they're doing damage or not. A white blood cell count may have diagnostic value after the first few days, for hardware trouble almost always causes a marked increase in their numbers. This procedure isn't infallible, either, for almost any kind of serious bacterial infection will cause a similar increase. Besides indigestion, hardware trouble may be confused with tuberculosis, pyelonephritis, Johne's disease, metritis, and liver infections.

TREATMENT. One of four things:

1. Standing the animal on an inclined platform and making it stay there constantly for at least three weeks. Raising the front feet has the effect of pulling the stomach and penetrating object back from the diaphragm until it can be walled off by Mother Nature to prevent further injury. About three out of four animals recover with such treatment.

   The platform is started by cutting a 2" x 6" beam so it is long enough to extend clear across the front end of the stall. It is then laid on the floor and turned up on its narrow side so that it fits close up against the bottom of the stanchion. Strong half-inch boards are secured and laid side by side until there are enough of them to completely cover the floor of the stall. These are cut so they are long enough to reach from the top of the 2" x 6" back to within a foot of the gutter. A 2" x 4" is then cut the width of the stall, turned on its narrow side and placed under the boards at the right place to give them added strength.

The boards are then nailed fast to the 2″ x 6″ and 2″ x 4″, after which cleats about an inch think are nailed across them at six-inch intervals to prevent slipping by animals.

2. Operating to remove the piercing object by surgery.

3. Removing "hardware" with an instrument consisting of a magnet and especially designed probang that permits dropping the magnet into the stomach and withdrawal with adherent metal.

4. Using an aluminum balling gun to make cows swallow strong 2 to 3-inch magnets. A combination of magnetic attraction and stomach movements will often retract imbedded metal.

PREVENTION. Largely a matter of keeping metal out of feeds and pastures. Grain can be passed over large magnets, but no practical method is known for removing "hardware" from roughage. H. K. Cooper has reported favorably—*Jour. Am. Vet. Med. Ass'n.* 125 (1954), 301—on the use of magnets as mentioned under *Treatment* for the prevention of hardware trouble. Magnets remain in the reticulum for several years, attracting metallic material, holding it, and keeping it from piercing the stomach wall.

Coccidiosis

CAUSE. Usually a single-celled parasite called *Eimeria zurnii*, although nine other supposedly less dangerous species of coccidia have been reported as affecting cattle. They are found in the digestive tract and give off eggs or oöcysts in the manure of host animals.

MEANS OF SPREAD. Entirely through the swallowing of oöcysts in feed or water that has been contaminated with manure from infested animals. The number that are swallowed largely determines the severity of symptoms. Oöcysts may be picked up from running streams below infected pastures, but are more commonly found in stagnant pools of water. The disease is favored by filth and lack of sanitation, but it sometimes appears under excellent conditions and the source of an outbreak may never be discovered.

SYMPTOMS. A thin bloody diarrhea is usually the most striking one, but a non-bloody type may appear in younger calves. The pulse is apt to be fast, sometimes approaching 100, and loss of blood is shown by paleness of the mouth and nostrils. Affected animals that are badly infested become thin and weak, often showing twitching and crazy actions before finally going down in a stupefied condition. Coccidiosis is commonest in animals between six months and two years old, although it may attack suckling calves or milking cows. Effects depend pretty much on the age and condition of animals, with the highest death losses in young and poorly fed beasts. Outbreaks may last only a few days or take weeks to subside in a herd. An attack usually gives increased resistance or complete immunity.

DIAGNOSIS. Tentatively made on the basis of a bloody diarrhea and the death of animals. Microscopic examination of manure that reveals oöcysts is positive proof of the disease. However, these may not be present in the beginning of an outbreak, nor shortly after recovery, either. Consequently, failure to find oöcysts doesn't necessarily rule out coccidiosis, especially if the typical symptoms are apparent. The disease may be confused with winter dysentery, shipping fever, poisoning, blackleg, or other troubles.

TREATMENT. Sulfaquinoxaline is one of the most promising drugs at this time, although sulfaguanidine and sulfamethazine have also been claimed as giving good results. Dosage is dependent on size and condition, but these remedies are commonly given at the rate of ½-1½ ounces daily to yearlings for a couple of days. They are best given as a drench or in capsules since medication of water may not insure proper treatment of all animals. Severely weakened animals may require transfusions of a pint to a quart of citrated blood to replace what they have lost and intravenous injections of a pint to a quart glucose solutions for food. Drugs may be needed to supply a protective coating for badly irritated intestinal linings. A 50-50 mixture of salol and bismuth subnitrate is useful for this purpose when given two or three times daily in 1 to 4 ounce doses. Dr. Brandenburg of North Dakota reports powdered catechu as being satisfactory. The dose is two tablespoonfuls in a pint of milk for each 400 pounds of body weight and animals are treated two or three times a day as needed. Straining can often be prevented by injecting 1 to 2 pints of mineral oil in the rectum.

PREVENTION. Best accomplished through pasture rotation and furnishing clean dry quarters for animals. Good feeding is important as is the daily disposal of manure and protection of drinking water against contamination. Wet spots should be filled, drained, or fenced off, regardless of whether they occur around a tank or in the middle of a pasture. Racks and troughs that are kept free of manure offer big advantages over feeding off the ground. Separation of calves according to age groups will avoid infestation of young animals by immune older ones that usually carry more coccidia. Premises are best cleaned up and disinfected after an outbreak, for under proper conditions oöcysts may remain dangerous for long periods.

Poisoning by Chemicals

CAUSE. Several possibilities on the average farm. (1) Fertilizers, chiefly nitrates. (2) Plant sprays like Paris green, lead arsenate, 2,4D, parathion, etc. (3) Paints containing lead. (4) Rodent poisons containing cyanide, arsenic, etc. (5) Ointments containing

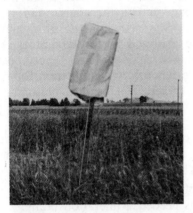

Fertilizer bags hung on fence posts like this may be eaten by cattle, who will be poisoned by them.

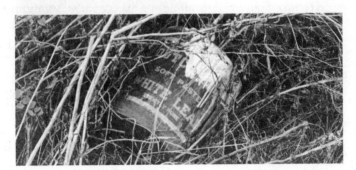

Old paint pail thrown into fence corner may be found by cattle to poison them years afterward.

mercury. (6) Seed treatments containing the same element. (7) Animal sprays containing DDT and lindane. (8) Medicines like copper sulfate, strychnine, carbon tetrachloride, etc.

SYMPTOMS. Largely dependent on the type of poison, amount eaten, size of animal, and amount of food in the stomach when eaten. Sometimes sudden death is the only one. Generally there are signs of pain and colic with fast breathing, rapid pulse, and sometimes slobbering or vomiting. Diarrhea and general weakness often causes animals to go down in a paralyzed condition. Occasionally there is grinding of the teeth and all kinds of crazy symptoms with evidence of delirium.

DIAGNOSIS. Usually a matter of checking places recently visited by animals and searching for poisonous materials they may have eaten or been given as medicine. This is because a diagnosis of poisoning should never be made unless the source and type of material can be demonstrated. Stomach contents or tissues like the liver and kidneys can be analyzed in the laboratory, but a request for a specific examination makes a fast report possible. Under the best of conditions a laboratory examination for poison is usually too expensive to be practical. Chemical poisoning may be confused with anthrax, lightning stroke, indigestion, or plant poisoning.

TREATMENT. Dependent on the poison but generally useless because of extensive damage already done in the body. The following are suggestions of a general nature:

1. *Nitrates*. 30-150 cc. of 1% methylene blue solution intravenously every hour as needed. Mineral oil orally.

2. *Arsenic*. Sodium thiosulfate 40-80 cc. 20% solution intravenously as needed. May be given orally in ½-1 ounce.

3. *Lead*. Epsom salts orally ½-2 lbs. Sodium citrate 12-24 oz. daily.

4. *Cyanide*. Methylene blue as for nitrates, sodium thiosulfate as for arsenic, or sodium nitrite 40-80 cc. 20% solution intravenously.

5. *Mercury*. Wash ointments off body. Sodium thiosulfate as for arsenic, or 100-500 cc. 20% sodium idodide intravenously.

6. *Copper*. Egg whites, milk, magnesium oxide 4 oz.-1 lb. orally.

7. *Strychnine*. Chloral hydrate ½-3 oz. well diluted with water orally.

PREVENTION. Keeping poisons away from cattle since they are particularly fond of the deadlier ones like nitrates.

1. Don't store fertilizers where animals can reach them.

2. Don't leave empty fertilizer bags along fences.

3. Don't dump surplus sprays in barnyards or cattle lots.

4. Don't throw paint pails into pastures or use them for feeding and watering animals.
5. Don't feed treated seed.
6. Don't put mercury compounds on the skin of cattle.
7. Don't use poisonous medicines carelessly.
8. Don't fail to follow directions for mixing sprays and dips.
9. Don't pasture ground recently sprayed or close to sprayed orchards, cabbage fields, etc.
10. Don't leave rodent poisons around barns or cattle sheds.

Poisoning by Plants

CAUSE. About 400 different species in the United States. Commoner ones are loco weed, bracken fern, nightshade, ragwort, horsetail fern, tarweed, cocklebur, larkspur, buttercup, and several types of lupines. Some, like the cocklebur, are poisonous only

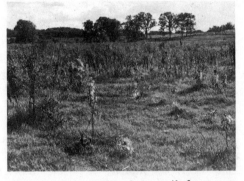

Burned-out pastures in the fall may cause cattle to eat poisonous plants they would otherwise leave alone.

at certain stages of development. Some, like horsetail fern, are more poisonous in hay than in the growing stage. Some, like saltbush, are poisonous because the ground they grow on draws up selenium to cause "alkali disease." Others are poisonous at all times under all kinds of conditions. Most cases of cattle poisoning occur either in the early spring when grass is scanty or in the fall after it has dried up. Under such conditions animals will eat plants that they would ordinarily leave alone. Sweet clover and prussic acid poisoning are considered separately in this book.

SYMPTOMS. Varied because of the large number of poisonous plants and their different toxic compounds. The symptoms given for chemical poisoning will serve equally well for plant poisoning, since outside of burning by chemicals there is no way of telling the two types apart.

DIAGNOSIS. Dependent on finding the causative plants. A diagnosis of "poisoning by some kind of a weed" is no diagnosis at all. It may be confused with the same troubles mentioned under the diagnosis of chemical poisoning.

TREATMENT. Aside from changing pastures or removal of troublesome roughage from the diet, none can be given. Once the offending plant is known, suitable medication can be supplied.

PREVENTION. Pretty much a matter of feeding animals well enough so they won't eat dangerous plants. Animals shouldn't be turned out too early in the spring when there is little grass and cattle are likely to eat anything that has a green color. Overgrazing of pastures should be avoided, since the time eventually comes when cattle have to choose between starving and eating objectionable roughage. Under crowded pasture conditions extra feed like hay and forage can be supplied to avoid poisoning. A knowledge of poisonous plants found in your area is also helpful, since such forage can be destroyed or avoided when it is recognized.

Ergot Poisoning

CAUSE. Several different poisonous factors contained in the fungus *Claviceps purpurea*. It is commonly known as "smut" and although usually thought of in connection with rye, it also grows on oats, barley, corn, dallis grass, and most other grasses.

SYMPTOMS. Either or both of two general types. One is the form which sees the sloughing of tissues from the lower legs and other body extremities, and this is the type usually reported. In many instances the tails drop off as completely as though they had been amputated with an ax. Leg lesions often resemble "girdles" placed on trees to kill them, and toes frequently slough away.

The other type is indicated by various forms of difficulty in movements. Animals may walk with a peculiar stiff-legged gait highly suggestive of lockjaw, and pronounced trembling of various muscle groups is often seen. Animals may fall when turning, go into convulsions, and have considerable trouble in regaining their feet. The appetite generally remains good and there are seldom any symptoms of general sickness. Animals usually have to eat smut-bearing feeds over long periods in order to produce symptoms. Growing grasses and plants need not be incriminated, for cases have been reported as following the feeding of ear corn, screenings, and certain types of hay that carried *C. purpurea*.

TREATMENT. Usually consists of doing nothing more than removing the causative feed from the diet. Most affected animals recover, although those in advanced stages of the nervous form often die.

PREVENTION. Entirely a matter of using care to provide good pasture and rations for cattle, since the animals don't eat the smutty feeds because they like them.

Halogeton Poisoning

CAUSE. Oxalic acid salts found in a plant called *Halogeton glomeratus*. This plant is a native of Asia and wasn't recognized in the United States until 1935, when it was seen in Nevada. Since that time it has spread rapidly and is now also known to exist in Utah, Idaho, Wyoming, and California. It may also be shipped in hay to other areas. It is highly resistant to drouth and grows readily on range lands where there is little other vegetation. Deaths are due to withdrawal of calcium from the blood.

SYMPTOMS. Much like those of milk fever, with animals often standing in a dejected attitude with the head hanging low as though they were half asleep. The beasts grow progressively weaker, stagger around, and finally go down in a paralyzed condition. They soon become unconscious, with breathing becoming slower and slower until death finally occurs without a struggle. Most cases are seen after the plants have dried up, since they have an especially bad taste when green. As a matter of fact, Halogeton won't ordinarily be eaten at any time if there's anything else around that's edible.

DIAGNOSIS. Through typical symptoms and availability of Halogeton on range when other feeds are scarce.

TREATMENT. None can be recommended at this time. Intravenous injection of calcium compounds has not been successful, although they should theoretically be helpful. However, the failure of treatment shouldn't be surprising, since irreparable damage has usually been done by the time symptoms are noticed.

PREVENTION. For complete safety, it's a matter of completely removing halogeton from the range. However, this hasn't proven too practical, since the job has to be done several times every year. Instead, the following practices are recommended for minimizing the danger of halogeton poisoning:

1. Feed animals well before turning them onto dangerous range, since they can stand more of the halogeton if it's mixed with

other feeds in the stomach.

2. Supply extra feeds when ranges have reached the point where little vegetation is available. In addition to providing a diluting factor, such feeds will also keep animals from getting extremely hungry so they'll eat dangerously large quantities of the plant.

3. Keep animals moving on the range so they'll have a better chance of finding something to eat besides halogeton. This is helpful in another way, for cattle can eat considerable halogeton if they get it a little at a time. If they eat large amounts in a short time they're pretty good bets to lie down and die.

4. Research has shown that sheep fed alfalfa pellets containing 5% dicalcium phosphate, are protected against halogeton poisoning, and it may also be effective in cattle. This amount is about ten times that ordinarily used in feeds. The chemical apparently ties up the oxalates in the intestines or is absorbed to replace calcium removed by the poison.

Soybean Oil Meal Poisoning (Stockman Disease)

CAUSE. Some still-unidentified poisonous factor which exists in trichloroethylene-extracted soybean oil meal. It has a cumulative effect and requires feeding of the meal for long periods before damage is done. The dangerous compound was first recognized at Iowa State College in 1948, and caused extensive cattle losses in Montana, Minnesota, North Dakota, and other states during the winter of 1951-52. The poisonous factor does not exist in soy bean oil meal that has been extracted by other methods.

SYMPTOMS. Not likely to be seen before animals have been on the meal for at least 30 days. Occasionally, beasts die suddenly without showing any previous signs of sickness, but most of them start by showing a profuse discharge from the nostrils. They go off feed, become weak, lose weight, and milking animals fall off to nothing in production. Body temperatures are likely to be high for a time, often approaching 109 degrees Fahrenheit. Some cattle show signs of indigestion like grunting, groaning, kicking at the belly, looking at the flank, grinding the teeth, alternate periods of constipation and diarrhea, and the appearance of small blood clots in the manure. In bad cases blood may be discharged from the mouth, nostrils, and all other body openings, with evidence of jaundice often appearing in the final stages. In some cases large swellings may appear where pockets of blood have formed under the skin and in muscles, usually in the throat or flank region.

Most animals die within a few days after symptoms are shown, but some linger on for weeks, with deaths continuing to occur in a herd for several months after feeding of the meal has been discontinued. Young animals and high-producing dairy cows are especially susceptible, and the death rate is high among cows in late pregnancy. There are apparently no complete recoveries and about eight out of ten animals that show symptoms can be expected to die, with the death rate seemingly dependent on the amount of meal that cattle have received daily.

Opening a dead animal will show bloody areas of various sizes throughout the body, and occasionally large hematomas under the skin of the flank or back. Clots of blood and ulcers may be found in the digestive tract, and hemorrhagic spots usually show up on the surface of the liver, kidneys, heart, thoracic wall, and lining of the urinary bladder.

DIAGNOSIS. Definite only in the laboratory, usually through the feeding of suspected meal to test animals or baby chicks. Toxicologic tests can also be made on the meal, but they are both expensive and time-consuming. A tentative diagnosis can be made on the basis of long-term feeding of moderate to large quantities of the meal in combination with typical symptoms and post-mortem findings. Under field conditions this trouble might be confused with bracken fern poisoning.

TREATMENT. None can be recommended as likely to help, although several have been tried, including blood transfusions, antibiotics, and sulfas.

PREVENTION. Unless new sources of the causative agent are discovered, entirely a matter of avoiding the feeding of soybean oil meal that has been extracted with trichloroethylene. This should not be too difficult unless a change in manufacturing methods is made, since all of the dangerous meal was withdrawn from the market and soybean oil meal production with trichloro-ethylene discontinued in 1952.

Lupine Poisoning

CAUSE. Various species of the plant genus *Lupinus* (wild bean), most of them growing in the western United States. Poisoning is due to alkaloids which are quickly eliminated by the kidneys. Accordingly, effects do not build up, and animals may eat large amounts over a long period if they do not exceed the poisonous limit at any one time.

SYMPTOMS. The earliest ones are increased excitability and uncertain, staggering movements. These may appear within a few hours after eating the plants. Animals may then go down in a paralyzed condition and die, sometimes within 12 to 48 hours. The breathing and heart rate are increased, but no fever is shown. Most cases occur during the late summer or fall.

The plants *L. sericeus* and *L. laxiflorus* are recognized as causing a different kind of symptom in a trouble called crooked calf disease which is discussed in another part of this book. It has been reported from South Dakota and Nebraska to the Pacific coast, north to Canada, and south to Utah.

DIAGNOSIS. Usually through a history of cattle having been pastured on ranges where lupine plants were available.

TREATMENT. None reported as having been successful.

PREVENTION. Entirely a matter of pasture management. See Poisoning by Plants elsewhere in this book.

Cottonseed Poisoning

CAUSE. A poisonous compound known as "gossypol" which is found in cottonseed products and evidently varies according to different soil and climatic factors. Although the gossypol is almost completely destroyed during manufacture, cottonseed oil meal and cake may still contain enough of it to cause trouble for cattle under certain conditions.

SYMPTOMS. Excessive watering of the eyes is common, with poor eyesight as shown by animals bumping into fences and stumbling over objects in front of them. The eyes may even be kept closed much of the time and complete blindness may eventually occur. Convulsions are frequently seen, along with such troubles as stiffness, lameness, loss of weight, and panting for breath after the slightest exertion. Deaths may occur, but the death rate usually isn't high if the diet is corrected. Calves under four months of age are most likely to be affected, since adult cattle are the most resistant of all farm animals in regard to cottonseed poisoning. There is little danger when older animals are on fair pasture or getting plenty of good hay, but symptoms of poisoning may easily develop when cottonseed products form almost the complete ration for long periods of time.

DIAGNOSIS. Usually through a history of faulty feeding that allowed too much cottonseed meal or cake in the ration. The trouble may easily be confused with deficiencies of vitamin A and various of the trace elements.

TREATMENT. Consists of remedying the ration and removing cottonseed products from it at least for a while.

PREVENTION. Largely a matter of avoiding the feeding of cottonseed products in large amounts for any considerable length of time. Such feeding is permissible only when it is supplemented with free-choice minerals and plenty of good pasture or hay. Calves less than four months old shouldn't receive any kind of cottonseed products in their rations.

Prussic Acid Poisoning (Hydrogen Cyanide Poisoning)

CAUSE. Certain plants in which prussic acid is formed through combination of a glucoside, amygdalin, and a ferment, emulsin. These compounds are both harmless alone, but unite when plants are damaged by cutting, trampling, wilting, stunting, frosting, bruising, or other causes. Danger is greatest when the plants are in the

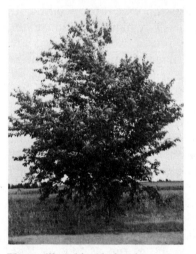

short, dark-green stage of fastest growth, while there is little or none in the same plants after they have reached a height of eighteen inches or more. Consequently, hay or silage made from short plants is likely to be poisonous while that from mature plants is generally safe. Plants grown on good soil are more dangerous than those from poor ground, and prussic acid content may be increased by heavy application of nitrogen fertilizers when soils are deficient in phosphorus. Trouble is commonest with sudan grass and other members of the sorghum family, but flax, chokecherries, arrowgrass, Christmas-berries, wild cherries,

Plants like this choke-cherry tree can cause prussic acid poisoning when the leaves are damaged or wilted.

velvet-grass, and laurel are sometimes involved, too. Death is actually due to suffocation because the exchange of oxygen and carbon dioxide is prevented in the body cells.

SYMPTOMS. Largely dependent on the amount of poisonous plants eaten, but often death within a few minutes. Affected animals may stagger a little and act sleepy before suddenly dropping dead. Severe muscular twitching is sometimes seen, while fast labored breathing and frothing from the wide-open mouth is invariably seen because of threatened suffocation. Animals that go down may grind their teeth and turn their heads into a flank like cows with milk fever. The breath generally has an almond-like odor and blood is likely to have a bright cherry-red color because of a change from hemoglobin to cyanhemoglobin.

DIAGNOSIS. Generally through a history of poisonous plants that have recently been eaten. Symptoms of suffocation, an odor of almonds about animals, and the peculiar cherry-red blood color will help to confirm the diagnosis. It may be confused with anthrax, blackleg, lightning stroke, milk fever, choke, and chemical or plant poisoning of other types.

Dr. A. A. Case of the University of Missouri recommends the use of the sodium picrate test as an aid in diagnosis. It is started by dissolving 5 grams of sodium carbonate in 94.5 cc. of distilled water, and then adding 0.5 gram of picric acid. It is best to place the resulting stock solution in a glass-stoppered brown bottle. If stored in a dark place this solution will remain fully active for many years. Typical cases of acute prussic acid poisoning are usually fairly easy to recognize, but diagnosis may be difficult in subacute cases where animals have eaten only small amounts of slightly poisonous forage. Dr. Walter Gibbons of Alabama has described the use of the sodium picrate solution for identifying such cases. To make this test, a small amount of liquid is obtained from the rumen of an afflicted animal by using the stomach tube. A drop of the sodium picrate solution is applied to a blotter or pieces of filter paper, and this is touched with a drop of the rumen liquid. A color change from yellow to red occurs when cyanide is present. If the color changes in less than 10 minutes, the animal has probably eaten enough to kill it. Suspected forage or rumen contents from sick or dead animals can also be tested for HCN with the sodium picrate solution. The test is run as follows: Use a small hand food chopper to thoroughly grind up about half a cupful of stalks or leaves or bark and then pack them lightly in a small glass jar that has a reasonably tight-fitting lid. Add 5 to 10 drops of chloroform to the chopped forage or rumen contents (considered already ground), wet a strip of filter paper with the picrate solution, apply the lid tightly so the strip hangs down inside the jar, and place in the sun, on an automobile motor or radiator, or some other warm place. A positive reaction is indicated by a color change from the picric acid yellow to shades of pink through red. The more HCN that is present, the quicker and darker the color change. Material should be watched for at least two hours before calling the test negative, but in some cases color changes will appear in a few minutes. Filter paper strips are best but are not absolutely necessary, for tissues, white paper towels, and white blotters have all been used in field emergencies. The test can also be run overnite at room temperature instead of placing the jar of suspected forage in a warm place. The chief difference is in the speed of reactions. It will be best to have the stock solution made up by a druggist, since the picric acid is explosive. If it must be made up at home, handle the picric acid in small amounts and keep it away from fire and protein solutions.

TREATMENT. Any of the following:

1. Sodium nitrite, fresh 20% solution, 40-80 cc. intravenously.
2. Sodium thiosulfate, 20% solution, 40-80 cc. intravenously.
3. Combination of above solutions, 20-40 cc. of each intravenously.
4. Methylene blue, 1% solution, 75-150 cc. intravenously.

At least one investigator believes that the intravenous injection of 10 cc. of a 20% solution of sodium nitrite followed immediately by 30 cc. of a 20% solution of sodium thiosulfate is the most satisfactory treatment for prussic acid poisoning.

Doses may be repeated in a few minutes, and a smaller third dose given if needed. Artificial respiration should be given whenever possible and continued as long as the heart beats. A high death rate will probably result regardless of the treatment used, since prussic acid is one of the most powerful poisons known.

Solutions and tablets for making up solutions or to be given by mouth and composed of combinations of methylene blue, sodium nitrite, and sodium thiosulfate may be obtained from your veterinarian. These solutions have proven highly effective, and it has been claimed that if given intravenously to a prussic acid-poisoned animal before the heart stops beating, the animal can be saved. A high death rate is to be expected regardless of the treatment used, since prussic acid is one of the most powerful poisons known.

PREVENTION. Largely a matter of eight "don'ts":

1. Don't use too much fertilizer that is heavy with nitrogen,

especially when soils are deficient in phosphorus.

2. Don't pasture plants that are short, or cut them for hay at that stage. Let them get at least eighteen inches tall first.

3. Don't pasture plants that have been stricken by drouth and remained small, regardless of age or color.

4. Don't pasture new second-growth that springs up after frosts or cuttings. Let it get at least eighteen inches tall first.

5. Don't pull cattle off dangerous pastures even overnite, for they soon lose their ability to withstand prussic acid.

6. Don't forget that cattle are much less likely to be poisoned by prussic acid if they are filled with hay before being turned into potentially dangerous fields.

7. Don't take chances with suspicious forage. Your veterinarian can test it with the picrate solution, or you can try it out by first turning in two or three of the less valuable animals.

8. Don't let cattle graze dangerous fields too closely, for it increases their chances of eating poisonous early plant growths.

Algae Poisoning (Water Bloom)

CAUSE. The common slimy green algae or "water bloom" found in drinking places of all kinds. When this material decomposes it gives off a powerful poison that has not yet been identified. It is extremely unstable and may be missing in water within a couple of days after formation. It is claimed that the poison is no longer present in surroundings when decomposing algae has reached a particularly bad-smelling stage.

SYMPTOMS. Evidently dependent on the quantity of algae and the amount of water drunk by animals. Sudden death is not unusual and finding dead or dying animals may be the first indication of trouble an owner has. At other times cattle stagger, appear weak in the hind quarters, and go down. Some may be found lying down and breathing deeply as though asleep, only to be sent into convulsions by the touch of a hand. In such seizures the head is apt to be jerked backward.

DIAGNOSIS. Generally based on deaths and symptoms at a time when winds have massed large quantities of algae along shore lines where animals drink. Trouble appearing after sudden accessibility to tanks or troughs that have been unused and accumulating algae for some time is also sufficient to cause suspicion of this type of poisoning.

Under farm conditions this trouble might be confused with prussic acid or hydrogen cyanide poisoning. However, in algae poisoning the blood is not bright red as in prussic acid poisoning. Suspected water or algae can be tested in the laboratory by feeding it or injecting it into laboratory animals to see if it causes symptoms. No chemical tests are known.

TREATMENT. With the exact cause unknown, it's rather difficult to prescribe treatment for this type of poisoning. However, the intravenous injection of 60 cc. of thionitrite and oral administration of thionitrite tablets every four hours, together with ½ gallon each of mineral oil has been reported as effective in the case of 18 animals showing typical symptoms of algae poisoning.

PREVENTION. By:

1. Cleaning and scrubbing water tanks once a week during hot weather.
2. Draining or fencing off pools of stagnant water.
3. Watching shore lines of lakes and ponds for accumulations of algae that can be brought in by winds at any time.
4. Watering cattle somewhere else when they appear.
5. Letting them return when the algae has reached the stage when it smells to high heaven.

In tanks, algae can be controlled by using powdered copper sulfate at the rate of 1 ounce per 8000 gallons of water, or 1 level teasponful per 150 gallons of water. Algae can be kept from reforming in tanks by placing copper sheets or shavings or even empty copper cartridge-cases in the water. These will remain effective for a long time unless the copper becomes covered with slime. Copper sulfate and sodium arsenite are both good for controlling algae in ponds. Workers at the University of Kentucky recommend that:

1. Copper sulfate be used at the rate of eight pounds per million gallons of water. It may be applied as a spray or by the drag-net method. The latter method calls for placing the copper sulfate in a loosely woven sack and towing it through the pond on ropes. The powdered form is used and dragged through the water until it is all dissolved. The first application should be made in the spring when the algae appear, and from three to five applications may be needed in a single season. If ponds contain skin-fish like catfish, treat one end at a time so they can escape concentrated areas. Scale fish are less sensitive.

2. Sodium arsenite be preferably used as a solution. One or two treatments applied as a spray in May or June at the rate of four to six parts per million parts of water will generally control algae. Whole ponds are not treated with this chemical, but usually only the areas infested with algae.

Fluoride Poisoning (Fluorosis)

CAUSE. Fluorine in combination with various chemicals. This element has some beneficial effects when given in small doses, but can cause serious trouble when animals get excessive amounts. There are five common sources of fluorides in large amounts:

1. Plants made dangerous by air-borne fluorides in areas around some types of industrial operations and aerospace studies using certain propellant fuels.

2. Water with high fluoride content, sometimes because of contamination with industrial wastes.

3. Feed supplements and mineral mixtures with excessive amounts of fluorides, sometimes in combination with phosphorus compounds.

4. Plants growing on soils high in fluoride content.

5. Rodent killers, insecticides, and sodium fluoride used for removing worms from swine and then left where cattle can reach them.

SYMPTOMS. Dependent on whether the poisoning is acute or chronic. The acute type results from the eating of compounds like those listed in No. 5 under CAUSE, and signs of trouble may appear within half an hour after they have been swallowed. They include such things as restlessness, excitement, refusal of food, reduced milk production, stiffness, slobbering, vomiting, diarrhea, weakness, dullness, and convulsions. Opening a dead animal will show a dark-colored blood and bloody inflammation of the digestive tract.

The chronic type is the one seen most often in cattle, and results from long-term ingestion of fluorides. The earliest symptoms shown are likely to be loss of weight and intermittent lameness in connection with stiffness in movement. An examination of the front teeth will show discoloration ranging from mottling to brown and actual blackening with evidence of extreme wear. The degree of poisoning can often be estimated by the appearance of the teeth. Evidence of fluoride poisoning is also likely to be shown by the bones of the legs which are often roughened so the lesions can be seen or palpated beneath the skin. In advanced cases they may become soft and rubbery.

DIAGNOSIS. Definite only in the laboratory through a combination of urine analysis for fluorine and x-rays of various bones. However, a tentative diagnosis can often be made on the basis of visible or palpable bone irregularities, together with discolored and badly worn front teeth in combination with a history of long exposure to possible sources of fluorine.

TREATMENT. Although no complete antidote is known for fluorosis, some compounds can lessen the damage that fluorides may cause. Aluminum chloride, aluminum sulfate, calcium carbonate, calcium aluminate, and defluorinated phosphate have all reduced the effects of fluorine in animals. For example, heifers fed aluminum sulfate in an experiment deposited 30 to 42 per cent less fluorine in their ribs than did heifers on the same feed without the aluminum sulfate.

PREVENTION. Feeding the compounds mentioned under TREATMENT can be tried in areas where fluorosis is a problem. If roughage that is high in fluorides must be fed, it should be combined with hay that has a low fluoride content. Similarly, if the drinking water is unavoidably high in fluorides, the roughage should be of low fluoride content. Fields that are high in fluoride content are best used for growing cereal or nonroughage crops like soy beans because grain does not take up fluoride from the soil to the extent that forage does. If raising crops under this plan will result in a shortage of roughage, the roughage should be imported from low-fluoride areas. Any phosphorus included in feed or mineral mixtures should be low enough in fluorine so that the total dry feed does not exceed 30 parts per million of fluorine.

Salt (Sodium Chloride) Poisoning

CAUSE. Basically a lack of water. It is most likely to occur when animals with a restricted water supply are starved for salt and then suddenly are given access to loose salt or brine solutions. Large quantities of salt placed in boxes or at one end of an open feed trough have caused trouble when a rain formed a concentrated solution of salt.

Solutions of salt are considered more dangerous than the same amount of salt in loose form, although some cases of poisoning from brine have been shown to be due to nitrites in the brine instead of salt. A new danger has appeared in recent years because high concentrations of salt have been mixed with various protein supplements to limit consumption of the supplement by range stock. Such supplements usually contain about 25% salt, and conceivably could cause trouble when fed to cattle that did not have access to plenty of water.

SYMPTOMS. The first ones are usually diarrhea and colic as shown by kicking at the belly and restlessness. Animals are dehydrated and very thirsty, which is only natural because a lack of water was probably an original cause of the poisoning. They urinate frequently, become stiff, finally go down in a paralyzed condition and die, often within 6 to 20 hours after eating the salt or drinking the brine. Opening a dead animal will show reddening and inflammation of the digestive tract as the principal lesion.

DIAGNOSIS. Can usually be made on the basis of symptoms and a knowledge of insufficient water in combination with the sudden availability of salt or brine. The diagnosis can be confirmed by laboratory tests that show high levels of sodium and chloride in the blood of affected animals.

TREATMENT. Immediately supplying large amounts of water. If animals are down, they may be unable to swallow, so the water is best given through a stomach tube. It will also prove helpful to give animals a quart or so of mineral oil to protect the lining of the digestive tract.

PREVENTION. Almost entirely a matter of management to provide plenty of water at all times in a familiar location, and salting cattle regularly so they have no chance to become ravenously hungry for it. Barrels or boxes that have contained salted meats or fish should be kept out of pastures so that cattle have no chance to drink out of them following rains. Care should also be used to see that animals have no chance to drink brine solutions that are being discharged from refrigerating plants, dairies, packing houses, etc.

Kerosene (Coal Oil) Poisoning

CAUSE. Drinking coal oil or being "drenched" with it as all or part of farm remedies. Sometimes the regular drinking water is contaminated with kerosene, either deliberately or by accident, or partially empty containers are left where cattle can reach them. In our own practice we once saw several yearling heifers that were affected after a storage tank for a heating system sprung a leak that permitted the formation of a pool of kerosene in a dry lot. Most cases are the result of similar accidents that make kerosene available for cattle.

SYMPTOMS. Affected animals go off feed, run moderate fevers, strain, have a diarrhea, and slobber ropy saliva. The eyes water, and the lining of the mouth is inflamed. The urine is dark and has an odor of kerosene, as does the breath. Opening a dead animal will reveal an odor of kerosene in the stomach contents, and there will generally be solidification of the lungs to show pneumonia. The pneumonia is caused by gases from the kerosene passing through the lungs.

DIAGNOSIS. Largely through the odor of kerosene in the breath and urine. However, the other symptoms described will help to establish the cause of trouble.

TREATMENT. Aimed at getting the kerosene out of the digestive tract as soon as possible. Rumen stimulants like nux vomica and tartar emetic are indicated, and if cases are caught early the rumen should be flushed. This is because the coal oil will float on top of the rumen liquid and so can be moved out of the stomach. Antibiotics should be given to protect against secondary infections, particularly those involving the lungs.

PREVENTION. Entirely a matter of keeping kerosene out of the reach of cattle, and avoiding its use as a medicine.

Urea Poisoning

CAUSE. Almost always due to improperly mixed feeds. It may also be due to the use of too much urea, access to the urea premix by cattle, lumping of the urea premix, and the feeding of either properly or improperly mixed feeds in large amounts to cattle that are unaccustomed to urea. Under these conditions the rumen bacteria which use the breakdown products of urea are not numerous enough to do a complete job, and free ammonia is absorbed to cause poisoning.

SYMPTOMS. Excessive slobbering with frothing at the mouth, staggering, weakness, bloating, trembling, and grinding of the teeth are common. Gasping and labored breathing are likely to be noted, while paralysis of the front legs, knuckling of the rear fetlocks, and convulsions may also be seen. Opening a dead animal is likely to show inflammation and reddening of the stomach lining, and there may be congestion of the lungs, either with or without bleeding in the organs. Death usually occurs within a few hours after symptoms are first shown.

DIAGNOSIS. Either through a laboratory analysis of the suspected feed or a feeding experiment on some of the less valuable animals. A feed sample of 10 to 20 ounces is usually enough for testing. A diagnosis can also be made by testing a blood sample, but many laboratories are not prepared to run blood ammonia levels.

Under field conditions urea poisoning might be confused with poisoning by mushrooms, plants, lead, mercury, and other metals. However, excessive slobbering by affected animals can cause suspicion of urea poisoning, and a herd history involving urea feeding or a change in the urea-containing feed may also help to indicate the true nature of the trouble.

TREATMENT. Suspected feed should be removed immediately. Dosing animals with an acidifying agent like vinegar is indicated, for the released ammonia is absorbed from the digestive tract and produces alkalosis. This type of treatment should be continued until symptoms are no longer shown.

PREVENTION. Almost entirely a matter of mixing feed properly and following directions in regard to using the premix. Recommendations once called for feeding urea to cattle at the rate of 1% of the total dry matter; 3% of the concentrate mixture; or to the extent of supplying ⅓ of the total protein equivalent of the concentrate mixture.

It has recently been shown that 90 to 100% of the protein in a ration can be supplied by urea if readily available carbohydrates are also fed. In this connection it has been recommended by some authorities that ½ pound of dehydrated alfalfa leaf meal be fed each animal daily to help in the utilization of the urea. It might be pointed out that this practice could easily lead to more trouble resulting from improper mixing of feeds.

Lead Poisoning

CAUSE. Generally through the eating of lead as a part of paints, varnishes, glazes, storage batteries, plumbing fixtures, boiled linseed oil, and various kinds of agricultural sprays. It may also be inhaled with gases from mines and smelteries, or with dust from lead-bearing soils. Absorption through the skin is unimportant as a cause of trouble, and it is unlikely that poisoning will be caused in cattle by the drinking of water carried through lead pipes. Trouble is usually the result of an owner's carelessness, and in one of our own cases several calves died after licking paint from an old sign that had been moved into a calf pen as protection against a concrete wall during the winter. Lead poisoning is generally regarded as the most important of all poisonings affecting cattle.

SYMPTOMS. Early ones consist of bawling with a changed

voice, trembling, and frequent urination. Advanced cases are characterized by evidence of brain involvement as shown by walking in circles, champing, twitching of the ears and muzzle, pushing into objects like fence posts, and blindness. Going off feed, dropping in milk production, and choking may also be seen. Although constipation is the rule, a diarrhea may occur. Chronic cases show wasting away, generalized weakness, and stiffness of various joints. Staggering, attacks of colic, and convulsions are common, and in some cases a pustular eruption of the skin may occur, along with abortion and sterility problems.

Opening a dead animal will usually show the digestive tract to be ulcerated and inflamed, and the intestinal lining may be grayish-black due to the formation of lead sulfide. The liver is likely to be pale and putty-like in consistency, and the kidneys shrunken with bloody spots on the surface.

DIAGNOSIS. Definite only in the laboratory through tests differentiating it from other diseases and showing tissues to contain lead in toxic amounts. Under field conditions the trouble might be confused with either rabies or circling disease. However, fever usually occurs in rabies cases while absent in lead poisoning. Convulsions that go along with lead poisoning are seldom seen in rabies, and only in the late stages of the disease when they do occur. The bellow of rabies is hoarser than the one often emitted by lead-poisoned animals. Animals affected with circling disease are usually duller in appearance and do not show the muscular twitchings associated with rabies and lead poisoning.

TREATMENT. Tranquilizers or something like chloral hydrate is indicated for quieting animals as soon as possible. Sodium sulfate or magnesium sulfate (Epsom salts) should be given by mouth because either one will combine with lead in the digestive tract to form insoluble salts incapable of being absorbed.

The most promising medicinal agent is calcium disodium ethylenediaminetetraacetate which removes absorbed lead from the tissues. It must be given repeatedly for several days. However, treatment with this drug may cause severe pain because of the sudden withdrawal of lead from the tissues, so care must be used so animals with chronic lead poisoning are not overtreated.

PREVENTION. Almost entirely a matter of being careful to keep lead-containing compounds out of the reach of cattle. Non-leaded paints can be used, and farm sprays containing lead should be managed so that residues on plants, equipment, and containers cannot be licked off by cattle. Such things as peeling paint, paint flakes, and old paint scrapings should always be remembered as possible causes of lead poisoning and treated accordingly.

Larkspur Poisoning

CAUSE. Two general groups of the genus *Delphinium* which grow on the Great Plains westward over the Rocky Mountains to the Pacific coast. The low-growing larkspurs are one to two feet high and include about 12 species of plants that are poisonous to some degree. They grow chiefly at the lower elevations and appear in the spring before grass appears. Cattle naturally eat them readily at such a time. Much of the poisonous quality is gone by the time the plants bloom in May, and the tops die completely by late June.

The tall larkspurs are three to six feet high and include about six species which grow at higher altitudes. They bloom in late summer, but remain poisonous for some time afterward. Accordingly, poisoning from tall larkspurs can occur from late summer to early fall.

SYMPTOMS. Depend on the quantity of larkspur eaten. Small amounts cause animals to go off feed and show evidence of increased excitability. They are also likely to become constipated and stagger or stumble when moving about. Larger amounts produce symptoms like slobbering, vomiting, bloating, convulsions, and death due to inability to breathe.

DIAGNOSIS. Usually through a history of the animals having been pastured on ranges where larkspur plants were available.

TREATMENT. Begins with keeping animals as quiet as possible. Half-wild range animals may be better off if no treatment is attempted. Quieter cattle can be given pilocarpine hydrochloride (2 grains) and physostigmine (1 grain) subsutaneously per 500 pounds of body weight. Constipation can be remedied by something like mineral oil or epsom salts, and bloat can be given appropriate treatment as described elsewhere in this book.

PREVENTION. Entirely a matter of pasture management to either eliminate or avoid the dangerous plants. For example, cattle might be kept off the lower pastures until May and moved off the higher pastures before late summer. Other measures listed under Poisoning by Plants in this book may also prove helpful.

Sore Mouth (Aphthous Stomatitis, Mycotic Stomatitis)

CAUSE. Unknown, but generally believed to be a fungus that lives on plants like clover, alfalfa, and similar legumes. In most cases a white mold-like growth can be found on the heads of suspected plants. Outbreaks usually occur in the late summer or fall after wet weather has caused a rank growth of plants, and the disease is likely to disappear after the first frosts. It is likely that secondary infections with different kinds of bacteria often occur.

SYMPTOMS. Much the same as described earlier for foot-and-mouth disease. However, the most characteristic symptom is shown by the formation of yellowish rotting spots and ulcers of various sizes on the lining of the cheeks. In bad cases the feet, teats, and even the skin of the back may show lesions. On the other hand, in mild cases sometimes only a few minor raw areas will appear on the lips. In cases of this type affected animals may appear to be stiff and walk in a peculiar wooden fashion. There are few deaths, although affected cattle may develop a bad diarrhea that causes them to lose weight at an alarming rate. Opening a dead animal may show ulcers all the way down the esophagus, and severe inflammation of the entire digestive tract. Outbreaks may occur either in pastured or stabled animals, and the disease usually affects only 2 to 5 per cent of a herd.

DIAGNOSIS. Largely through the elimination of troubles showing similar symptoms. May be confused with foot-and-mouth disease, red nose, virus diarrhea, mucosal disease, X disease, and malignant head catarrh. In past years this disease has frequently been mistakenly diagnosed as vesicular stomatitis. However, vesicular stomatitis is likely to affect many more animals in a herd, and this point may be helpful in making a tentative diagnosis. In contrast to the 2 to 5 per cent of a herd that is usually affected with apthous stomatitis, vesicular stomatitis may affect from 5 to 90 per cent of a herd, with an average of about 30 per cent. The belief that this disease is a form of vesicular stomatitis is not supported by experiments involving a study of lesions, transmission, and blood testing. On the other hand, mycotic stomatitis is probably the same as the condition called muzzle disease (papular stomatitis).

TREATMENT. The most important step is an immediate change of pasture or roughage. Ulcers in the mouth may be swabbed two or three times daily with astringent solutions like 3% alum or 2%

potassium permanganate. Ulcers on the teats and other exposed parts of the body can be treated daily with sulfathiazole, zinc oxide, scarlet oil, or various kinds of antibiotic ointments such as are used for the treatment of mastitis.

PREVENTION. In some cases the mowing or periodic clipping of pastures has apparently been effective.

Allergic Stomatitis (Clover Disease)

CAUSE. Essentially unknown, although it seems to be related to the eating of certain plants. The disease has been reported following the pasturing of cattle on red clover, Dutch white clover, and ladino clover, but clover pastures have not been involved in all outbreaks. In Australia, where it is known as "aphis disease," trouble has followed the feeding of lucerne or alfalfa. The condition is most likely to be seen in the spring or fall, and has been blamed on damaged forage. Since it is known that moldy forage can cause light sensitization, it is reasonable to believe that damaged forage can also cause allergic stomatitis.

SYMPTOMS. In mild cases cattle slobber, show inflamed nostrils, and may have a few small crusted lesions around the muzzle. Skin lesions may appear on the dewlap, legs, belly, and udder. These skin lesions appear first as small swellings that soon become wet with serum. The hair eventually falls out to leave a red area like moist eczema which is finally covered with a crust. An examination of the mouth will show reddening of the mucous membranes and small eroded areas. These raw areas heal rapidly, and recovery usually occurs in a short time.

In severe cases the mouth and skin lesions are worse. Ulcers may develop on the lips, tongue, and various parts of the mouth, and these are soon covered with a yellowish membrane. The eyes often water, and skin eruptions may occur over the legs, udder, and much of the back, oozing serum which forms crusts. Lameness may result, but recovery is usually fast and uneventful.

DIAGNOSIS. Largely a matter of differentiating this condition from other types of stomatitis and diseases causing similar symptoms. A history of pasturing on causative plants will sometimes indicate the true nature of trouble. Under field conditions it might be confused with troubles like light sensitization, diphtheria, red nose, foot-and-mouth disease, vesicular stomatitis, and mycotic stomatitis.

TREATMENT. Begins with the removal of cattle from suspected pastures and keeping them out of sunlight, which may be all that is needed. In severe cases, antihistamines may prove helpful, and corticosteroids have been reported as of value in getting animals back on feed a little faster. Solutions as recommended for other forms of stomatitis are indicated, and skin lesions can be treated with carron oil, calamine lotion, or various oily compounds and ointments.

Stomatitis (Inflammation of the Mouth)

CAUSE. Several different ones, including beards from plants like barley, foxtail, and needle grass, and injuries due to the rough use of a balling gun or the sharp edges of back teeth. However, trouble is often caused by burns from chemicals such as creolin which are given in capsules that accidentally break in the mouth. Continued use of drugs like iodides can produce the condition, and so can pasturing on certain plants like clovers. Attacks of indigestion may be followed by stomatitis, and infection may spread into the mouth from abscesses in the throat or cheeks. Finally, the condition may appear in connection with other diseases like pharyngitis and laryngitis.

SYMPTOMS. The commonest ones are excessive slobbering and partial or complete refusal to eat. Smacking of the lips may result in an accumulation of foam at the corners of the mouth. An examination will show mouth tissues to be red and swollen, and sometimes the existence of causative factors like plant awns or wounds. There may be grayish-yellow spots in areas of the mouth, and affected animals may have a foul-smelling breath or show a slight tendency toward bloating.

DIAGNOSIS. Usually on the basis of a mouth examination which shows typical lesions, and sometimes the awns or injuries which are responsible for the condition. Symptoms might cause it to be confused with troubles like choke, rabies, wooden tongue, or various of the contagious vesicular diseases such as foot and mouth disease or other types of stomatitis.

TREATMENT. Usually confined to washing the mouth with mild antiseptic solutions like 2% potassium permanganate, 10% argyrol, or 5% hydrogen peroxide. When awns are involved, they should be removed and the resulting lesions touched with silver nitrate. When stomatitis is caused by plants, antihistamines can be given, and animals should be removed from suspected pastures.

Roundworms of the Digestive System

CAUSE. Roundworms or nematodes of several different kinds. These parasites may represent species like *Haemonchus, Ostertagia, Trichostrongylus, Bunostonum, Strongyloides, Cooperia,* and *Nematodirus. Ostertagia* (one-fourth inch), and *Trichostrongylus* (one-fifth inch), *Cooperia,* and *Strongyloides* are so tiny and hair-like that they are difficult to see, while the adults of *Haemonchus* vary in length between three-fourths of an inch up to 1½ inches in length. The others fall between these limits, *Bunostonum* up to three-fourths of an inch, and *Nematodirus* one-half to 1 inch.

LIFE CYCLE. Eggs are passed in the manure by infested cattle, hatch, and develop to the infective stage within about 5 days under favorable conditions. The larvae then crawl up on grass blades or stems of roughage when they are wet with dew or rain. They are eventually swallowed with such feed, burrow into the lining of the stomach or intestines, grow to maturity in about three weeks, and start laying eggs of their own. An entire cycle can be completed in less than a month, and every infested animal adds more larvae to pastures and feeding grounds that may already be heavily infested. In the case of permanent pastures this can go on year after year, for neither the eggs or the larvae of most species are killed by winter freezing. To make matters worse, healthy-looking carrier animals often continue to pass worm eggs all the time. With minor variations, most of the stomach and intestinal roundworms have the same life cycle, and some larvae may remain in the lining of the digestive tract for long periods of time.

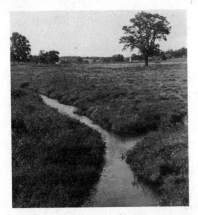

Streams like this one furnish fresh water in permanent pastures but they also furnish shade and moisture which are ideal for the propagation of internal parasites.

SYMPTOMS. Anemia that is shown by pallor of the lining of the various body openings is one of the most important. It varies in degree, but usually is severe in heavy *Haemonchus* infestations. Anemia associated with trichostrongyle infestations probably results from failure of the animal to absorb enough food materials, for these parasites do not remove very much blood from hosts. Swelling in the upper throat region often shows up to produce a condition called "bottle jaw" in parasitized cattle. Indigestion is common, and a severe watery diarrhea usually goes along with heavy infestations of *Ostertagia* and *Trichostronglus*. Depending on the type of worms causing trouble, the manure may also contain shreds of mucus and varying amounts of blood. By way of contrast, Haemonchus infestation may produce little or no diarrhea, and there may actually be periods of constipation. Other common symptoms include rough hair coat, failure to gain, loss of appetite, emaciation, and weakness.

Cattle are sometimes killed by the parasites, and if a dead animal is opened the worms can sometimes be found in the stomach and intestines. However, the tiny ones like *Ostertagia* can easily be missed, so it will be advisable to mix some of the intestinal contents with water in a glass dish that is then set on a piece of black cloth or paper. Examination with a magnifying glass will often show movement of the mixture before the worms are actually seen. Inflammation and swelling is often evident in the lining of various parts of the digestive tract, and so are nodules from which worms can sometimes be pressed out with a knife blade. The lining may also show tiny bloody spots and grayish areas which are really small abscesses where larvae have burrowed. In addition, small blister-like structures and variable amounts of mucus may cover much of the stomach and intestinal lining. Such an examination is best made of an animal that has died recently so that the worms are still moving and easier to see. Young animals usually show the worst symptoms, since one attack by worms appears to give a considerable degree of resistance.

DIAGNOSIS. Can often be tentatively made on the basis of anemia and poor weight gains by young animals, for these sometimes appear before eggs of the parasites are present in the manure. A definite diagnosis can be made either by finding the worm eggs in the manure under a microscope or an examination of animals after death. However, it must be remembered that the number of worm eggs being passed in the manure cannot be depended on to indicate the severity of infestation. When animals have been treated with phenothiazine, few or no eggs at all may be present, because this drug interferes with egg production by the female worms. Under field conditions infestation with round-worms might be confused with Johne's disease and coccidiosis.

TREATMENT. Phenothiazine is probably the safest and most effective of remedies for most of the roundworms. The usual recommended dose is two-thirds of an ounce for each one hundred pounds of body weight, with weak animals never getting over a half-ounce dose, and no animal receiving more than two ounces at any one time. However, the maximum dose can be increased to four ounces without danger of poisoning if the cattle are not showing symptoms of weakness or severe anemia. Repeated treatments may be required in badly infested herds, and only results will indicate how often the animals should be treated and the appropriate length of intervals between treatments.

When calves or only a few animals are to be treated, it is best to withhold feed for 24 hours, although the animals may have all the water they want. The proper amount of phenothiazine is then given in bolus form or mixed with water and given as a drench. When feeder cattle or large numbers of animals are to be treated, the phenothiazine is best given with regular ground-grain rations. Since a regular two-ounce dose per animal will generally cause cattle to refuse the feed, the drug should be distributed over a ten-day period.

This is easily done by first multiplying the number of cattle by two in order to get the number of ounces of phenothiazine needed. The result is divided by ten to get the number of ounces needed daily. This can be weighed out in a glass container, and the level marked with a glass pencil to serve as a measure for subsequent treatments. The daily dose is then premixed with a bushel of the regular grain. Half of this is given morning and night, first scattered on top of the silage, and then covered with the regular grain allowance. Furnishing phenothiazine free-choice in a salt or mineral or protein mix won't do a good job alone, but after most of the worms have once been removed, the free-choice mixtures will serve to keep worm infestation at a harmless level.

Continuous low-level feeding of phenothiazine may be combined with regular treatment as a more efficient means of controlling roundworms. Following heavy dosage that removes most of the worms, the low-level feeding will inhibit the laying of eggs by females, interfere with the development of larvae, reduce the hatchability of parasite eggs, and help to keep the worm population at a low count. Animals on low-level phenothiazine feeding should get 0.5 gram per 100 pounds body weight, and not more than 2.5 grams daily for a period of not over 90 days. Even in these small amounts, phenothiazine may make salt, minerals, or ground feed so unpalatable that animals won't eat enough of it and this has always represented something of a problem for owners. In recent years, though, phenothiazine has been combined with other ingredients to form granules that are odorless and readily eaten when mixed with regular grain rations. In this form the phenothiazine can also be fed in doses large enough to remove the worms and thus eliminate the need of treatment with drenches or boluses before low-level feeding is started. Phenothiazine is not recommended for lactating dairy cows because it may cause a red color in the milk.

As an alternative treatment for such animals, copper sulfate may be used. It has been given with good results in the following dosages:

1. Six ounces of a 2% solution as a single treatment, or
2. Two to six ounces of a 0.5% solution given twice weekly for four to six weeks.

In recent years there has been a great deal of research on new remedies. Several organic phosphate compounds have been demonstrated as highly successful against stomach worms, but they have not been widely used because of the danger of poisoning.

Methyridine is another new drug which is effective against roundworms of cattle. It has been reported as more effective against intestinal roundworms than those found in the stomach. Although it can be given by injection under the skin, it appears to be more effective when given to cattle by mouth.

One of the most promising new drugs is thiabendazole. When given at the rate of 40 to 50 milligrams per pound of body weight, it has been shown as effective against the adult roundworms of most species. It does some good against larval forms on the mucosal surface, but appears to be ineffective against those that have burrowed into the lining. It has the added advantage of being safe, and from 4 to 8 times the recommended dose can be given before evidence of poisoning appears.

Another new drug, bephenium hydroxynaphtholate, has been found effective in removing *Nematodirus,* and various of the piperazine salts have been used with good results. Newer remedies also include parbendazole and 1-tetramisole. A vaccine has been prepared for the control of *Haemonchus* infestation, and considerable research is being carried on in this field. Other effective treatments will probably be developed in the near future.

Regardless of what is used, repeated treatments will probably be required to correct severe infestations. This is particularly true of mature cattle that are carrying large numbers of larvae or immature worms. Not only animals showing symptoms, but the entire herd should be treated. This will decrease the build-up of infestation in pastures, and also prevent the development of severe symptoms in animals that are becoming heavily infested. Individual conditions will determine how often the herd should be treated.

Animals showing severe symptoms will require extra treatment in the form of remedies to control diarrhea and solutions to replace important body fluids that have been lost through dehydration. In severe cases blood transfusions may be indicated to save the lives of animals. In addition to supplying desirable treatment and good rations, affected animals should not be returned to heavily infested pastures before most of the parasites they are carrying have been destroyed. Otherwise they may become reinfested so quickly that the treatment does little good.

PREVENTION. A matter of observing a few "don'ts" like these:

1. Don't neglect regular treatment for this practice cuts down the worm population.
2. Don't run calves on the same pasture year after year.
3. Don't forget that good feeding helps to prevent infestation.
4. Don't overcrowd animals on pastures, especially in wet areas.
5. Don't pasture old and young animals together.
6. Don't tolerate mudholes or wet places in pastures.
7. Don't feed hay and grain off the ground.
8. Don't forget to isolate animals showing severe symptoms from the rest of the herd.

Flatworms of the Digestive System

CAUSE. Tapeworms or cestodes that usually belong to one of two principal varieties. One is called *Moniezia expansa* and the other *Moniezia benedeni*. They are much alike in appearance, being white, ribbonlike, and segmented. *M. expansa* is much more common, and may reach a length of fifty feet and be a couple of inches wide. Another tapeworm, *Thysanosoma actinioides*, better known as the fringed tapeworm because of a fringed rear border of its segments, is infrequently found in cattle. It is shorter than the *Moniezias* and is often found in the main bile ducts of the liver as well as in the small intestine.

LIFE CYCLE. The life cycle of flatworms is different from that of roundworms, for these parasites require an intermediate host. In the case of *M. expansa*, free-living oribatid mites commonly known as beetle mites or "grass mites" act as the intermediate host. These tiny mites exist in large numbers on pastures, and eat the eggs containing the larval form of the tapeworm. Inside the mite the larva develops into the next larval stage, known as the cysticercoid, in a period of six to sixteen weeks. The mites live in the humus layer of soil, and frequently migrate onto pasture plants, especially in the morning when grass is wet with dew.

Cattle swallow infected mites with pasture plants, and the cysticercoids escape from the mites in their digestive tracts. The head of the tapeworm then attaches itself to the lining of the small intestine and segments grow outward from it, with those furthest from the head being the oldest. The tapeworms become mature in about a month, and then begin to shed segments and eggs with manure to start the cycle all over again. Although the life cycle of *M. benedeni* is not definitely known, parasitologists of the Soviet Union have reported that oribatid mites are also the intermediate host for this species. The life cycle of *T. actinioides* is unknown.

SYMPTOMS. At various times diarrhea, loss of weight, convulsions, and even deaths have been reported as due to tapeworm infestation. However, it is likely that other internal parasites, feed deficiencies, and various types of disease have usually caused these symptoms, for experimental work indicates that tapeworms have little, if any, bad effect on the health of infested animals.

DIAGNOSIS. Easiest through finding worm segments in the manure.

TREATMENT. Usually lead arsenate, in doses ranging from one-fourth to 2 grams per animal according to size and condition. This drug can be mixed with phenothiazine. A suspension of diphenthane is used by most veterinarians for the removal of tapeworms. It is as effective and much less dangerous than the arsenate.

Liver Fluke Disease (Liver Rot)

CAUSE. Four species of liver flukes live as parasites in cattle.
1. *Fasciola hepatica.* This is the commonest and most important of the liver flukes, not only in the U.S., but all over the world. It has been found in practically all ani-

mals, including man, and has been reported in 22 of the United States. It is most prevalent in the southeastern and southwestern states, the Rocky Mountain states, and the Pacific coast states.

2. *Fascioloides magna.* This is a natural parasite of deer, elk, and moose. It is currently restricted to the states bordering Canada and a few localities in other states where it has become established in wild animals. Reports indicate that it is increasing in cattle, and that these animals are more severely infested than their natural wild hosts.

3. *Fasciola gigantica.* This fluke does not exist in the continental United States, but is found in Hawaii. Here it has become established in the low coastal areas, and is reported as being the most important parasite of both beef and dairy cattle in this state.

4. *Dicrocoelium dendriticum.* This is the so-called lancet fluke, which at present is limited to a small area in central New York. However, it is only logical to expect that it will eventually spread to other states.

LIFE CYCLE. Eggs are passed with manure by infested animals, and are capable of surviving winter freezing. Under favorable conditions these hatch in about two weeks into swimming larvae called miracidia. The miricidia must enter a water snail host within 8 hours or they will die. Once inside the snail, they go through growth changes, multiply greatly, and in about 40 days leave the snail as a brood of so-called cercariae. These soon attach themselves to grass blades or other vegetation and encyst there as a brown or creamy spot about the size of a pin head. In this form they can live for long periods unless they are exposed to sunlight or dry winds. When eventually eaten by cattle, the parasites leave their cysts, burrow through the intestinal wall, enter the abdominal cavity, and find their way to the liver. They penetrate this organ, grow to maturity, and start laying eggs of their own. The complete cycle may be completed in about four months, and the flukes may remain in cattle for two or three years. With minor variations, the life cycle is the same for all of the *Fasciola* flukes.

The lancet fluke is different. After passage with manure from an infested animal, the egg does not hatch until after it has been swallowed by a snail. This particular kind of snail is not a water snail, but lives on high, dry land. The snail passes the cercariae as slime balls which must be swallowed by a second intermediary host, which is a species of ant. The parsitized ant must then be eaten by an animal before infestation occurs.

SYMPTOMS. Much the same as described for stomach and intestinal worms, except that diarrhea may not always appear. Bloody droppings are unusual, but animals have poor appetites, lose weight, become pot-bellied, rough-coated, and sunken-eyed. Breeding troubles are common, and deaths are not unusual, particularly in the fall when pasture conditions are poor. If a dead animal is opened, the liver is apt to be seen as swollen and sprinkled with bloody areas. Small holes may exist from which young flukes and fluid destroyed liver tissue can be squeezed. Thickened bile ducts can sometimes be seen as ridges, and when they are slit open large numbers of the dark, flat, leaf-like flukes may be revealed. In especially bad cases the liver may be very hard, with bile ducts enormously thickened and blocked by lime-like deposits that resemble stone. Evidence of secondary bacterial infection is often visible, with abscesses of the liver and other parts of the body.

DIAGNOSIS. Usually through microscopic examination of manure that reveals the eggs of flukes. These are most conveniently separated by letting them settle out of solution instead of floating them to the top as done with worm eggs.

TREATMENT. One of the best is made by mixing a pound of finely ground hexachloroethane, two ounces of bentonite, one-half teaspoonful of white flour, and a pint and a half of water. This should be well-shaken before use, with the dose being 20 cc. for every hundred pounds of body weight. Fasting is not required before treatment, and calves under three months of age need not be dosed. Extremely weak animals should be handled carefully and given half the recommended dosage. Such treatment will not completely eradicate flukes, but using it each spring and fall will greatly reduce the number of parasites and improve the health of cattle through decreased infestation. None of the compounds that have been used for the treatment of *Fasciola* are effective against lancet flukes.

PREVENTION. In combination with the twice-a-year treatment, wet pastures should be avoided and drained whenever possible. Infected ground should not be used as a source of hay. In order to destroy snails it is sometimes practical to treat land with copper sulfate. This is best sprayed on as a 1 to 2% solution and to avoid possible poisoning, cattle should be kept off the grounds until after a rain has fallen. Some of the new compounds are more effective snail killers than the copper sulfate, but they are more poisonous for fish and other forms of life. As a practical preventive measure, cattlemen with a fluke problem will do well to consider keeping a few ducks or geese as snail hunters.

The lancet fluke is more difficult to control than the *Fasciola* which have a water snail as the only intermediate host. This is because the dry land snail and the ant which are the hosts for the lancet fluke are found in rough, rocky pastures in cattle-raising regions, thus making control programs both ineffective and very expensive.

Botulism (Forage Poisoning, Lamzietke, Loin Sickness)

CAUSE. A poison produced by at least six different strains of an organism called *Clostridium botulinum* when it grows in decaying vegetable or animal matter. It must be emphasized that infection is not involved in this trouble, for the germ is found practically everywhere, including the digestive tract of cattle, without doing any harm whatever. The poison produced varies according to the type of the organism, and requires a specific antitoxin for treatment. The three common names given to this disease represent little more than a difference in geographical area and the means by which the poison gets into animals, for the symptoms are much the same for all of them.

Lamzietke occurs in South Africa and is a form of botulism which results from a depraved appetite caused by a deficiency of phosphorus. Affected cattle eat decaying carcasses containing botulinum poison in their efforts to get the needed phosphorus.

Loin disease has been reported from Texas, and is the same trouble with the same cause and means of entry as given for lamzietke.

Forage poisoning has been traced back to the ingestion of spoiled hay, silage, and corn fodder as well as drinking water in which animal or vegetable matter has decomposed.

SYMPTOMS. Several cattle are usually affected in an outbreak. They show weakness and paralysis that grows worse and worse until they finally go down. The throat muscles may be affected so swallowing is impossible and the tongue may hang from the mouth while slobbering and discharging from the nostrils are also commonly seen. Animals remain fully conscious as a rule, and the temperature and pulse are usually normal while the respiration rate is increased. The head is often tipped to one side in a peculiar attitude while the gait is apt to be stiff and uncertain. Constipation is a common symptom, while animals sometimes seem blind and go through all kinds of crazy actions. Deaths may be sudden or result after a week or two, but there are few recoveries. Opening a dead animal isn't apt to show much of anything in the way of abnormalities. Beasts that happen to recover are sometimes unsteady in their movements for six or eight weeks.

DIAGNOSIS. Definite in the laboratory through electrophoresis, fluorescent antibody tests, or the injection of laboratory animals. A field test can be made by feeding suspected material to animals of small value from a different area and waiting to see if symptoms of botulism develop. Isolation of *C. botulinum* germs means nothing, because they are found practically everywhere. Symptoms without history of materials eaten might cause botulism to be confused with troubles like acetonemia, circling disease, rabies, and various kinds of poisoning.

TREATMENT. Specific antitoxins can be prepared, and they have prevented deaths of laboratory animals which had been injected with botulinum toxin. However, antitoxin has given poor results when used in the field, and its value at this time is questionable. No other drugs, antibiotics, or biological products have been shown as having any effect against botulism.

PREVENTION. Botulism can be largely prevented by avoiding spoiled feeds and seeing that drinking water is not contaminated with decaying vegetation or dead animals. In the case of lamzietke or loin disease, prevention is simply a matter of supplying a mineral mixture free choice to provide an adequate supply of phosphorus.

Abscesses of the Salivary Glands

CAUSE. Pus formation after infection by several different kinds of bacteria. Usually started by a bruising of the outer jaw or wounding of the mouth lining by roughage stems or beards from plants like barley or foxtail.

SYMPTOMS. Swelling in the location of the salivary glands around the lower jaws. This may be either thin or thick-walled, hot or normal, painful or not, depending on location and stage of development. Sometimes the animal isn't bothered at all, but at other times the abscess may prevent swallowing and cause the beast to lose weight and appear off feed. General symptoms are also inconstant, for there may or may not be increased pulse, respiration, and temperature.

DIAGNOSIS. Definite by drawing pus from the swelling with a hypodermic needle and syringe. Sometimes feeling fluid contents and a thin place in the wall where "breaking" will eventually occur is helpful in making a diagnosis. May be confused with a bruise, hematoma, wooden tongue, or lumpjaw.

TREATMENT. Alternate hot and cold applications may help to bring the abscess to a "head" so it will rupture. Soaking the swelling daily with iodine may help to retard secretions and reduce inflammation. Thick-walled structures may need to be opened surgically, with care being used not to cut any of the salivary glands so non-healing wounds will result. Regardless of whether abscesses

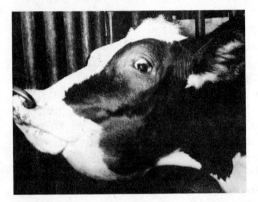

Calf with swollen jaw due to an abscess.

are opened or "break" naturally, it is advisable to wash them out immediately afterward with a 1% solution of potassium permanganate. Penicillin ointment such as used for mastitis treatment can then be introduced daily to aid healing.

Peritonitis

CAUSE. Anything responsible for infection inside the abdominal cavity or that part of the body which is covered by peritoneum under the skin and muscles. (1) Hardware trouble. (2) Injuries to the uterus through calving, artificial breeding, etc. (3) Blows or penetrating wounds. Often incurred through such things as castration and rectal examinations. (4) Parasites like flukes and worms. (5) Diseases like tuberculosis, actinobacillosis, etc. (6) Indigestion in the form of food impactions. (7) Torsion of uterus, intussusception, incarceration. (8) Caustic poisons that may eat through walls of digestive tract. (9) Rupture of bladder or abdominal abscesses.

SYMPTOMS. Somewhat dependent on cause, but droopiness and

rapid loss of weight are common. The temperature is likely to remain normal, with a fast pulse and irregular, shallow breathing. Pain is likely to be evidenced in the abdominal region and animals frequently lie down a great deal of the time.

DIAGNOSIS. Usually on the basis of symptoms and an examination that may show the cause. For example, torsion of the uterus or intussception may be revealed through a rectal exploration.

TREATMENT. Dependent on the actual cause. Sometimes no practical remedies are available.

Adhesions

CAUSE. Infection of any kind that can cause various body organs to grow fast to each other instead of remaining separated in a normal manner. Such infections are usually grouped under the heading of peritonitis. Hardware trouble is one of the commonest causes in cattle, with trouble involving the reticulum and adjoining structures like the diaphragm, lungs, liver, spleen, and other stomachs. The various causes listed for peritonitis may cause adhesions between the intestines and other organs.

SYMPTOMS. Often none at all. At other times animals may decline in milk production, lose weight, and become "picky" about eating without apparent cause. Involvement of the lungs or diaphragm may cause evidence of abnormal breathing. Evident symptoms are probably due to pain caused by pulling in areas of adhesions. Opening a dead animal may reveal a single extensive adhesion or a great many widely separated ones.

DIAGNOSIS. Definitely made only by surgery that exposes the adherent areas.

TREATMENT. Surgery that involves freeing the structures that are grown together.

Liver Diseases

CAUSE. Several that are mentioned in this book. In general, they act to obstruct the flow of bile in a normal manner. (1) Parasites like flukes. (2) Inflammation of the duodenum lining that closes the entrance of the bile duct. (3) Pressure on the bile duct by tumors and tubercules. (4) Abscesses due to bacterial infection following hardware trouble, foot rot, fluke invasion, etc. (5) Damage by specific diseases like anaplasmosis, tuberculosis, etc. (6) Fatty degeneration due to unknown causes as with acetonemia. (7) Shrinking or enlarging of liver by plant poisons like ragwort and lupines. (8) Poisoning by chemicals like copper, lead, and mercury.

SYMPTOMS. Chiefly jaundice as shown by yellowing of the eyes, mucous membranes, and sometimes even the skin itself. The extent of jaundice and the darkness of color sometimes indicate the severity of trouble, but the jaundice may not always appear. Kicking, convulsions, paralysis, and other nervous symptoms are often seen, and the urine may become dark-colored. Other symptoms depend pretty much on the nature of primary trouble. Pain is often shown high in the right flank over the liver.

DIAGNOSIS. A definite one is often impossible. However, the appearance of jaundice and "crazy" actions together is usually enough to suggest the existence of some kind of liver disorder.

TREATMENT. Entirely dependent on the cause. None can be recommended in certain cases of fatty degeneration.

Liver Abscesses (Necrobacillosis of the Liver)

CAUSE. Usually a germ called *Spherophorus necrophorus,* the same one that causes foot rot and diphtheria in cattle, although other types of bacteria may be involved at times. Regardless of the exact type, germs reach the liver after getting into the bloodstream following infection in various parts of the body. Many cases are believed started by "hardware trouble" when a metal object pierces the stomach wall. Others may follow attacks of mastitis, lumpjaw, wooden tongue, navel-ill, foot rot or infection of the uterus at calving time, and infrequently they have been caused by tuberculosis germs. Recent investigation has shown that when cattle are suddenly changed to grain feeding the rumen may become inflamed because of an excess of acidity. Causative germs may then get into the inflamed areas and be carried to the liver by the bloodstream.

SYMPTOMS. In the later stages animals may go off feed, run fevers up to 107° F., and milk cows may drop off completely in production. However, there are usually no symptoms other than a gradual loss of weight, although some animals will show signs of soreness in the right flank. The poor condition is sometimes puzzling, for affected animals may eat well at the same time they are steadily losing weight. The trouble seems commonest in beef cattle.

Opening a dead animal may show a single large abscess or a number of small ones on a diseased liver. If abscesses rupture, peritonitis may result, with symptoms of this trouble, or sudden death may occur if abscesses rupture into one of the large blood vessels of the liver. The ailment is important even when animals are passed for human consumption, for abscessed livers have to be "tanked" in packing plants, and this loss to packers is absorbed either by the owner in the form of lower live weight prices or by the consumer in the form of higher prices for the beef he takes home.

DIAGNOSIS. Seldom made in the living animal, although the gradual loss of weight may cause an abscessed liver to be suspected. This trouble may be confused with others like Johne's disease, hardware trouble, tuberculosis, acetonemia, chronic peritonitis, and impaction of the fourth stomach.

TREATMENT. None likely to be practical, since most cases are rather bad before they show symptoms that cause an abscessed liver to be suspected, and most owners prefer to sell such animals "subject" to postmortem inspection rather than spend money on treatment that is apt to prove of doubtful value. However, the intravenous injection of sulfamethazine at the rate of 1 grain per pound of body weight plus oxytetracycline at the rate of 2 mg. per pound has proved effective and might be tried in the case of valuable animals.

PREVENTION. Largely confined to good management practices. The following measures are recommended:
1. Disinfect navels of calves at birth to prevent navel-ill.
2. Do everything possible to keep animals from eating materials that will result in hardware trouble.
3. Follow preventive measures designed to reduce the incidence of foot rot in herds.
4. Treat cases of lumpjaw and wooden tongue early before germs have a chance to reach the liver.
5. Use uterine capsules to control infection in cows that fail to "clean" within 12 hours after calving.
6. Test cattle at least every five years for tuberculosis.
7. Change feed lot cattle gradually from roughage to grain in order to avoid excessive fermentation which produces a high concentration of acid in the stomach so that the lining of the organ is badly inflamed.
8. Do the same thing with dairy cows that are being changed over to grain and brought to "full feed" after freshening.
9. Fatten cattle on a ration in which the proportion of concentrates to roughage is 2:1 or lower.

Liver Degeneration

CAUSE. Usually disturbances of metabolism associated with the intake of feed. This is well illustrated by acetonemia, where the primary lesion is generally fatty degeneration of the liver. In beef cattle the condition usually appears in fat animals that have been fitted for show or sale in too big a hurry, and it is often complicated by advanced pregnancy. In beef and dairy cows alike, the primary cause is often under-feeding or actual starvation in the late part of the gestation period. Being off feed for a lengthy period of time from any cause will induce some degree of liver degeneration. Continuous high fever for several days will produce the condition, and so will toxemia due to infectious diseases like pyelonephritis or metritis. Chemical poisoning by phosphorus, lead, arsenic, or copper compounds will cause liver degeneration, and so will poisoning by plants like certain species of Crotalaria and Senecio. Light sensitization, mold poisoning, and allergic stomatitis will also cause liver degeneration.

SYMPTOMS. When liver degeneration is due to acetonemia, the symptoms will be as described for the various forms of that disease (see p. 000). The icteric index will range between 25 and 50. See Jaundice.

When the condition appears in fat cattle being fitted for show or sale, signs of indigestion and loss of appetite may be shown for a week or two in the beginning. Animals become progressively duller, finally stop eating entirely, and put in a great deal of time lying down. They generally show signs of pain by grunting, groaning, and kicking at the belly. Temperatures usually remain normal, but the pulse rate is likely to go over 100. The icteric index ranges between 25 and 100, is usually over 50, and the Ross test for ketone bodies is positive. Only a small amount of dark, mucoid manure is passed.

When malnutrition in late pregnancy is the cause, animals go off feed, appear weak, stagger when walking, and show various degrees of stiffness and paralysis. Affected animals are invariably emaciated and in poor condition. The lining of the mouth and other body cavities is pale, and sometimes will show evidence of jaundice. Other symptoms as noted under pregnancy disease may also be shown.

DIAGNOSIS. Made on the basis of history, laboratory results, and the elimination of other diseases. It may be suspected in fat cattle when the pulse rate is high while the temperature remains normal, there is evidence of pain, jaundice is shown, the Ross test is positive, and there is no response to treatment.

When starvation is the cause, evidence of malnutrition in combination with advanced pregnancy is always a significant factor. A positive Ross test and signs of soreness over the liver in the right flank can be considered as supportive evidence of liver degeneration.

Under field conditions the trouble might be confused with others like liver abscesses, hardware disease, displaced abomasum, and acetonemia. The use of laboratory facilities to establish the icteric index and obtain a white blood cell count will help to establish a differential diagnosis.

TREATMENT. Useless when degeneration is well advanced, for none of today's miracle drugs are capable of rebuilding vital organs like the liver. Cortisone injections have been reported as helpful when the condition is caught in time, and so has oral dosing with 2 ounces of choline chloride daily. Some of the starved pregnant cows may be saved by blood transfusions, feeding of a good quality ration, and the intravenous injection of electrolytes and a 5% dextrose solution.

PREVENTION. The measures suggested for the prevention of acetonemia are also recommended for the prevention of liver degeneration. In the case of show cattle, it is especially important not to hurry their conditioning.

Hyperkeratosis (X-Disease)

CAUSE. Highly chlorinated naphthalene. The four highest numbers of the chlorinated naphthalene series can cause this disease, but the less chlorinated naphthalenes do not. About 1 gram of penta- or hexachloronaphthalene per 300 pounds of body weight will destroy an animal or make it worthless. Trouble may be caused either by skin contact or eating the naphthalene. Most cases in the U.S. have resulted from the use of lubricants containing highly chlorinated naphthalenes in feed pelleting machines. Other cases are believed to have been caused by the naphthalenes in various oils, lubricants, roofing compounds, lumber preservatives, etc., that are often kept on the average farm. Calves may develop the disease after nursing cows which have eaten the harmful naphthalenes.

SYMPTOMS. Depend on whether animals have been exposed through direct contact or eating of the naphthalenes. Those following skin exposure through direct contact are largely limited to thickening and wrinkling of the skin, for only slight internal lesions result from such contact.

The first symptoms likely to be noted after the naphthalenes have been swallowed are slobbering and watering of the eyes. Close examination will reveal circular red areas in the mouth and nostrils. As time goes on the animals become dull, go off feed, and lose weight. In a month or so the skin begins to thicken on the neck, cheeks, and shoulders. Such thickening eventually spreads over most of the upper two-thirds of the body. The skin between the hind legs around the scrotum or base of the udder usually thickens, but the lower legs remain normal in appearance. No symptoms of itching are shown unless lice and mites or bacterial infection of the skin becomes involved.

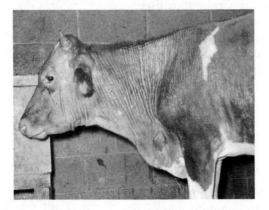

Bull with X disease, showing characteristic thickening and wrinkling of the skin.

In the final stages the skin appears dry and wrinkled, with considerable loss of hair from affected areas. Horn development stops in calves and the horns of older animals may become greatly indented at the base. Young animals frequently develop pneumonia, and may show evidence of a diarrhea. Calves may be carried a month or so beyond the normal due date and then delivered dead or so weak that they die within a few days. Large doses of the naphthalenes may cause abortions. In any case, the birth of calves is often followed by pyometra. Mastitis and acetonemia are also common after effects, and so are breeding troubles in both cows and bulls.

Opening a dead animal will usually show raised nodules of

various sizes in the mouth, on the tongue, and in the esophagus. Cysts are likely to be found in the pancreas, gallbladder, and kidneys.

DIAGNOSIS. Entirely through elimination of diseases causing similar symptoms, and a history of exposure to materials that may contain highly chlorinated naphthalenes. This disease might be confused with other troubles like lousiness, mange, malnutrition, virus diarrhea, malignant head catarrh, and various other types of poisoning.

TREATMENT. None can be recommended, although large doses of vitamin A have been shown as capable of temporarily raising the blood level of vitamin A. Sulfas and antibiotics can be given to control secondary infections. Removing the causative material and feeding good hay will often be followed by recovery of affected animals, but it may take up to two years to occur. This is because the naphthalenes may remain in an animal's body for a long time after the source of poisoning has been eliminated.

PREVENTION. The following recommendations can be made:

1. Keep old oil drums, grease cans, and similar containers where cattle have no chance to lick at them.

2. Do not allow cattle around areas where tractors are drained or machinery is serviced.

3. Arrange facilities so that no drainage from grease racks and machine sheds get into areas where cattle run.

4. Keep cattle away from sources of asphalt, roofing compounds, flaking creosote paints, and materials like those used to coat the inside of silos.

5. Be cautious about using commercial feeds that have been reported as possible causes of X-disease. If in doubt about the truth of such stories, request information from state officials or local veterinarians.

6. Remember that highly chlorinated naphthalenes can persist for years in or on contaminated materials, and treat suspicious materials accordingly. This applies particularly to things like treated lumber and fence posts.

Slobbering (Salivation, Ptyalism, Sialosis)

CAUSE. Several different causes are possible, since this is a symptom, not a specific disease. It is seen most often in connection with various forms of stomatitis or choking on foreign objects. It may also result from indigestion, burns and other injuries to the mouth, bad teeth, infection like wooden tongue and foot and mouth disease, the eating of certain plants, sour silage or spoiled feeds, hardware disease, torsion of the abomasum, or growths in the upper digestive tract. Chemical poisoning by mercury, iodine, lead, copper, and arsenic will induce excessive salivation, and so will the injection of drugs like lentin and arecoline. Poisoning resulting from botulism and algae can cause slobbering because of pharyngeal paralysis, and the same thing can happen in the case of diseases like rabies and mad itch or pseudorabies.

SYMPTOMS. Obvious as drooling or excessive salivation. Sometimes the saliva is ropy and foamy, and at other times it is water-clear. Other symptoms will depend on the nature of the primary cause.

DIAGNOSIS. A matter of eliminating the various possible causes to arrive at the true nature of trouble. A review of the accompanying symptoms will prove helpful in this respect, and so will a history of recent feeding, maintenance practices, and the number of animals involved.

TREATMENT. Depends on the primary cause. Once this is corrected, the slobbering will probably cease.

Intussusception or Telescoping of Intestine

CAUSE. Unknown, although tumors and weakening of intestinal walls by parasites have been suggested. The intestine folds into itself in telescope fashion to shut off the blood supply as well as passage of manure. Usually occurs in the ileum.

SYMPTOMS. Sudden appearance of pain as shown by kicking at the belly, twisting of tail, bawling or groaning, standing with hind feet in the gutter, or laying down. The pulse is often well above 100, although the temperature usually remains about normal. Breathing is apt to be irregular and catchy. Bowel movements are usually lacking entirely, with the rectum filled with blood that looks like tar. Pain is apt to disappear after the first day or two, but unrelieved animals usually die in about a week.

DIAGNOSIS. Through the typical symptoms and a rectal examination that often reveals a large firm mass in the right flank. May be confused with hardware trouble, indigestion, and incarceration.

TREATMENT. Surgical. If done within the first few hours the intestine can sometimes be pulled back into normal position. In cases of longer standing the telescoped area is removed and the cut edges of the intestine are sewed together to permit normal bowel movements again. Operations have been reported as successful when done as late as the fourth day after appearance of symptoms, but chances for recovery are increased by early attention.

Incarceration of Intestine

CAUSE. Passage of an intestinal loop through a tear in the peritoneum or by being choked off by fibrous cords. In cattle this usually happens through the draping of intestines over areas of adhesion. This obstructs normal passage of manure to the anus.

SYMPTOMS. Almost exactly the same as just given for intussusception.

DIAGNOSIS. A rectal examination may reveal the presence of adhesions beneath the intestines at the narrowest point.

TREATMENT. Surgery to relieve the strangulation through breaking down adhesions or otherwise as needed.

Nitrate Poisoning

CAUSE. Nitrates or nitrites in feeds, water, or fertilizers. This trouble was first reported in the U.S. in 1937 under the name of "oat hay poisoning." Study since then has shown that oats, wheat, corn, barley, cane, or sorghums of all types, together with alfalfa and many pasture grasses have a tendency to concentrate nitrate under drouth conditions. These plants may remain dangerous even after they have been made into hay or silage. Common weeds that occasionally carry large amounts of nitrate include pigweed, chickweed, Jimson weed, smartweed, velvet weed, sunflower, bull nettle, giant ragweed, Johnson grass, groundcherry, lambsquarter, and black nightshade. Surface water stored in ponds may contain dangerous amounts of nitrates or nitrites, either through natural processes or drainage from lots and fields. The same thing is true of shallow wells. It is generally believed that any amount of nitrate over 0.5 per cent in the total rations may possibly cause trouble, and even with good rations, any amount over 1.5 per cent of nitrate in the total rations is dangerous. This may happen when no one part of the ration is dangerous, but a combination of feeds will result in raising the nitrate content to a dangerous level. For example, alfalfa or clover may contain 0.6 per cent nitrate, and the silage another 0.7 per cent nitrate. A common form of nitrate poisoning is caused by ammonium nitrate or sodium nitrate fertilizers. These may be stored where cattle can get to them, empty fertilizer bags may allowed to blow into pastures, or fertilizer spreaders may be left in cattle lots. In some cases trouble has followed fertilizing fields without removing the cattle, or turning animals into fields immediately after they have been fertilized.

Although referred to as "nitrate poisoning," the nitrates are relatively nonpoisonous when compared with nitrites, and it is the reduction of nitrates to nitrites that actually causes trouble. The nitrite is easily absorbed from the digestive tract, and combines with the hemoglobin of the blood to form methemoglobin. This interferes with the oxygen-carrying capacity of the blood so that cattle may suffocate, showing symptoms much like those of prussic acid and corn stalk poisoning.

It is well known that some plants contain a substance which under certain conditions is able to reduce nitrates to nitrites. This fact may explain some mysterious cases where previously harmless forages suddenly became poisonous. For example, experiments have shown that oat hay moistened with rain or snow and exposed to air may contain dangerous amounts of nitrites afterward. This reduction reaches a peak in about 20 hours after moistening. Such an occurrence is possible only when the forage already contains considerable nitrate.

SYMPTOMS. Apparently largely dependent on the amount of nitrate exceeding 0.5 per cent in the ration. When poisoning is severe, symptoms are those of suffocation, including gasping, staggering, and frothing at the mouth. In addition, animals may urinate frequently, bloat, and kick at the belly. In milder cases the signs of nitrate poisoning may vary from normal-looking cows which abort or produce dead full-term calves to seemingly healthy animals which have an unthrifty appearance and lowered milk production. Many of this latter group will have a history of sore feet, lameness, and digestive upsets suggestive of hardware trouble. Total rations containing over 1.5 per cent of nitrate will often cause breeding troubles.

DIAGNOSIS. Difficult to make when symptoms alone are considered. However, certain characteristics of blood from suspected animals may help to distinguish between prussic acid poisoning, corn stalk poisoning, and nitrate poisoning, all of which show similar symptoms. In puzzling cases, the following information may have diagnostic value:

1. Prussic Acid—Fresh blood has a peculiar cherry-red color.
2. Nitrate—Fresh blood has a chocolate-brown color.
3. Corn Stalk—Heating a blood sample until it clots and then allowing it to cool will cause it to turn a bright pink color.

TREATMENT. Largely dependent on the symptoms shown and

the type of animal affected. Methylene blue solutions given intravenously at the rate of about 2 grams of methylene blue for each 500 pounds of body weight will be effective in cases where the animals have not eaten excessive amounts of the nitrate. As an alternative, methylene blue or sodium thiosulfate tablets may be given orally. These tablets and the solution may be obtained from your veterinarian. Doses of mineral oil may help to counteract the caustic action of nitrate salts, and drenching with vinegar may also prove helpful. In the case of animals showing mild symptoms, they can often be helped by adding molasses and vitamin A to the ration, even without a change of other feeds. In the case of wild animals, quiet and rest will probably do more good than any kind of treatment, which is certain to agitate the cattle.

PREVENTION. Pretty much a matter of following management procedures designed to keep nitrates away from cattle. However, there will be times when it will be advisable to check water and certain feeds for nitrate content. Testing materials are available through veterinarians, and if you do not have one in your area you can have your druggist mix one recommended by Dr. Arthur Case of the University of Missouri.* It is made as follows:

Mix a full-strength reagent by dissolving 500 mg. of diphenylamine in 20 cc. of water, then cautiously adding concentrated sulfuric acid to make 100 cc. This mixture is cooled and stored in a brown bottle. Since this reagent is very dangerous, it must be handled carefully and kept out of the reach of children.

The field test is usually made with half-strength reagent made by mixing equal parts of the strong reagent and 80 per cent sulfuric acid. The full-strength reagent can be used to detect nitrate in small amounts as is likely to be the case in pond water. The half-strength reagent is both reliable and adequate whenever the nitrate content is high enough to be dangerous.

If nitrate is present a blue color develops rapidly when the reagent is applied to test material. The depth of color and the speed of reaction helps to indicate the amount of nitrate that is present. A greenish color indicates that the material should also be tested for nitrites. Colors other than blue or green can be ignored as far as nitrate tests are concerned.

Dr. Arthur Case also recommends the diazotization test for nitrite.* The A solution is made by dissolving 500 mg. of sulfanilic acid in 150 cc. of 20 per cent glacial acetic acid. The B

* Journal of the American Veterinary Medical Association, April 15, 1957, page 326.

solution is made by dissolving (with gentle heat) 200 mg. of alphanaphthylamine hydrochloride in 150 cc. of 20 per cent glacial acetic acid. Each is stored in a dropper bottle away from light.

The test for nitrite is performed by adding 2 cc. of the unknown water, plant juice, or extract to 2 cc. of the A solution; then adding 2 cc. of the B. solution; and gently mixing. The development of various shades of rose-pink to dark rose-red indicates the presence of nitrite. If man or animals have to use the water or forage that reacts to this test, a quantitative test for nitrite should be run to determine exactly how much nitrite is present.

On cornstalks or other large plants, it is easier to slash the stalks and apply the test solutions, three or four drops at a time, directly to the pith. Drouth-stunted corn may have so much nitrite present that the color becomes a dark rose-red within seconds after the B solution is dropped on the test spot. This test may be used in combination with other diagnostic procedures when outbreaks of suspected cornstalk poisoning are being investigated.

In addition to tests for the elimination of dangerous feeds and water, owners may also help themselves to avoid cases of nitrate poisoning by:

1. Adding molasses and vitamin A to rations in order to reduce the toxicity when the nitrate content of the total ration is not over 1.5 per cent.
2. Examining the fertilization program to reduce the danger of using too much nitrogen, especially during drouth years.
3. Using irrigation whenever possible to reduce nitrate concentration by plants during dry growing seasons.
4. Making routine use of the nitrate and nitrite tests on hay, silage, and pasture plants that grow during drouth years.

Bracken (Brake) Fern Poisoning

CAUSE. Generally one of two types of fern, either *Pteridium latiusculum Maxon* or *Pteridium aquilinum Kuhn.* The former plant is native to eastern United States and Canada, while the latter is widely distributed in North America. This trouble was first noted in England in 1893, and in the United States in 1920. These ferns are also known by the names of eagle fern and hog brake. They are unpalatable, and usually will not be eaten unless cattle are badly starved because of short pastures, although certain animals seem to acquire a taste for them. Even in times of drouth, the ferns are likely to have an inviting bright green appearance. The poisonous principle of bracken is unknown, but it is often considered as likely to be the same as the one causing trouble when cattle are poisoned with trichloroethylene-extracted soybean oil meal. The plants remain dangerous even after they are dried and made into hay. The chief identifying feature of bracken ferns is the separation of the stem into three distinct parts.

SYMPTOMS. Occur only after the ferns have been eaten for 30 days or more, and may appear two or three weeks after cattle have been removed from pastures containing bracken. Under this latter condition, owners sometimes find it hard to believe that the ferns are responsible for trouble. A high fever is characteristic, with temperatures ranging between 106 and 108 degrees, and animals becoming noticeably anemic. Two types of the disease are usually recognized.

The digestive type is the commonest, with animals acting droopy, going off feed, and bleeding from the eyes, nostrils, vagina, and anus. The respiratory type shows many of the same symptoms, and in addition, there is swelling in the throat region, snoring sounds, and fast, difficult breathing. Opening a dead animal is apt to reveal a great deal of bloody fluid in the abdomen and thoracic cavity, together with blood clots and other evidence of bleeding in the digestive and uro-genital tracts. Practically all cattle will die within 12 to 72 hours after first showing symptoms, and in some outbreaks the finding of one or two dead animals in the pasture has been the first indication of trouble. Cases usually appear in the northern states during the fall months when drouth and over-grazing has destroyed pastures. In the south and southeast, cases may appear during the dry early summer months as well as in the fall. Trouble usually stops appearing after the first fall frost.

DIAGNOSIS. Usually on the basis of symptoms, lesions, and the availability of bracken ferns in pastures. Under farm conditions this trouble may be confused with others like shipping fever, red nose, leptospirosis, anaplasmosis, trichloroethylene-extracted soy bean oil meal poisoning, and bacillary hemoglobinuria. In doubtful cases a differential white blood cell count will prove helpful, for none of the diseases mentioned except leptospirosis will cause such a marked reduction in the number of white blood cells.

TREATMENT. None recognized for acute cases. Less serious cases may possibly be helped by blood transfusions, with at least a gallon of blood being given daily until improvement occurs.

PREVENTION. Largely a matter of supplying animals with extra feed during critical pasture periods, either in the form of hay or green forage crops. When dangerous pastures must be used, the ferns can be destroyed with suitable sprays, or owners can try the system reported by Boddie* as being used by Scottish farmers with good results. These owners believe that they have avoided losses among their hill cattle by removing them to ground free of bracken at three-week intervals. This system may be improved by allowing succeeding groups of cattle to overgraze fern areas, and regularly removing them to fern-free pastures. Following this practice over a period of years reduces the fern growth below the danger point at the same time poisoning is prevented by the alternate grazing plan.

Selenium Poisoning, Blind Staggers, Alkali Disease

CAUSE. An element which is found in the soil and water of certain areas, and is then taken up by various plants. The selenium content of these plants depends upon at least five things:

1. The chemical form of selenium in the soil.
2. The amount of selenium in the soil.
3. Whether the selenium is available to deep-rooted or shallow-rooted plants.
4. The type of plant.
5. The stage of growth.

The two chemical forms of selenium are known as the organic and inorganic. The organic form is readily available to crop plants, while the inorganic is not because it is practically insoluble in neutral or alkaline soils. However, the inorganic is made available by the so-called "converter" plants.

Some of the wild range plants have an unusual ability to absorb the inorganic form of selenium, and when they die they leave the selenium in the organic form which is readily available to all plants. Converter-type plants include milk vetch, winter fat, snow-on-the-mountain, prince's plume, saltbush, and woody aster.

This trouble is probably better known by the names of "blind staggers" and "alkali disease." Blind staggers usually represents the acute form of poisoning which is characterized by staggering, blindness, and a high death rate. Alkali disease represents the chronic form which takes a slower course and causes fewer deaths. Incidentally, the chronic form has nothing to do with alkali, which is harmless to cattle in concentrations up to about 1½ per cent in the drinking water. The term "blind staggers" is also misleading, because affected animals may neither stagger nor be blind.

SYMPTOMS. Cattle in the early stages are picky about eating,

* Veterinary Record, 59 (1947), pages 470-486.

wander away from the herd, and have fits of trembling. As time goes on, animals have a tendency to wander in aimless circles and try to walk over obstacles rather than around them. The front legs seem to be weakened, with the head often pushed against solid objects for support. Although animals are completely off feed, they will often eat dirt or rotten grass. In the final stages they are almost completely blind, with the eyelids swollen and inflamed. They may groan, kick at the belly, slobber, and grind the teeth. Convulsions are common, and paralysis of the throat muscles may prevent swallowing. Death occurs in about 90 per cent of these acute cases.

Animals suffering from the chronic form are first noticed as appearing dull, refusing feed, growing thin, and seeming somewhat stiff in their movements. A little later on they may become severely lame. This isn't surprising, for there is painful swelling and cracking of the skin around the tops of the hoofs, together with deformities of the hoofs themselves. These may become extremely long and roughened, or even be sloughed off entirely. In many cases the horns appear roughened, too, and most of the long hair is lost from the switch of the tail. Extremely sore feet may prevent walking and cause animals to move about on their knees. Calves may be born showing such symptoms, and those sucking affected dams may also be poisoned. Affected females may suffer from breeding troubles or become completely sterile.

DIAGNOSIS. On the basis of typical symptoms in combination with hoof and horn changes accompanied by loss of hair from the switch. Under farm conditions the chronic form of this trouble might be confused with circling disease, ergot poisoning, sporadic bovine encephalomyelitis, fescue foot, trace element deficiencies, lead poisoning, and lightning stroke.

TREATMENT. Begins with immediate removal from dangerous range or a change of rations to eliminate causative feeds. Many animals will recover following such a procedure without anything else being done. When practical, though, animals should be given something like epsom salts to act as a laxative and help clear the digestive tract of poisonous material. Animals that are down or in a seriously weakened condition may require the injection of sugar solutions directly into the jugular vein.

The inclusion of arsenic in salt mixtures for range cattle has been claimed as helpful in selenium areas. If it is used, recommendations must be followed closely, and mixing must be thorough, for arsenic is a powerful poison, itself. Authorities state that the final mixture should contain 25 parts per million of arsenic in the form of sodium arsenite. This means 1.9 grams (about one-fifteenth of an ounce) per 100 pounds of salt.

PREVENTION. Almost entirely a matter of avoiding the feeding of roughage or grain that contains selenium, since no practical way is known of removing it from feeds or the soil. Fortunately, cattle ordinarily do not eat plants that contain harmful amounts of selenium, so elimination of weeds, and other range improvement measures should prove helpful. In addition, overgrazing must be avoided, and extra feed should be provided in times of drouth so animals are not forced to eat plants they otherwise would leave alone. It has been claimed that animals can be safely grazed on dangerous range if plenty of grass and other selenium-free forage is available. However, the presence of converter plants on such range can make this something of a gamble, too. The feeding of a high-protein ration has been reported as giving a certain degree of protection against the poisonous effects of selenium.

When Cattle Have Diarrhea

There are at least 22 different causes of diarrhea in cattle:
1. COCCIDIOSIS, caused by several species of coccidia.
2. WORMS, either tape or round varieties.
3. SPOILED FEEDS like heated grain, dusty hay, or moldy silage.
4. OVER-EATING on various feeds, chiefly grain.
5. TOO MUCH SALT, especially when animals haven't had it for some time.
6. TOO MUCH MOLASSES in feed.
7. FEED CHANGES, usually involving pastures or green crops.
8. PLANT POISONING.
9. CHEMICAL POISONING.
10. TRACE ELEMENT DEFICIENCY.
11. HARDWARE TROUBLE.
12. TWISTING OF THE UTERUS in pregnant cows.
13. METRITIS or inflammation of the uterus.
14. MASTITIS.
15. STOMATITIS due to various types of infection.
16. PNEUMONIA.
17. SHIPPING FEVER.
18. VIRUS DIARRHEA of either the New York or Indiana type.
19. RED NOSE or IBR.
20. MUCOSAL DISEASE.
21. WINTER DYSENTERY.
22. JOHNE'S DISEASE.

When Cattle Have Sore Mouths

Cattle occasionally slobber, are "picky" about eating, or show other signs of having a sore mouth. At least 17 different troubles can cause such symptoms.

1. Lumpjaw. Although a bone disease, it may be accompanied by ulceration of the gums.
2. Wooden Tongue.
3. Diphtheria.
4. Mycotic Stomatitis.
5. X-Disease.
6. Light Sensitization. Slobbering may occur even though mouths aren't sore.
7. Virus Diarrhea.
8. Mucosal Disease.
9. Red Nose or IBR.
10. Foot and Mouth Disease. Although not likely to be seen in the U.S., it is well to keep it in mind as a possibility.
11. Vesicular Stomatitis. Chiefly important because it might be confused with foot and mouth disease.
12. Blue Tongue. Although generally considered as exclusively a disease of sheep, it can also affect cattle.
13. Anthrax. It may cause symptoms of sore mouth in the early stages, but other more serious signs soon identify it.
14. Snake Bite. The tongue may be so badly swollen that it protrudes from the mouth.
15. Mouth Injuries. Generally caused by plant awns or "beards" that become imbedded in mouth tissues. Some cases are due to cuts, and an occasional animal gets a piece of binder twine looped around the base of the tongue.
16. Burns from chemicals and medicines.
17. Bad teeth. Symptoms are usually due to teeth that are painfully cracked or broken. However, they sometimes grow too long and have sharp edges which then cut into the lining of the cheeks.

Any time there's evidence that sore mouths are due to a contagious disease, owners will do well to call a veterinarian at once. In areas where veterinary service isn't available, help can be obtained from livestock officials in the state capital.

About Mold Poisoning

At one time or another moldy hay and grain has been blamed for everything from diarrhea to abortions and even death of various farm animals. This isn't likely to be true in most cases, for experiments have shown that moldy feed seldom causes serious trouble. Many of the deaths blamed on molds are really due to toxins produced by botulism bacteria in spoiled feeds instead.

Experiments at South Dakota over a two-year period showed that the feeding of moldy corn was not noticeably injurious to sheep, cattle, or swine. Reports from Purdue and the University of Maryland indicate that there is little danger of causing trouble by feeding moldy corn to poultry.

The feeding of moldy corn has often been reported as a cause of vulvo-vaginitis in swine, but none of the feeding trials with it has caused the condition. Until some kind of an experiment involving moldly corn consistently produces vulvo-vaginitis in a reasonable number of experimental animals, there can be no definite proof that mold is the causative factor.

In spite of reports like those just mentioned, stockmen will do well to be a bit careful with moldy feed. Authorities recognize about 15 common kinds of mold that occur in hay and silage, with several of these being very dangerous. One is a green mold that is extremely poisonous for cattle, sheep, and swine, and will also affect horses. Another is gray-black, and belongs to the Aspergillus group. It is often found inside corn nubbins as well as in hay and silage, and is very poisonous for cattle, sheep, and swine. One of the most dangerous silage molds known is red with a white or blue interior. The so-called "pink mildew" mold of corn is also capable of causing poisoning like ergot.

Considering the seemingly conflicting evidence, the average stockman is likely to be badly confused in regard to what he should do with various types of moldy feed. It is impractical to have each batch of such feed tested in a laboratory, but the owner can easily run a simple test right on the farm. A few of the less valuable animals can be fed large amounts of the suspected feed for a week or ten days. If no suspicious symptoms are noted in this time, small amounts of the same feed may then be fed to the entire herd while the first group of animals continues to receive it in liberal quantities. Damaged feed of any kind must be fed with caution, since some types of mold poison have a delayed action so that symptoms are slow in appearing. Then after they do show up, the symptoms may grow worse in a hurry, and end in death for animals within a few days.

All moldy feed needn't be thrown away, but neither should it be considered as harmless until it has been proven as such. It may be difficult to say that certain symptoms are due to mold poisoning, too. Abortions in a certified Bang's-free herd may be caused by something like leptospirosis or vibriosis or iodine deficiency instead of moldy feed. Similarly, a diarrhea may be due to something like virus diarrhea or winter dysentery or shipping fever instead of spoiled feed. Finally, deaths may be due to something like parasites or blackleg or lead poisoning, so you may have a little trouble in deciding just what is to blame for such troubles. Your best way of avoiding such diagnostic work consists of using extreme care when using moldy feeds. If you do that, you'll at least know that mold poisoning isn't causing livestock trouble for you.

Displacement of the Abomasum

CAUSE. Instead of lying to the right of the rumen or first stomach on the floor of the abdominal cavity, the abomasum or fourth stomach is doubled over on itself, crowded under the rumen, and forced up on the left side between the rumen and the ribs. The weight of the first stomach and doubling of the abomasum interferes with normal passage of food materials into the intestines and the animal sickens. This condition is most likely to appear in cows either a short time before, or a week or two after calving.

The actual cause of such displacement is not definitely known, but four possibilities are suggested:

1. As pregnancy advances, the unborn calf in the uterus may work down under the rumen instead of developing along the right side of the rumen and above the abomasum. Continued enlargement of the uterus in this position will naturally force the abomasum back on itself, and finally under and to the left of the rumen.
2. Cows that have milk fever, acetonemia, or mastitis are sometimes rolled so they are brought into position for more convenient treatment. Similarly, pregnant cows suffering from a twisted uterus are sometimes rolled to untwist the neck of the uterus. Such rolling might easily disturb the normal position of the abomasum.
3. When cattle are moved across the country in trucks or railroad cars, the sudden stops and starts may displace various internal organs.
4. Since most cases involve cows that have been eating large quantities of grain or ground forage for long periods, such feed may encourage displacement of the abomasum. If this

is true, we can expect to see more of this trouble in areas where the use of hay choppers is increasing.

SYMPTOMS. Almost exactly the same as described on page 199 of this book for the digestive form of acetonemia. Animals go off feed and lose weight at a rapid rate. They look dull, have a gaunt, tucked-up appearance, and usually show signs of being constipated. The temperature, pulse, and respiration rates are all likely to be within the normal range. The urine test for acetonemia will show a mild reaction. Treatment with acetonemia remedies usually results in improvement for a few days, followed by a recurrence of symptoms.

DIAGNOSIS. Pretty much a matter of distinguishing it from acetonemia. The following points may be of value:

1. Treatment with cortisone compounds is followed by prompt improvement in uncomplicated acetonemia cases, but has little effect on an animal with a displaced abomasum.
2. The urine test gives a pronounced color change when acetonemia is involved, but only a mildly positive reaction for a displaced abomasum.
3. The rumen can usually be felt in the left flank in a case of acetonemia, but not in a case of displaced abomasum because it has been pushed toward the middle of the abdominal cavity.
4. Sounds of rolling gas can often be heard under the ribs of the left side in cases of displacement, but are very unlikely in acetonemia.
5. Manure is likely to be scanty and hard in acetonemia cases, and scanty but soft or watery in cases of displacement.

In addition, displacement of the abomasum will need to be distinguished from hardware trouble, kidney infection, indigestion, and other conditions that sometimes show similar symptoms.

TREATMENT. Surgery is the only effective one known. The left flank is opened so the abomasum can be returned under the rumen and to its natural position on the other side of the body. The operation has a better chance of being successful if it can be performed after the cow has freshened. This is because the pressure of the pregnant uterus may prevent return of the abomasum to its proper position. If an owner decides not to risk the operation, it will be best to sell the animal for beef as soon as possible. Otherwise the cow will eventually die after starving herself into a skeleton-like condition.

Ulcers of the Abomasum

CAUSE. Not definitely known, but it is believed that the ulcers are probably closely related to abnormal acidity of the stomach contents. It is possible that stress factors like calving and the beginning of lactation might stimulate gastric secretions with more than a normal acid content. The character of the diet or a nervous disposition might also have an influence on stomach acidity.

SYMPTOMS. Somewhat dependent on the size and number of ulcers. Dairy cows may show symptoms of milk fever or acetonemia, and beef cows may go down in convulsions. In most cases affected animals are off feed and vaguely unwell for a period of days or weeks while the ulcers are developing. Many animals probably recover when the ulcers finally heal, but trouble becomes serious when the ulcer eats completely through the stomach wall. If the wall of a large blood vessel is eroded, animals may bleed to death in a short time. Otherwise animals usually suffer from peritonitis and a chronic bloody diarrhea that results in anemia and a gradual wasting away until they finally die.

DIAGNOSIS. Definite only through surgery that demonstrates the ulcers, but a tentative diagnosis can sometimes be made on the basis of anemia in combination with a chronic bloody diarrhea. The condition might be confused with others like hardware trouble, coccidiosis, internal parasite infestation, and various kinds of poisoning.

TREATMENT. In the case of valuable animals, an operation to repair the ulcers might be justified. Otherwise remedial measures would be limited to blood transfusions and treatment of the peritonitis, with chances of recovery being very poor, and dependent on spontaneous healing of the ulcers.

PREVENTION. Since the exact cause is unknown, no definite preventive measures can be recommended. However, assuming that increased gastric acidity is really an important causative factor, these two may be helpful:

1. Mix rations so that a heavy concentration of barley is avoided, since this grain seems particularly likely to cause rumenitis and inflammation of the other divisions of the bovine stomach.
2. Change feed lot cattle gradually from roughage to grain in order to avoid excessive fermentation which produces a high concentration of acid in the stomach. Do the same thing with dairy cows that are being changed over to grain and full feed after calving.

Molybdenum Poisoning, Molybdenosis

CAUSE. An excess of molybdenum in feeds or forage grown in naturally occurring molybdenum areas, or regions where molybdenum has been used in extra amounts as a fertilizer to stimulate the utilization of nitrogen. Effects will depend on the amount of copper available, for excess molybdenum interferes with the action of copper, which in turn causes interference with iron metabolism in the body. Molybdenum in young growing plants appears to be more dangerous than a similar amount of the element in cured hay or grain. If the copper value of feed is below 5 p.p.m. in fast-growing pastures, molybdenum in a concentration of 1 p.p.m. may be dangerous, while copper levels of 10 p.p.m. will usually prevent poisoning by molybdenum in concentrations up to 4 p.p.m. Experimental work has shown that molybdenum increases the loss of phosphorus from the body.

SYMPTOMS. Range all the way from simple failure to do well to serious conditions like anemia, severe diarrhea, loss of hair, extreme loss of weight, and mysterious fractures of the leg bones and shoulder blades. Colors may bleach out so that Herefords change to fawn, and Angus to gray. Mature animals may develop a pacing gait, with both legs on the same side moving forward together. Young animals may be affected with ricket-like symptoms of enlarged joints and beading on the ribs. Many calves will be born as monsters two or three months ahead of time. Animals of both sexes may be made sterile, and bulls are likely to remain permanently sterile. Females that do not come in heat or fail to settle when bred, usually respond to treatment so they are restored as breeders. Molybdenum poisoning has been blamed for heart failure in older animals which in some areas is known as "falling disease" or "quick death."

DIAGNOSIS. Made on the basis of suspicious symptoms occurring in areas where molybdenosis is a problem. It can be confirmed by the improvement of affected animals within a few weeks after treatment is started.

TREATMENT. An old remedy consists of drenching animals with one gram of copper sulfate in water for each 100 pounds of body weight, and 1 mg. of cobalt carbonate at weekly intervals. Treatment should not be continued for longer than two months, and may be stopped any time improvement warrants it. Injections of copper glycinate have also been effective, and supplementary phosphorus feeding is a valuable supportive measure. Female cattle that have partially or entirely recovered from molybdenosis can live out normal lives and produce normal calves, according to research results obtained at the University of Nevada. Such animals do not show evidence of spongy bone, but cattle severely stunted by molybdenosis never reach the same size as unaffected animals when all other factors are equal.

PREVENTION. In areas where the molybdenum content of forage is less than 5 p.p.m., the use of 1% of copper sulfate in salt has provided satisfactory protection, but 2% of copper sulfate will be necessary for higher concentrations of molybdenum. When cattle are not supplied with salt because of a high salt content in the feed or other reasons, it may be necessary to increase the amount of copper in the mineral mixture (as high as 1.25%), and to apply copper fertilizers to pastures. Injections of copper glycinate may also be used as a protective measure.

"Jaw and Tongue Trouble"

CAUSE. Not definitely known, but the trouble has been reproduced by feeding large quantities of mesquite beans in an experiment conducted by the Texas Agricultural Experiment Station. This ailment is prevalent in certain areas of Texas and Oklahoma. Considered as an excellent feed, mesquite beans have been widely fed by ranchmen, particularly under drought conditions. Research workers theorize that sugar in the beans changes the bacteria in the rumen so animals can no longer digest cellulose or efficiently synthesize vitamins of the B complex.

SYMPTOMS. Affected animals slobber so badly that the feed trough or salt box often contains several quarts of saliva. Animals chew continuously, often holding the head on one side, as though affected with a bad tooth. This chewing may continue for long periods without swallowing or bringing up any cuds. When cattle regurgitate, rumen contents may be spewed over a wide area. About a fourth of the affected animals protrude their tongues ½ inch to 4 inches. The tongue is not paralyzed since it can be used for licking, and at times affected animals will lick themselves almost continuously. About 10-50% of the animals will have soft swellings under the tongue or jaws. These swellings are sometimes quite large, and have a tendency to appear and disappear within short periods.

DIAGNOSIS. Through typical symptoms, especially when there is a history of animals receiving mesquite beans as a feed. It might be confused with troubles like bad teeth, wooden tongue, vesicular stomatitis, mycotic stomatitis, and plant awns in the tongue.

TREATMENT. None can be recommended at this time other than a removal of mesquite beans from the ration.

When Cattle Lose their Cuds

Back in Grandpa's day a great many stories were told of cattle that had "lost" their cuds. This was a bad business, indeed, for the poorest of stockmen knew that a cow was likely to become sick if she had nothing to chew on in her spare time. The most favored treatment consisted of replacing the natural "lost" cud with an artificial one. This could be almost anything, ranging from a greasy dishrag or chunk of salt pork to a lard-coated length of rope or well-oiled piece of leather. We don't know how many cattle were cured by such treatment, but we do know that both the ailment and remedy were well known not so many years ago.

Cattle seem to have grown more intelligent since then, for it's been a long time since we have run across any that had "lost" a cud. However, the animals do stop chewing them at times so they worry their owners as much as they ever did. The owners seem to have grown a little wiser with the years, too, for they no longer use artificial cuds at such times. That is because they figure that sickness causes cud-chewing to stop instead of cuds being "lost" to cause the sickness. Since practically anything that will make a cow sick will cause her to stop chewing her cud, it may be quite a job to decide exactly what kind of treatment is needed.

When Cattle Vomit

Several different conditions may cause cattle to vomit, and vomiting may occur either with or without other symptoms of trouble.

1. When it occurs as a herd problem, the feeding of silage (either corn or grass) is probably the commonest cause.
2. Highly acid foods. An example would be the last silage near the bottom of a silo which contains a great deal of liquid.
3. Rupture of the diaphragm.
4. Displacement of the abomasum.
5. Swelling that has partially or completely blocked the opening of the stomach into the intestine.
6. Warts or similar growths in the upper part of the esophagus.
7. The eating of indigestible material. Afterbirth is sometimes involved in these cases, and feed sacks are regularly reported as the cause of vomiting by cattle.
8. Torsion or intussusception of the intestines.

9. Hardware disease. Vomiting due to this cause is most likely to occur soon after eating or drinking.

10. Pieces of wire and other hardware can cause vomiting while simply lying loose in the stomach and without having pierced the stomach walls at all.

11. Sand and gravel can do the same thing after having been swallowed with dirty roughage.

12. Plants like sneezeweed or lily of the valley.

13. Overfeeding causes vomiting because stomach movements are slowed down so that large masses of the feed accumulate and ferment to produce a sour condition. Such trouble is often seen in cattle that are being changed from roughage to grain in feed lots, or dairy cows that are being brought to "full feed" too quickly after calving.

14. Damaged feed is frequently to blame for vomiting by cattle. Included in this class are such things as frozen grass, moldy silage, heated grain, and rotten straw. High-producing dairy cows or beef animals being finished off in feed lots seem to be particularly susceptible to damaged feed.

TREATMENT. Depends on the primary cause, so no single one can be recommended for all cases. When silage is the cause, discontinuing the feeding for a short time will stop the vomiting. The affected animals can then often be gradually returned to full feeding of the silage without recurrence of the vomiting. The same thing can sometimes be done when feeds other than silage cause trouble.

In many cases it will be desirable to give animals a good dose of a laxative like epsom salts or mineral oil for the purpose of cleaning out the digestive tract. Whatever you do, though, be sure that indigestion is to blame before you give a laxative to a vomiting animal. The chances are roughly two to one that the vomiting is due to something else, and will only be made worse by such treatment.

When no definite cause for vomiting can be determined, it may help to give antacids like baking soda or magnesium hydroxide daily for three days.

Perverted Appetite, Pica

CAUSE. Usually some kind of a mineral deficiency. However, cattle may have depraved appetites even when plenty of minerals are available. Under such circumstances calves often chew on wood, evidently for the sake of exercising their jaw muscles. Adult cattle may eat grease and oil, probably simply because there is something about the taste or smell that appeals to them. Similarly, it is well known that cattle have a natural liking for dangerous materials like lead paint and nitrate fertilizers. A lack of common salt is frequently the reason why cattle start eating filthy bedding that has been soaked with urine. On the other hand, young calves may start eating bedding and other indigestible materials for no good reason at all.

SYMPTOMS. Animals start eating materials that they would ordinarily leave alone. Range cattle seem particularly addicted to old bones. A perverted appetite may not be noticed in the case of animals that are affected with some other disease, although it often goes along with troubles like anaplasmosis, Texas fever, acetonemia, and rabies.

DIAGNOSIS. Offers no trouble, although the basic reason for eating such material is often somewhat in doubt.

TREATMENT. Usually through the furnishing of a mineral mixture on a free-choice basis. Supplying calves with whole oats instead of ground grain will often end their wood-chewing activities. It may be necessary to put wire basket muzzles on calves to break them of eating filthy bedding. It will also be a good idea to supply salt on a free-choice basis, preferably in a box separate from the mineral mixture. In some cases a change to better rations is indicated. Animals that are showing a perverted appetite because of some other disease should receive treatment for the primary cause.

PREVENTION. Pretty much through supplying salt and minerals separately on a free-choice basis in combination with feeding properly balanced rations. Old paint pails, worn-out batteries, and empty fertilizer bags should be destroyed or placed where cattle have no chance of getting at them. It will also be advisable to keep cattle away from machinery and places where oil has been drained from machinery, trucks, automobiles, and tractors.

Cattle Need Salt

Most people know that Stephen Babcock invented the test for butterfat in milk, but few of them know that he also did a lot of work to show the importance of salt for cattle. One of his tests involved dairy cows that were well-fed, but received no salt for a year. Eventually all of these animals broke down, with complete loss of appetite and cessation of milk production. Recoveries occurred rapidly when the cows were given salt again.

On the basis of these and other experiments made over fifty

years ago, salt-feeding recommendations were made which are still widely followed. Generally, they provide for three-fourths of an ounce daily for each 1000 pounds of body weight, and in addition, three-tenths of an ounce for every 10 pounds of milk produced daily. This means that good milk cows often won't get enough salt when it is furnished only as one per cent of the grain ration, and beef cows may also suffer under such a plan. If more salt is mixed with the grain, it may be made so unpalatable that animals won't eat it.

To avoid trouble it will be best to furnish the salt free-choice in addition to mixing one per cent with the grain. Cattle that want more salt can then get it without being compelled to eat dirt or filthy bedding. Such feeding is recommended for calves as well as older animals, and should be started as soon as they begin to eat grain. Opinions vary on the relative value of loose and block salt, but a recent experiment at Cornell University supplies some interesting information.

A three-year average showed that cows voluntarily ate about twice as much loose salt as block salt. However, the cows that received block salt got enough to meet their needs and did as well as those that ate twice as much loose salt. It was also shown that cattle have a definite preference for loose salt when they have a choice between it and the block variety. The extra loose salt was regarded as "luxury consumption" in all cases, or more than the cows really needed.

Similar experiments at Cornell have enabled authorities to estimate the salt requirements of cattle with more accuracy than provided by earlier studies. It was found that one-half an ounce daily wasn't quite enough for a milking cow over a long period, while 2 and 4 ounces daily were more than she needed. Continued work pin-pointed the requirement at about one ounce of salt daily for cows producing up to 12.000 pounds of milk annually, with this being in addition to that found naturally in her feed. Higher production would require a little more salt.

A recent Kansas experiment showed that steers receiving salt outgained those without it by 65 pounds each, and sold for fifty cents a hundred more. Based on the amount eaten by the steers during their growing and fattening periods, these differences would make the salt worth about a dollar per pound for feed.

Reports from other experiment stations indicate that cattle won't do well without salt, and that it can easily prove to be your cheapest feed and biggest money-maker. Putting it in feed probably won't be enough, and you have no way of knowing exactly how much individual animals will need for maximum returns. Accordingly, you'll do well to put out either salt blocks or loose salt in weatherproof boxes where your cattle can help themselves as they like.

Remember, though, don't suddenly supply salt free-choice to cattle that have been without it for a long time. Otherwise you may poison them. Instead, feed them individually an ounce twice-daily, and gradually increase this amount until they are accustomed to salt.

Black Disease (Infectious Necrotic Hepatitis)

CAUSE. An organism known as *Clostridium novyi* which produces poisons and seems closely related to fluke damage of the liver in that it is dependent on fluke disease for maximum growth. It can remain as spores in the soil for a long time, and is believed to multiply in the digestive tracts of healthy animals. It affects sheep as well as cattle.

MEANS OF SPREAD. Spores are swallowed with food or water, and then are carried to the liver by either the blood or fluke larvae. Here damage caused by the migrating flukes results in favorable growing conditions for the germs. In multiplying, the *C. novyi* produce poisons which damage the liver even more and this helps to spread the germs through the organ.

SYMPTOMS. Affected animals appear listless, lie down most of the time, and usually die within a few hours after becoming sick. As a matter of fact, the finding of dead animals may be the first indication of trouble, particularly in beef herds. Young cattle are affected most often, and the majority of cases occur in the late summer and fall. The body temperature of affected animals may be either normal or below normal.

DIAGNOSIS. Definite only through isolation in the laboratory of *C. novyi* or through fluorescent antibody testing. The isolation of *C. novyi* cannot be taken as positive proof because the germ is often found in apparently healthy animals.

Opening a dead animal will show yellowish areas of liver damage which tend to follow the track taken by migrating flukes. A straw-colored fluid is usually found in the body cavities, and there may be bleeding in the tissues just under the skin. Under field conditions black disease might be confused with liver fluke infestation, but sudden deaths should always cause black disease to be considered as a possibility.

TREATMENT. Generally useless because death occurs so quickly after symptoms are first shown. If any is given, it should be crystalline penicillin administered intravenously first to establish a high blood level immediately. This can then be followed by intramuscular injection of 3-million unit doses of penicillin in oil.

PREVENTION. The most practical is through vaccination with *C. novyi* bacterin or toxoid. In addition, a preventive program will be helped by using a fluke control program consisting of:

1. Avoiding or draining wet pastures.
2. Avoiding the use of hay from such land.
3. Treating such land with copper sulfate to destroy snails which act as hosts for fluke larvae. A recommended procedure is given under Liver rot.
4. Keeping a few geese or ducks on suspicious pastures. Along with the grass they eat, they will also pick up quite a few snails.

Animals which die from black disease should be burned or deeply buried in quicklime to prevent spread of the germs.

Torsion (Twisting) of the Cecum

CAUSE. Generally believed to be either:

1. Displacement by a calf in the uterus during late pregnancy which rotates the cecum when it is pushed aside, or
2. Lack of natural or peristaltic movements of the cecum which permits it to fill up with contents of the digestive tract. The added weight and size then makes it more likely to twist when animals lurch to their feet after lying down. Lack of peristaltic movements can be due to troubles like indigestion, contagious diseases, and hardware trouble.

Regardless of the exact cause, such twisting has the effect of preventing normal passage of ingesta from the cecum, just as twisting the top of a sack would prevent emptying of its contents.

SYMPTOMS. Much like those listed for intussusception, but not so severe. For example, colicky symptoms will be milder, and a small amount of soft or watery manure will be passed as in the case of displacement of the abomasum instead of none at all, or the pasty, tarry type passed in cases of intussusception. In addition, no blood is likely to be found in the rectum. The right flank will appear to be fuller than normal, and a splashing sound can sometimes be heard after a strong push in that area.

DIAGNOSIS. Positive by means of a rectal examination which

reveals the cecum as enlarged and hardened like a loaf of Vienna bread. Under field conditions symptoms might cause this trouble to be confused with others like hardware trouble, acetonemia, indigestion, incarceration of the intestine, or displacement of the abomasum.

TREATMENT. Surgery to empty the cecum of gas and fluid and correct the torsion is highly effective if cases are caught early. If circulation has been cut off for so long that gangrene has set in, it may be best to completely remove the cecum. No medicinal treatment can be recommended.

5.

MAMMARY TROUBLES

Anatomy of the Cow's Mammary System

The udder of the cow is supported by three different structures:

1. The skin is one of them and includes coarse tissue beneath it which helps bind the front quarters to the belly wall.

2. The lateral suspensory ligaments are two pairs of elastic sheets which support the sides of the udder. One pair lies just under the skin and originates from the subpelvic tendon. They pass down and forward over the udder on each side with the free ends finally being attached to the inside surface of the thighs. The second pair also originates from the subpelvic tendon, but these sheets practically cover the udder at a deeper level. They are chiefly different from the first pair by being attached at different levels by fibrous tissue which passes into the udder and becomes part of the inner structure of the gland. Both continue to the bottom of the udder where they become part of:

3. The median suspensory ligament which is formed by the union of two tissue sheets originating from the belly wall. This ligament divides the udder into right and left halves and is the principal support of the organ.

The right and left halves are each divided by a practically invisible fibrous wall which runs an irregular course through the tissues. Divisions as noted mean that each quarter of the udder is completely separated from all the others. This can be demonstrated by injecting colored material which defines the boundaries of individual quarters. Each of these quarters is ordinarily furnished with a single teat to permit drainage.

At the end of each teat is an opening that is variously known as the orifice or meatus and marks the lower end of the so-called "streak canal." This is really a short duct with a lining made up of longitudinal folds which fit together quite closely. It is completely

253

surrounded by a sphincter muscle which keeps it closed to retain milk in the quarter and prevent the entrance of bacteria.

The streak canal connects with the lower end of the teat cistern. This widens gradually, with a number of folds occurring where the enlargement begins. These folds are divided into smaller ones, and the entire structure is commonly known as the "rosette." Above this the cistern may develop into either a funnel-like or bell-shaped cavity, dependent on the rapidity of enlargement. The walls are covered with folds which sometimes contain pockets of various sizes.

The teat cistern connects with the gland cistern directly above it. This serves largely as a storage chamber between milkings and is made up of various-sized pockets into which the larger milk ducts empty. There are usually eight to twelve of these large ducts. Traced back, they branch and rebranch into literally thousands of smaller ducts with each of these eventually ending in so-called alveoli of milk producing glands. These glands are virtually bathed in blood and secrete milk from it.

Mastitis

CAUSE. Any one or more of several different bacteria. *Strepto-coccus agalactiae* is probably the commonest one, but other types of streptococci and staphylococci are involved as well as some of the coliform organisms in occasional cases. Sometimes these bacteria are normal inhabitants of healthy udders and do no harm until conditions are made just right for their growth and development. At other times they get into the udder through the teat orifices and cause trouble from the beginning. Things that permit bacterial growth in either case can be called contributing factors or secondary causes. There are several of them that can be given in the form of a list:

1. Dragging udders through dirty water and muddy barnyards and so allowing germs to come in contact with the ends of teats.

2. Insufficient bedding that permits udders to "catch cold" through lying on cold bare floors.

3. Filthy stable conditions that allow udders to become smeared with manure and dangerous germs.

4. Stalls of improper size. When too narrow they encourage teat and udder injuries through trampling by adjoining animals. When too long, the platform becomes dirty and

cows lie with their udders in manure. When too short, cows stand in the gutter to smear their udders with filth. This is one of the biggest causes of mastitis in the average barn.

5. Projecting nails, boards, bolts, etc., that are apt to injure udders.

6. Excessively deep gutters that bruise udders when cows back into them while being turned out.

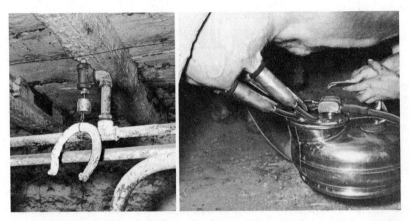

Left: Hanging weights on the safety valve of a milking machine will increase the vacuum but will also increase the incidence of mastitis.
Right: Pulling teat cups off cows before vacuum has been completely released from milking machine tends to suck the ends of the teats wrong side out to invite mastitis.

7. High doorsills that cause udder bruising when cows enter or leave the barn.

8. Kicks, blows, "hooking" by other cows, falling on slippery floors, and other assorted causes of udder bruises. Regardless of how such bruises occur, they are dangerous because they favor bacterial growth inside the udder.

9. Dirty milking practices that include squirting "bad" milk on the floor, "wet hand" milking, failure to wash udders, etc. Such things give germs a better chance to invade udders.

10. Faulty adjustment of milking machines. Pulsators may be set too slow or too fast. Vacuum may be too high because of weights on valves or too low because of plugged air hoses or pipe lines.

11. Improper milking practices like leaving machines on too long, milking at irregular intervals, and others that help to keep cows from being milked completely dry.

12. Pulling teat cups off cows before the vacuum has been completely removed. This practice tends to suck the teat orifices wrong side out so delicate tissues are exposed to bacteria.

13. Use of improperly sterilized milk tubes and udder instruments.

14. Allowing heifer calves to suck each other so the tiny udders have a chance of being ruined long before they produce any milk.

MEANS OF SPREAD. Most commonly through dirty milking practices. Teat cups and hands that aren't disinfected between cows may easily carry germs from infected animals to healthy ones. The importation of diseased cows may account for a mastitis outbreak in a clean herd, and the same thing is true of all the secondary causes just listed.

SYMPTOMS. The earliest one is usually abnormal milk from one or more quarters. Flakes and clots of different sizes may be seen, or the milk may be thick and stringy instead. Instead of a normal white color it is often yellow or even bloody. Involved quarters are frequently hot and swollen and often painful to the touch. The amount of milk from such quarters is greatly decreased, and frequently secretion stops entirely. In extremely serious cases cows go off feed, run high fevers, breathe rapidly, and show other symptoms of generalized blood poisoning. Such cases are commonly referred to as septic mastitis, and affected animals frequently die unless they are promptly treated. If infection isn't controlled milk-secreting tissues are generally destroyed and replaced with areas of scar tissue that can be felt as hard lumps when the udder is palpated. These lumps are incapable of ever producing milk, of course, and they never change back to normal tissues. Attacks of mastitis are likely to fluctuate and appear in waves to convince owners that cures have been effected without treatment of any kind. However, close observation of such cases usually reveals recurring attacks, and animals of this type are apt to be carriers of dangerous germs that are given off even during periods when the milk seems normal. Mastitis often results in lowered milk production and so-called "short milkers" because of udder damage that may not be easily noticed.

DIAGNOSIS. Usually based on the appearance of abnormal milk, either with or without udder swelling and decreased production by affected quarters. A strip cup is useful for demonstrating clots and flakes, and detection of abnormal milk is sometimes helped by using a few squirts from a healthy quarter. This is because normal milk and mastitis milk will seldom mix to hide an "off" color. The use of treated paper has been advocated as a test for mastitis milk,

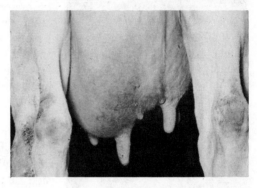

Badly swollen hind quarter due to chronic mastitis.

but it does no more than show an alkaline condition due to bacterial action. Only microscopic examination of milk will show the type of bacteria that is involved. An exception must be made in the case of the Hotis test, for it will detect Streptococcus agalactiae in milk.

As described by Hotis and Miller in 1936 the test consists of adding one-half cc. of 0.5% bromcresol purple solution to 9.5 cc. of milk that has been drawn into a sterile tube in an aseptic manner. This is then incubated for 24 to 48 hours at a temperature of 98 degrees Fahrenheit. The presence of *S. agalactiae* is shown by yellow deposits around the sides, or in the bottom of the tube.

Feeling of the udder may reveal hardened areas of scar tissue as evidence of past attacks and possible existence of dormant infection that has suddenly flared up again. Cows reported as having decreased production and being "short milkers" should be suspected of having mastitis even when milk doesn't show abnormalities in the strip cup. At various times mastitis may be mistaken for leptospirosis, shipping fever, X disease, and any of the causes given in this book for bloody milk.

TREATMENT. None that is satisfactory in all cases because of the many different types of bacteria that may be involved. However, the most important part of any treatment consists of immediate removal of grain from affected cows in combination with milking at hourly intervals. The frequent milkings remove bacteria before they have a very good chance to multiply and make infection worse, while removal of the grain lessens milk production at a time when the udder has to be considered as sick and unfit to work. Either hot or cold applications may also help.

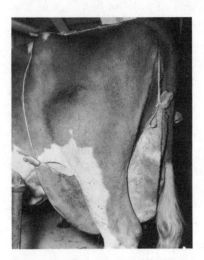

A sack properly tied over an udder to hold snow or cracked ice as a cold pack in the treatment of mastitis.

Cold applications are best made by using a beet pulp sack or material of a similar size and strength. A strong string or small rope is tied to each corner and the sack is placed under the udder. The strings on the front end are brought up over the sides and tied together at the backbone just in front of the hip bones. The ropes on the back corners are brought up between the hind legs, pulled up tightly on each side of the tail, and then tied to the first two strings where they meet on the backbone. The space between the sack and udder can then be filled in with snow or cracked ice. A satisfactory hot application is cheaply made by dissolving a couple of ounces of Epsom salts in a quart of water as hot as the hand can stand. Pieces of flannel or towels can be soaked in it and then applied to the udder, being changed every few minutes as cooling occurs. Vigorous but gentle massage is also recommended to stimulate circulation of blood in the udder which will help to remove the poisons of infection from the organ.

In recent years penicillin has come into widespread use against mastitis. It was originally provided as a powder which was mixed with sterile water and injected directly into the udder with a syringe. This form has been largely replaced by penicillin put up as ointment in tubes or in solid sticks or "bougies" which are inserted directly into affected quarters. Dosage varies between 100,000 units which is often sufficient in early cases up to several million units which may be required over several days in severe cases. Applications are generally continued until the milk has returned to a normal condition.

Aureomycin has also been widely used in the treatment of mastitis, and there seems little to choose between it and penicillin when infection is caused by streptococcal types of germs. Experiments indicate that aureomycin may be a little more effective against certain of the staphylococci, while both are inferior to streptomycin against coliform types of infection. Because farmers seldom bother to find out what kind of bacteria is causing mastitis in their herds, streptomycin has been offered in combination with penicillin as an ointment. In this way it is hoped that if one drug isn't the right one, the other may do some good.

At various times it is advisable to use drugs like sulfanilamide in oil, terramycin, gallimycin, tyrothricin, and others not generally available or practical when the exact type of causative germ is unknown. In cases of septic mastitis and extreme sickness it is generally advisable to give various of the sulfas intravenously for the sake of controlling infection that has often spread from the udder to widely separated parts of the body. Milk from treated quarters is best discarded or fed to pigs and calves for a few days after treatment has been stopped, since the presence of drugs in market milk is generally objectionable. The treatment of mastitis is usually believed as most successful during the dry period. Any of the regular drugs may be used for this purpose, but tyrothricin seems particularly effective in dry cows and is often used with good results. It has not been generally popular for use on milking cows because of its tendency to cause udder swelling after use. This is of no concern in dry cows, since the swelling seldom lasts for very long. The drying off of affected quarters has sometimes been recommended as a good procedure, since the quarters are then likely to be perfectly healthy when the cow freshens the next time. However, it is sometimes quite a job to get an infected quarter dried off without causing a great deal of trouble. Even if it is possible to get the quarter dried off, it is likely that the cow will be "light" in that particular quarter at the next freshening even though the milk seems normal again. A better practice consists of making infected animals into nurse cows for calves, since many of these animals freshen the next time with sound udders and normal production. It is likely that frequent sucking acts like hourly milking in the removal of bacteria before they have a chance to cause excessive udder damage. Cows with quarters so badly infected that calves won't suck them won't make suitable nurse cows, of course. This sort of procedure is recommended for cows that have constant recurring attacks of mastitis which never get extremely bad but are expensive to treat all the time.

PREVENTION. Pretty much a matter of avoiding the causes listed earlier. However, a few desirable points may be mentioned in regard to sanitary milking practices:

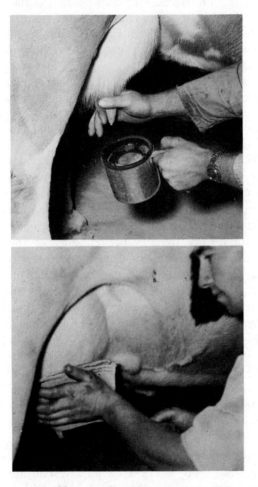

Regular use of a strip cup will aid in early detection of mastitis cases.

Washing udders with a chlorine solution before milking will insure cleaner milk and prevent a great many mastitis cases besides.

1. Use a strip cup at every milking and draw a few streams of milk from each quarter for examination before milking.
2. Affected cows should be isolated from healthy ones and grouped according to degree of infection. Healthy cows are then milked first, slightly affected next, and so on with the worst infected cows being milked last. Changes

may be made as needed in regard to location of the cows.

3. Wash udders with individual towels that have been dipped in a chlorine solution of 200 parts per million. When cloth towels are used they should be washed after use and left to soak in a chlorine solution until the next milking. Udders should be dried after washing and before milking is started. Paper towels have been demonstrated as practical in some herds for udder washing and may be discarded after a single use.

4. Using one of the so-called "fast-milking" programs can be depended on to decrease the incidence of mastitis in any herd. All cows can't be milked in the same length of time, so allowances will have to be made in this respect. Hand stripping may have to be followed at times in order to do a good job, for any degree of mastitis is apt to be made worse by leaving variable amounts of milk in the udder. With this being true, some animals may have to be entirely milked by hand, for occasional beasts just won't "let down" their milk to machines. Regardless of the modifications made necessary, all cows should be milked just as fast as possible to insure cleaner milking.

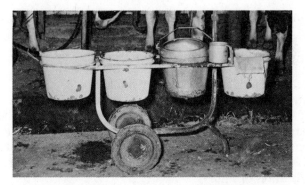

A portable cart like this one will help a fast milking program to aid in mastitis prevention.

5. Milking machines should be dipped between cows to prevent spread of germs. This is best done by using two pails, one containing clear water and the other a chlorine solution such as used for washing udders. Milk is washed off by first dipping in the clear water and disinfection

then accomplished by dipping in the chlorine. The clear water is best changed every four or five cows. It's true that dipping in the chlorine doesn't kill all the germs to be found in the teat cups. However, it at least washes away a lot of them and kills a few, so we consider the practice as having merit. Whatever view is held regarding the cause of mastitis, repeated trials have shown that cleanliness and disinfection at milking time always reduce the amount of trouble caused by the disease.

6. When hand milking is done the hands should be washed and disinfected between cows just as in the case of teat cups.

7. After milking is completed it is advisable to dip the ends of teats in chlorine solution such as used for washing udders at the start of milking. This can be done quickly by using about a half pint of solution in a shallow basin that is big enough to take the ends of all four teats at once. The chlorine can be used on 25-30 cows before being replaced with fresh solution.

Vaccination with various products has not been generally successful for either the prevention or treatment of mastitis. The same is true in regard to the feeding of certain minerals and vitamins that have been advertised for this purpose.

Injured Teats

CAUSE. Generally through trampling by other animals, but large-uddered cows will sometimes step on their own teats while trying to regain their feet after lying down. Barbed wire and glass are other common causes of udder injuries.

SYMPTOMS. Usually a badly mashed teat that is sore and swollen in addition to being torn. Cuts are likely to bleed badly and leave dangling pieces of skin. Milk usually leaks out if the streak canal or teat cistern has been opened. At times the skin is not broken and soreness or inability to get milk out of a teat may be the only indication of injury.

TREATMENT. Mainly concerned with preventing infection that is likely to result in mastitis. Wounds should first be thoroughly cleaned with water and a mild antiseptic. Hydrogen of peroxide is useful in deep wounds for its boiling action helps to bring out particles of dirt. When cleaning has been completed the injury should be carefully dried with cotton since water retards healing. If the streak canal or teat cistern has been opened the cut edges of these structures can be stitched together with catgut, although healing is generally unsatisfactory in a lactating cow because of the constant dripping of milk. At this point it is advisable to apply some kind of a healing agent to the wound, and the penicillin ointment commonly used for mastitis treatment is excellent for this purpose.

The edges of wounds that run lengthwise of the teat can be pinched together with the fingers and held in that position by strips of adhesive tape that are laid across them and around the teat. At other times they may be stitched or held with tiny metal clips made especially for closing wounds, although resultant swelling usually causes them to pull out. Wounds running around the teat are treated in the same way. If the cut is bad and has opened the streak canal or teat cistern, it may be best to cut off the dangling end of the teat and touch it with silver nitrate to control bleeding.

Raw surfaces on the end of the teat resulting from such amputation or other causes are particularly likely to cause mastitis and should be kept bandaged between milkings. This is easily done by folding gauze to form a small square and then laying two strips of adhesive tape across it at right angles to each other with the "sticky" side of one against the gauze. The bandage can then be placed on the end of the teat with the tape being carried up the sides to hold it in place. Another strip or two of tape can be laid

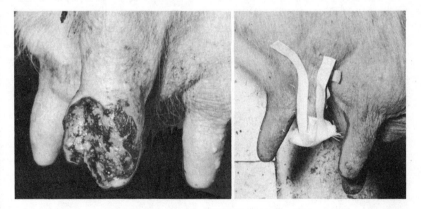

Left: Teat injury due to trampling by neighboring cow.
Right: Bandaging the end of an injured teat may be the means of preventing a bad attack of mastitis.

over them and around the teat if desired. When injuries are severe it may be desirable to use a milk tube until healing is well advanced. Such a procedure avoids further injury at milking time and allows the wound edges to grow together rapidly.

PREVENTION. Largely through providing well-bedded stalls of ample width that are protected against invasion by adjoining animals. Keeping premises clear of loose barbed wire and similar material will also prevent a great many teat injuries.

Milk Fever (Parturient Paresis)

CAUSE. Basically a deficiency of calcium in the blood due to its sudden withdrawal for colostrum at the same time that there is a delay in resorption of the mineral from the bones or its absorption from the digestive tract. The condition appears to be related to age (older cows are more susceptible); the calcium content, phosphorus content, and the acidity of the ration; and possibly the release of a hormone produced by the thyroid gland which interferes with calcium resorption from the bones. Body mechanisms that effectively prevent a calcium deficiency before calving apparently are not able to change quickly enough to prevent it following a sudden withdrawal of the mineral after calving. The lack of calcium may also be to blame for a deficiency of phosphorus in the blood because of a lowered absorption of phosphorus from the digestive tract and an increase in a hormone produced by the parathyroid glands.

SYMPTOMS. Food and water are completely refused, and the disease usually appears shortly before or after calving, although it may be seen weeks later. The earliest symptoms are usually staggering and an uncertain gait in combination with weakness and evident lack of coordination in the hind legs. There may be twitching of the muscles and various kinds of crazy actions, but affected animals usually get progressively duller and more reluctant to move

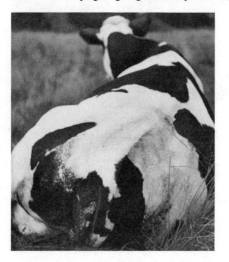

Typical S-curve of cow's neck indicating milk fever.

until they finally go down in a paralyzed condition. There is no passage of manure and urine in the latter stages, and a "downer" cow frequently turns her head around to the side in a characteristic position. At other times the head remains extended but with the neck bent into an S-shaped curve. Strangely enough there is seldom any fever, and the body temperature may actually be a little below normal. Bloating frequently occurs, especially if animals are allowed to stretch out flat on the ground. Milk fever is rarely seen in first-calf heifers.

DIAGNOSIS. Usually through the appearance of suggestive symptoms close to calving time or a history of milk fever attacks in former years. The diagnosis of this disease may be complicated by at least two factors:

1. It may appear in cows other than at calving time, especially during heat periods when eating is somewhat neglected. If available, a test for blood calcium will often prove helpful for the diagnosis of milk fever in such animals.

2. Many symptoms of milk fever are the same as for other diseases which may actually be causing trouble. These include acetonemia, hardware disease, mastitis, metritis, bloat, calf paralysis, fractured pelvis, grass tetany, railroad sickness, and heat stroke. In an emergency it may be necessary to give treatment for milk fever in order to establish a diagnosis. Improvement within a few minutes indicates milk fever, otherwise something else is to blame. However, it must be remembered that the intravenous injection of calcium preparations may kill a cow that does not have milk fever, so this can be seen as a risky business.

TREATMENT. Usually a pint of calcium gluconate solution warmed to body temperature and given intravenously very slowly. This is particularly important since rapid administration may result in sudden death through heart failure. The dose may have to be repeated, or an extra pint of calcium gluconate given under the skin to prolong the period of availability. When acetonemia exists in connection with milk fever as it often does, calcium gluconate may be combined with dextrose in a solution.

An older but equally effective treatment consists of inflating the udder with air to prevent further secretion of milk and additional loss of calcium from the blood. A milk tube and some kind of pump is needed, and extreme care must be used in regard to cleanliness. Each quarter is inflated separately and teats are tied off with strips of gauze to retain the air. These strips should be removed every two or three hours to permit circulation of blood or the ends of the teats may become gangrenous and drop off. Udder inflation may be repeated in six hours if considerable improvement isn't noted. This method is objectionable because a lack of sterile equipment often leads to infection that results in a bad case of mastitis.

Sick animals should be propped up in a normal position with bales of hay, etc., in order to prevent severe bloating. Drenching must never be attempted under any conditions. This is because swallowing is impossible and liquids poured down the throat are pretty sure to go into the lungs and cause fatal pneumonia. Aside from that, the medicines would do no good even if they were placed directly in the stomach, for milk fever can't be cured in that way. It is best to skip one milking completely, and animals should not be milked entirely dry for at least three days after treatment has been given. Calves should be removed from the cows and not permitted to suck them again during the three-day period. Failure to observe these precautions is likely to cause a relapse through encouraging milk production at a time when the cow is in an abnormal condition.

PREVENTION. There are no measures that will prevent all cases of milk fever. However, the following represent good management and are often helpful:

1. Give cows a dry period of at least six weeks.
2. Give animals plenty of exercise in late stages of pregnancy.
3. Feed light laxative rations two weeks before calving.
4. Remove calves from dams after they have sucked once.
5. Don't milk cows entirely dry first three days after calving.

Experimental work in regard to preventing milk fever has been carried on by both California and Ohio State University scientists.

The California work* is concerned with the relative amounts of calcium and phosphorus in the rations of dry cows. It was carried on by Drs. J. M. Boda and H. H. Cole in a herd of high-producing Jerseys that had suffered a high percentage of cases over a period of several years. They concluded that milk fever is a result of improper functioning of the parathyroid glands which supply calcium. It was theorized that these glands become relatively inactive while the cow is dry, and then they just can't get going fast enough when a lot of calcium is suddenly needed after calving. They reasoned that if most of the calcium was taken out of a dry

* Hoard's Dairyman, January 10, 1954, page 11.

cow's ration, the parathyroids might be forced to keep on working during the dry period and be fairly active at freshening time.

Their experimental work over a period of two and a half years indicates that a low-calcium, high-phosphorus ration fed to dry cows for about a month before calving time will prevent most cases of milk fever. The opposite type of ration, high in calcium and low in phosphorus, seems to encourage the occurrence of it.

The California low-calcium, high-phosphorus ration is made by mixing 800 pounds of ground barley, 500 pounds of wheat bran, 600 pounds of rolled barley, 100 pounds of cottonseed meal, 40 pounds of monosodium phosphate, and 10 pounds of salt. Each dry cow gets eight pounds of the above mix daily, along with eight pounds of oat hay or some other type of roughage similarly low in calcium. Such a plan of feeding means that the dry cows must be isolated in a barn or lot during the last month before calving.

The Ohio State work** involves the feeding of large amounts of vitamin D just before calving, and was reported by Drs. J. W. Hibbs and W. D. Pounden. This vitamin is needed by the body in order to make use of calcium and phosphorus, and supplying it enables the cow to draw extra calcium from her bones when it is suddenly needed for milk. The work was carried out in the Experiment Station herds, involving 48 mature Jersey cows which had previous histories of milk fever. No symptoms at all were observed in the 14 cows fed 20 to 30 million units of vitamin D daily for 5 to 7 days before calving. One of the 12 cows receiving 10 million units of vitamin D daily had an attack of milk fever. Fourteen of the remaining 22 cows which served as controls and received no vitamin D, had milk fever.

The feeding of vitamin D in the bigger doses maintained blood calcium at a higher than normal level during the critical period following calving. The vitamin apparently acted as a temporary substitute for the parathyroid glands, probably by increasing the absorption of calcium from the digestive tract. This results in a "buffering" effect against the sudden withdrawal of blood calcium brought on by the beginning of milk production. Experiments carried out in cooperation with the Ohio State Veterinary College showed that if the period of dosage is limited to five to seven days, no harmful effects are likely to result from feeding several million units of the vitamin daily. However, prolonged feeding of it is dangerous. Abnormal heart action and calcium deposits in the

** Journal of Dairy Science, *37*, 1955, page 65.

heart and blood vessels were among the bad effects noted. Accordingly, it is recommended that massive doses of vitamin D should not be fed for longer than seven days. Little protection was given against milk fever until the vitamin D had been fed for at least three days, and the protection disappeared within two or three days after such feeding was stopped.

This vitamin D feeding plan won't always work out on a farm, because there is no way of telling exactly when a cow is going to freshen. The breeding date will help considerably in estimating the time of calving, but no less than eight different factors may lengthen or shorten the normal gestation period by a week or so. About the best an owner can do is to try and time the vitamin feeding so it is started at least three days before and preferably a week before the calf is born. If it is started too early, the feeding will do no good in the event it has to be stopped two or three days before the calf is born; if started too late, it won't do any good, since it takes two or three days for the effects of vitamin D to show up.

A low calcium intake in the weeks before calving will often prevent milk fever if no other steps are taken. Accordingly, it is not yet certain that the administration of vitamin D in connection with such feeding will provide extra insurance against the trouble. At this time the following are suggested as preventive measures:

1. Limit the calcium intake to about an ounce daily for a few weeks before calving. It should be remembered that alfalfa hay has by far the highest calcium content of all common feed-stuffs, and that its use should be avoided in the feeding of cows in advanced pregnancy. Oat hay and corn silage are particularly low in calcium, and grass hays are also low in this mineral. All the common grains are low in calcium, and corn is lowest of all.

2. Do not include additives containing calcium in concentrate mixtures fed before calving.

3. Avoid the mixing of calcium supplements like dicalcium phosphate with salt for cows before calving. This is because the calcium intake may become quite high, especially during spells of hot weather when extra salt may be craved.

4. When a program of low calcium intake is followed, a ten-million unit dose of vitamin D may be injected intramuscularly two to six days before calving. There is little danger of adverse effects following such dosage, but it may not do a great deal of good, either.

5. If it is impractical to limit the calcium intake, the phosphorus intake should be adjusted so it is equal to or slightly higher than the calcium intake. In such cases the vitamin D treatment may give extra protection, but some undesirable side effects may also occur following its use.

6. Increase the calcium intake immediately after calving to 3 to 5 ounces daily. Dicalcium phosphate or limestone should replace sodium phosphate in the ration.

7. All changes, either in the type of roughage or amount of concentrates being fed, should be made gradually. Increases in amounts of concentrates should not exceed a couple of pounds daily.

Giving calcium gluconate before the appearance of symptoms is likely to be both impractical and dangerous. For one thing, there is no way of knowing ahead of time whether or not a cow is going to have milk fever. For another, the injection of calcium at such a time may actually do damage by upsetting the calcium: phosphorus ratio so that an attack of milk fever is actually encouraged or a cow is killed by overstimulation of the heart.

Grass Tetany (Grass Staggers, Wheat Poisoning)

CAUSE. Not exactly known, but some kind of an upset in metabolism produces a low magensium content in the blood. One authority has called it a "metabolic disease caused by the soil." The condition is evidently made worse by exposure of animals to cold, wet weather. Poor winter feeding also seems to be a predisposing factor, especially when rations have been low in roughage, or animals have been running on poor pasture. Under such conditions this trouble is known in some areas as "winter tetany," and does not seem to be dependent on green feed at all. A similar condition has been described in Norwegian cattle that had been fed on herring meal and poor quality roughage. Bad attacks have also been reported in beef cattle running on grass following rains in the late fall or early winter.

Some authorities believe that the magnesium deficiency is brought about by substances in the green feeds which make the mineral unavailable. Others contend that the deficiency is related to factors in the ration like low intakes of carbohydrates, protein, and dry matter, and high intakes of elements like potassium, phosphorus, nitrogen, and manganese. In some cases it appears that a shortage of calcium is also involved, so that even a low level of magnesium may be too much, and the faulty ratio can cause trouble. At the other extreme, too much calcium in proportion to magnesium might be expected to cause typical symptoms like convulsions.

SYMPTOMS. Generally much like those of milk fever, but often with twitching of muscles, grinding of teeth, and frequent urination that is more like the nervous form of acetonemia. Sometimes animals are sent into convulsions by a sudden noise or touch, with muscles becoming stiff and the third eyelid protruded as if they were affected with lockjaw. The temperature usually remains normal, although the breathing rate may be greatly reduced. A chronic type of this disease causes high-producing cows to gradually lose weight over periods of weeks or months. They are often thought to be "milking themselves down," for the appetite and milk production remain normal. Trouble is unsuspected until typical symptoms are shown, when poisoning may be blamed for convulsions and death. Symptoms vary widely according to severity of attacks, and there are several intermediary forms between the chronic and suddenly-appearing types. Attacks usually occur shortly after turning cattle onto lush grass in the spring or luxurious legumes later in the year. It is most often seen in heavy-producing cows, but is not always connected with lactation since dry cows and even young stock are sometimes affected. Most of the severe cases end in death unless prompt treatment is available.

DIAGNOSIS. Can usually be made on the basis of suspicious symptoms occurring after an extended period of feeding on poor rations or following shortly after animals have been turned into lush green pastures. Urine tests may be helpful, for urinary magnesium falls to extremely low levels during an attack of grass tetany. However, such testing is likely to be useless after treatment with calcium solutions. Sometimes the failure of calcium treatments will indicate the possibility of grass tetany. If animals are found dead, the disease must be differentiated from other possible causes of sudden death. Under field conditions grass tetany might be confused with milk fever, lockjaw, rabies, acetonemia, lead poisoning, lightning stroke, heat stroke, and various kinds of plant poisoning.

TREATMENT. Preferably a combined calcium gluconate and magnesium solution given intravenously in 500 cc. doses. In cases of emergency a 25 per cent solution of Epsom salts (magnesium sulfate) given subcutaneously may help, although the drug is not available so quickly and the lost time may mean the difference between life and death for an animal. Intravenous injections should be made cautiously as recommended for milk fever.

If at all possible, affected animals should be moved to a quiet place after treatment, and supplied with good quality legume hay. Relapses should be expected in severe cases, and can be largely prevented by subcutaneous injections of magnesium salts or magnesium oxide given by mouth at the rate of 2 ounces per day per animal for a week and then tapered off. Continued treatment may result in the eventual recovery of animals that do not respond immediately. Mild cases may require only the first treatment.

PREVENTION. Through inclusion of at least 0.2% magnesium in the dry matter of the ration. If the magnesium content is not known, about an ounce and a quarter should be added daily for cows. This is present in two ounces of magnesia (magnesium oxide), or four ounces of magnesium carbonate.

Magnesia is preferred for mixing with grain, and should be added to the amount fed. For example, if 14 pounds of concentrates are fed, then 20 pounds of magnesia should be added per ton. Similarly, if 7 pounds are fed, then 40 pounds of magnesia should be added per ton of concentrate.

Calves can be protected by feeding a half-ounce of magnesia every other day. The magnesium content of the ration can be raised by providing good clover or alfalfa hay, and such feeding is recommended for treated animals as well as for part of a preventive program.

If exposed animals are not given grain supplements, the magnesium can be mixed with equal parts of salt and provided on a free choice basis. However, it will not prove very helpful unless cattle are hungry for salt, since they seem to have no particular desire for magnesium. An alternative is to mix the magnesia with equal parts of molasses and put this out on a free choice basis. Most of the cattle will lick at such a mixture. Another procedure consists of dusting the pasture with about 30 pounds of magnesia per acre. This will ordinarily stick to plants for a couple of weeks or so. Experiments in Holland indicate that topdressing pastures with magnesium compounds instead of straight potash fertilizers will reduce the number of grass tetany cases.

It is believed that the feeding of balanced rations which include plenty of good quality roughage during the winter will help to protect cattle against grass tetany when they are turned to pasture in the spring. Some authorities believe that taking cattle off pastures at night and feeding them hay for the first two weeks of the pasture season is helpful in preventing this trouble.

Milk Sickness (Trembles)

CAUSE. Either white snakeroot, a plant which grows from the eastern United States westward to Oklahoma, or rayless goldenrod, a plant which grows from Colorado southward to Texas. Cattle are usually poisoned on pasture, but the dried plants are also poisonous although to a lesser degree than the green ones. The poisonous factor is transmitted through milk to calves and human beings. Animals may be killed either by eating small amounts of the plants for a long time, or by eating a large amount at one time.

SYMPTOMS. The first ones are trembling of the muzzle and legs, but the trembling soon involves most of the body muscles. The tremors are accompanied by loss of appetite, constipation, loss of weight, and weakness that eventually causes the animal to go down. In the final stages there is labored breathing, grinding of the teeth, and loss of consciousness which is followed by death. There is no fever. Symptoms may persist from a day or two to a week or so, depending on the amount of plants eaten. Calves that are nursing affected cows may also be poisoned and show symptoms.

TREATMENT. Begins with removal from the causative pasture. The animals may then be given supportive treatment like dextrose solutions and stimulants as indicated. Milk should be withheld from calves but the cows should be milked frequently to speed up excretion of the poisonous factor.

PREVENTION. Entirely a matter of pasture control to eliminate the causative plants. Measures listed under poisoning by plants in this book will prove helpful.

Mammillitis

CAUSE. A virus. Although known in Great Britain since 1966, this disease was unknown in the United States until 1969, when it was diagnosed in Minnesota. It probably exists in other states.

MEANS OF SPREAD. Not definitely known, and the way it is originally introduced into an area is also unknown. Herds on adjoining farms often become infected, but isolated outbreaks have also been reported. Milking machines and milkers' hands have been blamed for spread within a herd, but isolation of infected animals and washing of udders has seldom proved effective in preventing spread. It has been suggested that biting flies may cause undetected skin reactions in other parts of the body and that this then gives considerable resistance to mammary infection. This would explain the semi-immunity of older cows in many outbreaks, with the flies thus becoming spreaders of the disease.

SYMPTOMS. The first one may be chapping of the teats of older cows that evidently carry some degree of resistance to the disease. This may then spread to cause serious symptoms in susceptible newly calved heifers or adult animals. However, in most cases the first symptom is the sudden appearance of blister-like vesicles on the udder and teats, particularly at the base of the teats. When these lesions appear, the entire teat is apt to swell, develop a translucent appearance like milk glass, and sometimes turn blue in color.

Within a short time the vesicles rupture to leave one of two different kinds of ulcers. Some of them are deep and painful which may cover an entire teat and remain raw for weeks. Others remain soft and are soon covered with a thick brown scab which bleeds profusely if broken.

In less severe forms swollen plaques instead of vesicles develop on the udder and teats, and ulceration is shallow. Such lesions remain dry, and do not appear to be very sore, although the skin of the teat may turn blue-black in color.

Milk production may fall off by 20% or more, the milk is likely to be contaminated with blood, and cows resent being milked. In addition, serious mastitis complications are almost sure to go along with this disease. Outbreaks seem to be commonest during the late fall or early winter, and only milking cows or those recently turned dry are likely to be affected. Mild cases may last for only a week or so, but the severe ones may persist for two or three months. The general health of affected animals remains good unless secondary infections like mastitis develop. Some degree of immunity evidently develops after an attack, although one recurrence has been reported 13 months after the first infection.

DIAGNOSIS. Definite only through laboratory tests, although a tentative diagnosis can often be made in severe cases on the basis of the deep ulceration following rupture of the vesicles. Under field conditions mammillitis might be confused with cowpox, pseudo cowpox, and papular stomatitis.

TREATMENT. None satisfactory, but mild ointments and oily

preparations may be used to help healing of the ulcers. In case of an outbreak, spread can be controlled to some extent by milking the older and unaffected cows first, and the infected animals last.

PREVENTION. No preventive measures can be given at this time, but research work on calves indicates that it might be practical to vaccinate animals with the live virus on parts of the body other than the udder. This would correspond to the resistance tentatively credited to biting flies. Such vaccination would be extremely undesirable unless the disease became a problem in certain areas, and would require official permission by state and federal regulatory agencies.

Acetonemia or Ketosis

CAUSE. Essentially unknown, although an accumulation of so-called "ketone bodies" and a deficiency of sugar in the blood are responsible for the symptoms. The "ketone bodies" are waste productions of digestion that are evidently increased by a lack of carbohydrates in the diet. This may result from almost anything that will cause a cow to draw on her body fat at a rapid rate. For example, an animal may go "off feed" for some reason or other at calving time and be forced to live off her body reserves instead of nutrients ordinarily furnished by feed. Lacking carbohydrates needed for complete digestion, considerable of the "ketone bodies" accumulate in the system to cause acetonemia.

The same sort of thing may happen when cows have been producing heavily for a few weeks, even though they have been eating well all the time. In such cases the animals just haven't been able to eat enough to meet the demands of milk production while maintaining their bodies. Consequently, they "milk down" and may develop acetonemia if the fat is drawn off at too rapid a rate. The well-known fact that excessive fat is quickly used up by fresh cows probably explains why many of our well-fitted show animals are subject to the disease shortly before or after calving. Grass ensiled at the wrong stage may result in silage containing an excess of butyric acid so it is capable of causing acetonemia. As in the case of milk fever, a disturbance of metabolism is suspected of being the basic cause of acetonemia.

SYMPTOMS. Dependent on one of the three recognized forms:
1. *Digestive.* Usually a marked decrease in milk production accompanied by a severe loss of weight in an extremely short time. Animals may go completely "off feed" or be

"picky" about grain while continuing to eat hay and silage about as usual. The symptoms usually appear gradually and aren't noticed until they really become serious. Animals often appear to be "bound up" although a diarrhea is not unknown. Arching of the back, lowering of the head, dullness, and a sleepy expression are characteristic. Temperatures are usually normal, although extremely high fevers have been reported at various times. This form is commonly seen a month or six weeks after freshening, but may even appear before calving.

2. *Milk Fever.* So-called because this type shows the same symptoms listed for milk fever under that disorder. Animals appear wobbly on their feet and eventually go down in a paralyzed condition. When such symptoms are shown it is practically impossible to tell acetonemia from milk fever. As a matter of fact, both acetonemia and milk fever may affect a cow at the same time, and such a doubling-up of diseases often occurs.

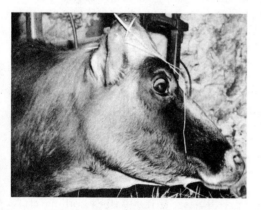

Cow with typical wild-eyed expression often seen in the nervous form of acetonemia.

3. *Nervous.* Delirium and crazy actions that may include almost anything. The expression is wild, bellowing is common, and people may even be attacked. Animals may jerk out of stanchions and appear blind to the extent of running into walls and fences. They may grind their teeth, lick themselves, walk in circles, lean forward in stanchions, or roll their eyes. Sometimes they stagger, slobber, suck their tongues, and stand with their legs spraddled or crossed. Frequently there is violent twitching of muscles and occasionally even convulsions.

Any or all of these symptoms may appear in a given case, for there is no sharp line drawn between the three different forms. Loss of appetite and lowered milk production is common in all of them, although cows sometimes continue to milk heavily even when they have been made extremely thin by the disease. Dairy cows and heifers are usually affected, with attacks coming either shortly before freshening or several weeks afterward. Affected cows frequently give off a body odor of acetone, which is sweetish and somewhat like chloroform. The same odor can frequently be detected in milk or urine from the animals, too.

DIAGNOSIS. Chiefly on the basis of symptoms, with the so-called Ross test used to confirm suspicions. Ready-mixed solutions are available through veterinarians so owners can run their own tests. A few drops of the solutions mixed with a sample of urine will show a color change to some degree of purple when "ketone bodies" are present in abnormal amounts. The darkness of color and rapidity of color change will often serve to show the severity of an attack. In mild cases the color may be little more than pink and take nine or ten minutes to develop, while in severe ones the urine may become almost black in a few seconds. Tablets with concave surfaces are also available from veterinarians for running the test. They are used by simply adding a drop of urine to one of the depressions and watching for color changes in the tablet.

Although more expensive, a testing powder may be compounded at home for testing suspected urine. It is made by mixing one part of finely powdered nitroprusside with 100 parts of pure ammonium sulfate. It is used with sodium hydroxide flakes for the acetone test. A pinch of the compound is dissolved in a teaspoonful of urine and a small flake of the sodium hydroxide is then added to see if a purple color develops.

A reaction to the test alone does not furnish definite proof that acetonemia is the primary disease. It really does nothing more than indicate the use of considerable body fat at a time when there is a shortage of sugar that is available for use in digestive processes. Under these conditions a large number of perfectly healthy cows will be found as reactors to the urine test. Reactions may also be due to various types of illness that have made cows go "off feed" and dependent on body reserves for continued life. Consequently, the test must be regarded as only a handy tool that must be used in connection with other symptoms. In its various forms acetonemia may be confused with indigestion, hardware trouble, circling disease, rabies, metritis, and other ailments.

TREATMENT. Sterile sugar solutions given intravenously in 500 cc. doses are probably the most practical in uncomplicated cases. One or several doses of 40-50 per cent solutions may be needed for complete recovery. A pint of stock molasses or a pound of cane sugar given orally every day is usually recommended as treatment in connection with the solutions given intravenously. Such feeding may be continued as long as needed, but the amount may have to be reduced in the event scouring develops. An ounce of chloral hydrate dissolved in a quart of water and given once or twice a day will help to quiet delirious animals, and is also claimed as useful in freeing glycogen from the liver to provide a natural sugar for use in digestive processes.

If above treatments fail, other remedies may be tried. These include vitamin A, cobalt, insulin, pituitary extract, epsom salts, cortisone, and ACTH. Glycerin has also been recognized as a treatment for acetonemia. A similar compound, propylene glycol, has been reported from the University of Georgia as being effective in several cases. It has the advantage of being much cheaper than glycerin. The recommended dosage is four ounces given orally twice daily, with improvement being expected in two or three days.

In work at Wisconsin and Cornell University, Dr. L. H. Schultz has reported beneficial results from the use of either sodium acetate or sodium proprionate. These are given orally, either mixed with grain or as a drench, with the sodium proprionate appearing as a little more effective than sodium acetate. Since both are rather unpalatable, cows may refuse to eat grain rations containing these compounds in suitable amounts and so make drenching necessary. The recommended dosage calls for about a half pound daily of either the acetate or proprionate. The feeding of smaller amounts, such as a tablespoonful or two, three times a day, isn't likely to do any good at all, and it seems likely that many failures with these compounds have been due to unduly small doses. They may be obtained as calcium acetate and calcium proprionate, and appear equally as effective as the sodium salts. However, the calcium compounds aren't so soluble as the sodium salts, and aren't so popular because of this fact.

Whatever treatment is used, it may be advisable to remove only part of the milk or stop milking entirely for a few days to aid recovery. This practice is recommended only in the case of cows with healthy udders, since mastitis may otherwise result. When grass silage with a particularly bad odor is being fed, treatment will often be helped by withdrawing the silage for a few days. Most acetonemia cases recover after varied courses and lengths of time, but occasional animals aren't helped by any kind of treatment and waste away to skin and bones while drying up completely.

PREVENTION. No recommendations can be made that will prove 100% effective in all cases, but any of these may prove helpful:
1. Give cows 2-4 ounces daily of sodium propionate.
2. Feed cows so they aren't excessively fat at calving time.
3. Bring cows to full feed quickly after calving.
4. Feed poor quality grass silage very sparingly.
5. Avoid making abrupt changes in types of roughage.
6. Be sure that the ration contains at least 14% protein.

Drs. G. M. Umberger and W. S. Boley of Harveyville, Kansas, recently reported favorably on the use of an iodine compound over a one-year period in a dairy herd with a history of much ketosis. During this year the iodine compound was added to the daily ration of each cow, beginning the day after she calved and continuing for 30 days. The complete report was published in the October 1956 issue of the *North American Veterinarian* (vol. 37, no. 10, page 841), and follows in part:

Ketosis had been a serious problem in this herd for several years. During the 1953 season, seven (41 per cent) of 17 cows developed clinical ketosis within a week after calving. In 1954, there were 11 cases (46 per cent) among the 24 cows calving. With one exception, all the cows that had ketosis in 1953 had it again in 1954. One cow had it three years in succession.

The iodine compound was added to the ration beginning in November, 1954. At this time the grain feed consisted of soybean oil meal, bran, ground milo, ground oats, and 1 per cent salt. Later the soybean oil meal was replaced by a 32 per cent concentrate. The iodine compound was added to the ration in these three ways:
1. Feeding salt. Added at the rate of ½ pound per 100 lb. salt and made available free-choice to the cows on pasture.
2. Grain feed. Mixed with salt (¼ lb. per 100 lb. salt) and this mixture was incorporated as 1 per cent of the grain mixture.
3. Postpartum supplement. As each cow calved she was given 1 tablespoonful of the iodine compound daily in her feed. At first these daily doses were continued for only 10 days. But when two cows developed ketosis right after discontinuance of the compound, the period of supplementation was extended to 30 days, after which no more ketosis developed.

As shown by this report, there were only two cases of ketosis in 24 calvings in 1955, and these two cases occurred after the owner stopped the daily feeding of the iodine compound. Even so, the incidence of ketosis fell from 46 per cent to 8 per cent when iodine was added to the feed. On the basis of what is known about the stimulation of the thyroid by iodine, and through it the anterior pituitary gland, there is good reason to believe it also increases the output of various hormones. Accordingly, any action from the feeding of an iodine compound seems comparable with the action of ACTH, cortisone, and other hormones that help to maintain normal blood sugar levels. The compound used in the Kansas herd is the same one mentioned in this book as useful in the prevention and treatment of foot rot, and can be obtained through your veterinarian.

From a practical standpoint it seems advisable to do everything possible to keep animals from going "off feed" close to freshening time. Sometimes it's pretty hard to decide whether cows have gone "off feed" because of acetonemia or have developed acetonemia because of being "off feed."

Railroad Sickness or Transport Tetany

CAUSE. Essentially unknown but a deficiency of calcium in the blood is definitely involved. It is brought about by transportation in hot trucks or railroad cars without food and water for long periods. The most susceptible animals seem to be those in good condition that have recently been removed from pasture and are in advanced stages of pregnancy.

SYMPTOMS. Much the same as for milk fever or the nervous form of acetonemia. Attacks usually develop shortly after unloading, but they may occur while animals are still in transit. Food is generally refused entirely, but there may be extreme thirst. Animals under five years old and less than seven months pregnant are seldom affected, and the disease appears almost entirely during the summer months. Stricken cows may improve within a few hours, especially if they give birth to calves during an attack. Those that show no improvement within three days generally have poor chances of surviving, and under any conditions the death rate is usually high.

DIAGNOSIS. Generally through symptoms in connection with advanced pregnancy and recent shipment. May be confused with milk fever, acetonemia, shipping fever, and diseases with similar symptoms.

TREATMENT. The same as given for milk fever, although the percentage of recoveries cannot be expected to be equally high. Chloral hydrate as given for acetonemia is useful for quieting violent animals.

PREVENTION. Moving animals off pastures and keeping them in barns for a couple of days before shipment is regarded as helpful. The beasts should then be loaded as quietly as possible and given plenty of room in well-ventilated quarters. The feeding of hay throughout the trip and frequent watering is desirable, and it has been reported helpful to keep cows in lots or pastures for a short time after they are unloaded.

Suppurative Dermatitis

CAUSE. Several different types of pus-forming bacteria which infect the skin of the udder. May start in chafed or "scalded" areas or be introduced through materials like barley straw and green sawdust that are used for bedding.

SYMPTOMS. A painfully raw and bad smelling area of the udder. Commonly appears where the halves rub together or against the inside of the hind legs, but may affect any part of the organ. In advanced cases there may be actual rotting of the flesh and deep penetration of tissues. Investigating the source of a bad odor frequently leads owners to a trouble not previously suspected.

DIAGNOSIS. Usually through the appearance and smell of raw areas in locations subject to friction and "scalding." May be confused with mange, light sensitization, or "blowing" by flies.

TREATMENT. Chiefly by keeping affected areas clean. They are best washed thoroughly with mild soap and warm water before each milking, afterward being carefully dried with a soft cloth or towel. The sores can then be well-soaked with white lotion, an old remedy that is made by mixing 6 drams of zinc sulfate and one ounce of lead acetate in a pint of water. Ready-mixed tablets that require only the addition of water to make white lotion, can also be obtained from veterinarians. Since the ingredients settle out on standing, this preparation must be well shaken before each usage. The white lotion is generally preferred over ointments because it dries quickly and kills germs without collecting dirt. Miracles must not be expected in advanced cases, for the infection is often hard to conquer and may require weeks of diligent attention.

PREVENTION. Principally a matter of keeping stables clean. Cows with large udders are particularly susceptible to chafing and should be regularly examined for early symptoms of trouble. Treatment with white lotion may be started as soon as they are discovered.

Sore Teats

CAUSE. Often chapping due to exposure of wet teats to cold and wind. Also from sunburn, freezing, fungi on plants, overstrong disinfectants, irritation by flies, and infection by various types of bacteria found in mud and filth.

SYMPTOMS. Usually "stepping" and kicking by cows because of pain at milking time. Investigation may reveal bleeding cracks or irritated areas of the teats.

DIAGNOSIS. Usually through the appearance of the affected areas. Must be distinguished from the small red swellings and pustules associated with the two types of cowpox which are discussed elsewhere in this book.

TREATMENT. The same procedures and remedies suggested for use against the false type of cowpox are equally effective against the various causes given for sore teats.

PREVENTION. Entirely a matter of management designed to eliminate the causes. A coating of sulfathiazole ointment applied after each milking is particularly effective for protecting teats against mud and wet pasture plants that may be causing soreness.

Bloody Milk

CAUSE. Several different ones that may be listed as:

1. Udder injuries through falls, kicks, "hooking," etc., that rupture small blood vessels and permits blood to mix with milk.
2. Congestion at freshening time that has the same effect.
3. Mastitis attacks that may do the same thing while causing destruction of tissue.
4. Diseases like bacillary hemoglobinuria and leptospirosis.
5. Drugs like phenothiazine have been reported as giving milk a red color to make it appear bloody when it really isn't.
6. Feeds like beets, pokeberries, etc., may do the same thing.
7. Certain types of bacteria growing in cans and other types of equipment may also give milk a red color resembling blood.
8. Warts and cuts on the outside of the teats may bleed enough to give milk a bloody color.

TREATMENT. Dependent on the cause. When due to udder congestion or injuries, the following are recommended:

1. Milking every three or four hours until the milk regains a normal color. It may take several days for the results of such treatment to become apparent.

2. Bathing and massaging the udder with a hot salt solution for a few minutes after every milking. Some of the standard udder balms and liniments may be substituted for the salt solution if desired.

3. Removal of the grain ration and replacing it with laxative feeds like bran until the milk clears up.

Cases that fail to respond under such treatment may be helped by intravenous injection of a pint of 2% formaldehyde solution or thromboplastin and gelatin compounds available through veterinarians.

PREVENTION. Largely a matter of correcting everything that may possibly cause udder injuries. This includes such things as high door sills, deep gutters, and others mentioned as causes of mastitis. Light feeding of laxative rations and plenty of exercise before calving will do a lot to prevent the appearance of bloody milk at freshening time. Exercising animals alone when they are approaching calving time may help. Such practice is designed to prevent udder injuries through accidents or fighting.

Udder Congestion, Udder Edema

CAUSE. Not definitely known, but essentially a collection of fluid, chiefly lymph, under the skin. It is closely related to high milk production, and the weight of the gravid uterus, increased capillary pressure, stepped-up physiological activity, and change of hormone dominance at freshening time are all recognized as contributing factors. During the period shortly before freshening, a considerable amount of extra blood is sent to the changing udder through arteries. Under normal conditions blood sent to the udder is promptly returned through veins, so no accumulation of fluid occurs. Under the conditions of impending milk production, pressure is lowered in the veins so blood cannot be returned as fast as it is sent in by the arteries. This results in a gradual accumulation of fluid in the tissues of the udder and belly, particularly in heifers that are developing an udder circulation for the first time. Heavy grain feeding was once believed to be a cause of udder edema, but tests at the University of

Illinois showed that this was not true. Workers found that cows, fed 12 pounds of grain daily, had no more edema than those receiving no grain. Similarly, heifers eating 9 pounds of grain daily had no more edema than those eating only hay and silage. Accordingly, most authorities now believe that this condition is largely due to the inheritance of a tendency to heavy milk production.

SYMPTOMS. Mainly a greatly distended udder that may even interfere with walking and movement of the hind legs which may occur several weeks before, and persist for nearly as long a period after calving. At times the serum and lymph that has invaded the tissues, spreads out under the skin to cause swellings along the belly which greatly enlarge the navel region and extend as far forward as the front legs. The milk may be bloody, and excessive weight may tear loose the fibrous attachments which hold the udder up against the body.

DIAGNOSIS. Made on the basis of swelling of the entire udder at calving time which has a tendency to gradually disappear after milking is started. It may be confused with chronic edema, or udder congestion due to mastitis, injuries, or abscesses. In chronic edema the swelling is usually confined to the rear quarters, and may extend up the back of the udder. Udder swelling due to mastitis, injuries, or abscesses is usually limited to only one or two quarters and may persist for long periods.

TREATMENT. Exercise, preferably alone to avoid danger of injury, is good with whatever other treatment is used. Other old remedies include things like massaging the udder for a half hour twice-daily with a mild non-blistering liniment or ointment, bathing the udder frequently with either a hot solution of Epsom salts or cold water, and placing the udder in a suspensory packed with chopped ice. All of these treatments are logical and eventually effective, but they take valuable time so they may not be used often and long enough for best results. Accordingly, many owners have turned to the use of drugs, recently demonstrated as effective in reducing udder edema by stimulation of the kidneys and elimination of the excess subcutaneous fluid through increased urine secretion. These are usually given as either a drench or bolus, and certainly represent a more convenient and faster method of treatment than any of the older ones. All of these drugs have been used effectively in the treatment of simple udder congestion: chlorothiazide (Diuril), hydrochlorothiazide (Vetidrex), acetazolamide (Vetamox), and various corticosteroids.

PREVENTION. Plenty of exercise both before and after calving is likely to be helpful, as in the case of treatment. As mentioned earlier, cutting down on the grain ration will not help to prevent udder edema. According to recent experiments, the milking of cows and heifers before calving has no value in preventing congestion of the udder, either. However, some authorities have pointed out that the pre-milking in the experiments was done only for a week or so before freshening, while many dairymen believe that it has to be started at least three weeks before calving, if it is to do any good.

Rupture of Prepubic Tendon

CAUSE. Usually an injury of some kind but may also result from excessive abdominal weight in advanced pregnancy or the condition known as hydrops amnion. The tendon is either broken or pulled loose from its attachments to the pubic bones.

SYMPTOMS. Dropping of the fore part of the udder and a huge swelling ahead of it which is because a great part of the internal organs are no longer held up in their normal positions. This is to be expected, for the chief supporting muscles of the belly are attached to the tendon and when it gives way all the supported structures also collapse. The condition may be confused with ruptures in the thin part of the rear belly wall which permit part of the intestines to escape under the skin.

TREATMENT. None available.

"Holding Up" Milk

CAUSE. Usually started by fear of the milking act or unusual occurrences causing disturbance in the barn at milking time. Changes in feeding or barn routine will encourage it, as well as things like sickness, pain, heat periods, removal of a calf that has been sucking, or washing udders too far in advance of milking. After occurring for a while it may become a habit. The trouble is poorly named, for a cow has no choice, and can no more "hold up" her milk than she can control the beating of her heart.

SYMPTOMS. Failure to give the expected amount of milk although the udder seems full. An increased yield is usually given at the next milking. Once it has become established as a habit, cows are apt to go dry after a short lactation period.

TREATMENT. Entirely a matter of eliminating the cause. Feeding at milking time may distract the attention enough so that milk will be yielded. Once well-established as a habit, it is doubtful if anything will help.

PREVENTION. Chiefly a matter of milking animals so they aren't hurt or scared while it is being done. This is particularly important in the case of first-calf heifers that are being broken to milk. When done properly animals usually learn to enjoy having their full udders emptied and cooperate in getting the job done. Since cows are creatures of habit, frequent changes in barn routine are to be avoided.

"Breaking Down" of Udder

CAUSE. Basically an inherited weakness of the coarse tissue which lies under the skin and helps bind the front quarters to the belly wall. Continued heavy production is a secondary factor that over a period of several years puts an extra strain on the weak tissue and causes it to gradually break away from its attachments.

SYMPTOMS. A depression of varying depth and width that extends around the tops of the front quarters and lowering of the udder because of broken attachments. In advanced cases the skin may appear to be the only fastening of the fore quarters. The condition causes no pain and does not interfere with production, being chiefly in the nature of an undesirable blemish and departure from accepted type.

TREATMENT. None available.

Milk Stones or Milk Calculi

CAUSE. Not definitely known, but suspected to be some type of udder infection that results in the formation of "stones" composed of calcium, fat, casein, and sometimes blood. These are usually found free in the teat cistern, but are sometimes attached to its walls by fibrous strings. Sometimes called a "spider."

SYMPTOMS. Occlusion of the streak canal that prevents passage of milk after a few squirts have been drawn. Manipulation of the teat will permit another few squirts and then the stoppage will recur. Having sharp irregular edges, manipulation of the "stone" may cause evidence of pain. It acts on the principle of a ball valve, and must get into a certain position in order to cut off the flow of milk. Stones may sometimes be felt with the fingers, particularly after they have entered the streak canal.

TREATMENT. The smaller "stones" can usually be squeezed out through the teat orifice by manipulation with the thumb and fingers. Cows may need to be restrained or a local anesthetic used on the teat to prevent kicking while this is being done. Stones that are attached with fibers will probably have to be cut loose with a special narrow-bladed knife that is introduced through the teat orifice. Larger stones may require nicking of the sphincter muscle on the inside to permit their passage through the streak canal.

"Blind" Quarter

CAUSE. Usually an injury that has resulted in the rosette or sides of the gland cistern growing together so milk can't enter the teat. Commonly due to calves sucking each other and chewing on

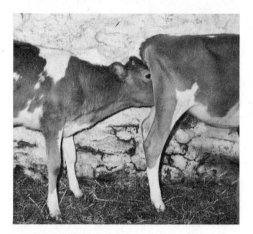

Heifer calves that suck each other may ruin tiny udders long before they produce any milk, and cause "blind" quarter.

the tiny udders. Infection of various kinds will have the same effect and sometimes much of the secreting tissue is grown together as well as the sides of the cistern. A defect of development may also leave a thin membrane across the bottom of the gland cistern to keep milk from coming down into the teat.

SYMPTOMS. No milk can be obtained from the quarter and none can be felt in the teat. The upper part of the quarter may appear to be full of milk or the entire quarter may be misshapen and plainly incapable of producing milk. This condition is not to be confused with occlusion of the streak canal, for in those cases the teat can be felt as full of milk.

TREATMENT. None available when parts of the quarter have grown together. A membrane across the gland cistern can be opened up by entering the teat orifice with special instruments.

"Hard Milkers"

CAUSE. Usually infection or injuries that have thickened the lining of the streak canal and narrowed the passageway through it. Occasionally the condition is inherited and is due to extremely strong sphincter muscles.

SYMPTOMS. All four teats are likely to milk hard when the trouble is inherited. Mastitis or injuries may cause ordinarily easy-milking cows to suddenly show up with one or more teats from which milk can't be obtained without a tube. This sort of thing is often seen in fresh cows that went dry in good shape and suffered trouble during their dry periods that was unsuspected by the owner.

TREATMENT. Surgery that is done at milking time when the teats are full so the correct amount of cutting can be done. The operation consists of nicking the sphincter muscle until the desired ease of milking is attained. Cutting too deeply may cause cows to become "leakers." It is advisable to infuse the udder with 100,-000 units of pencillin after every milking for at least three days and teat dilators are advisedly used during the same period to keep the cut edges from growing together as tightly as before.

PREVENTION. The same measures as given for preventing teat injuries under mastitis in this section.

Leaky Teats

CAUSE. Usually an inherited weakness of the sphincter muscles that makes streak canals incapable of holding milk in the udder. May also follow injuries to teat ends and unskilled surgery performed on hard-milking cows.

SYMPTOMS. Leaking of milk at all times or when only a little milk is in the udder. Not serious when it occurs near milking time in high-producing cows, for considerable pressure exists in the udder a few hours after milk has been withdrawn. Cows that don't leak under such conditions are usually classed as hard-milkers.

TREATMENT. Surgery that removes a tiny V-shaped piece of the sphincter muscle is the most satisfactory. This has the effect of constricting the muscle and squeezing the streak canal shut as healing occurs. It is advisedly done while cows are dry. A less successful method consists of injecting a drop of Lugol's solution in four different places around the circumference of the teat orifice. Resultant swelling usually stops leakage, but the treatment may have to be repeated every time inflammation subsides.

Teat Fistula

CAUSE. Usually an injury that has cut into the teat cistern and failed to heal completely because of constant dripping of milk over wound edges. Sometimes follows the removal of extra teats.

SYMPTOMS. Leaking of milk through an opening other than the natural orifice of the teat.

TREATMENT. Surgery that is performed during the dry period is the most successful, since the opening is stitched shut to insure complete closing. Burning of the hole with caustic potash or silver nitrate is an alternative method, with closing supposed to occur through healing of the burn wounds. It is not generally successful when used on larger fistulas.

Warts on Teats

CAUSE. A virus.

SYMPTOMS. Typical warty growths on the teats. Sometimes they resemble dry slivers of wood, but are capable of becoming irritated to the extent of bleeding and soreness. When occurring near the ends of teats they may be factors causing mastitis outbreaks.

TREATMENT. Surgical removal while the cows are dry is the most practical. Resultant wounds can be touched with silver nitrate to control bleeding. Daily soaking with castor oil or vinegar has also been claimed as effective for removing warts from teats.

Udder Abscesses

CAUSE. Usually a bruise infected with pus-forming bacteria.

SYMPTOMS. Swellings of various sizes that may appear anywhere on the udder but are commonest on the back part of the rear quarters. In the early stages these swellings are usually hard, red, and painful, but they eventually become soft as they fill up with pus. Patches of skin are apt to peel off because of severe fever during the early stages. The abscesses may become localized and do no particular harm or infection may spread all through the body to cause generalized blood poisoning. In either case the abscess usually breaks, sometimes followed by the sloughing of an entire quarter.

TREATMENT. Hot and cold packs may help to bring the abscess to a "head." Those that localize are best opened and drained when they reach the soft stage. An opening made in both the top and bottom of an abscess will permit washing it out with a 2% solution of potassium permanganate for a few days to guard against infection. Animals showing serious symptoms of generalized blood poisoning will merit intravenous use of mixed sulfas and intramuscular injections of million-unit doses of penicillin. If not promptly and properly treated they are very likely to die.

PREVENTION. Eliminating the causes of udder injuries.

Beating that Summer Milk Slump

We've been having that summer slump in milk production for so many years that it is generally accepted by owners as inevitable. This isn't surprising in most areas, for a combination of hot weather, flies by day, mosquitoes by night, and burned-out pastures make it seem logical. Hot weather may not only cause a slump in milk production, but may also result in a lowered fat content. Anyway, research at the University of Missouri showed that the test is likely to go down as the temperature goes up.

We can control flies and mosquitoes by spraying, and furnish shade to help protect cattle against extreme heat. We can help still more by supplying the cows with plenty of cool fresh water. The water is important in three ways:

1. It lowers high body temperatures that keep cattle from eating. Since they don't sweat very much, cows suffer more from heat than human beings or horses, and milk production goes down accordingly in hot weather.
2. It is a solvent that carries food to the body tissues and moves away waste products. Blood itself is composed of over 80 per cent water, so a lack of water means lowered vitality of a cow.
3. It helps digestion in cattle by softening feeds so that fermentation is made more effective. A lack of it interferes with digestion, and inefficient digestion naturally means less milk.

In addition to these more commonly considered factors, summer feeding also has quite a bit to do with the way cows maintain milk production during this season. According to the books, a cow can produce up to 30 pounds or more of milk daily on grass alone. However, in order to do it, she will need to eat about 125 pounds of grass a day. A big cow can eat this much, but she'll need better than average pasture so that she doesn't have to graze more than eight hours per day. Since cows won't eat much during the hot days, this good pasture should be available at night when most of the grazing is done. Cows that produce at high levels on pasture alone must have exceptional pasture. Otherwise milk cows will need supplementary grain in order to maintain summer production.

With the foregoing requirements in mind, owners will find that the following management practices will help to beat that summer milk slump:

1. Spray regularly for control of flies and mosquitoes.

2. Supply clean cool water at easily-reached places so that cows won't go half a day between drinks.
3. Provide at least one shady place big enough for all cows to loaf during the hot part of days.
4. Reserve the best pastures for night grazing.
5. Rotate and clip pastures regularly to provide constant new growth. A temporary electric fence can be moved around to divide a field into strips for alternate grazing.
6. When good pastures aren't available otherwise, fields can be sowed with something like sudan grass so that green feed becomes available during the late summer.
7. As an alternative, some of the first hay crop can be made into silage for late summer feeding.
8. Emergency crops like soy beans can be sowed for cutting and feeding green during the late summer.
9. Keep good hay in a rack in the pasture all the time. This practice will also provide extra insurance against bloat when dangerous crops are being pastured.
10. Furnish extra grain during the pasture season and increase it without waiting for milk production to fall off as a warning that additional feed is needed.
11. Remember that milk production can be held up only if cows get feed enough to support it at the expected level. Those lush spring pastures don't last very long under the summer sun.

Preventing Off-Flavors in Milk

A recent investigation showed that there are five main causes of a bad odor or "off-flavor" in milk. Contrary to popular belief, it has been conclusively shown that the milk doesn't absorb bad odors or undesirable flavors after it has been drawn from the cow.

They often get in because fumes were breathed by the cows shortly before milking time. One experiment showed that a strong garlic odor was present in a cow's milk two minutes after she had inhaled garlic fumes for ten minutes. Similar results have been obtained with commoner bad odors present in dirty, poorly-aired barns. In one case a poorly ventilated loafing shed was found to be causing trouble, even though the milking barn itself was spotlessly clean. If the barn smells bad, there's a good chance that the milk will smell bad, too.

In other cases the bad odors and flavors get into milk because of feed recently eaten by the cows. During the winter months such smells and tastes are apt to be caused by various kinds of roots, roughages, and silage, and in the pasture season the milk may have a "grassy" flavor or have an odor from obnoxious plants like wild onion or dog fennel. Concentrates seldom affect milk flavor.

Bad odors and tastes may also be caused by an enzyme called lipase which is present in all milk and has the function of breaking down butterfat. There is usually only a little of this lipase in milk, and its action is generally stopped by cooling. However, the milk of some cows contains an exceptionally strong lipase that continues acting even after the milk has been cooled. Such milk is generally given by cows in the latter stages of their lactation period. Even when milk contains only normal small amounts of lipase, its activity is aided by stirring or shaking warm milk, and can be helped still more by cooling the milk, warming it, and then cooling it again.

This lipase activity may be to blame for some of the bad odors and tastes that occur on farms where pipe-line milker installations are used. Vertical sections of tubing known as "risers" are often necessary when pipelines are extremely long and run from one part of a barn to another. Since they are connected to the pipe by right-angle elbows, there is often a great deal of turbulence in these sharp turns which break down the fat globules just like violent stirring or homogenization. Experiments at Cornell University have shown that shooting air through pipelines to clean out the milk will occasionally give the milk a rancid flavor, too. Workers at Michigan State University have reported that leaky valves in pipelines cause acid to be formed in milk, giving it a bad taste. There is also a possibility that foaming and churning in the farm milk tank may sometimes be responsible for bad odors and off-flavors in milk.

Disinfectants and other bad-smelling products may get into the milk from unclean hands or dirty utensils, while bad flavors sometimes come from various udder ointments. The various anti-biotics have little influence on milk flavor, but a medicinal taint may result when phenol-bearing ointments come in contact with chlorine used in washing udders or utensils.

Once the chief causes of bad odors and off-flavors are recognized, a great deal of trouble can be prevented if you will:

1. Keep barns clean and well-ventilated.
2. Feed cows after milking instead of before.
3. Take cows off pasture a couple of hours before milking.

4. Turn dry cows into new pastures a few days ahead of the milking herd. This allows them to eat troublesome weeds before they have a chance to affect milk.
5. Clip pastures, with a check plot several feet square being used to determine the best time for doing it. Troublesome plants are hoed off in this plot until they fail to start up again, and then the entire pasture is clipped.
6. Eradicate troublesome weeds completely by killing them with a recommended spray, and then reseeding the pasture.
7. Refrain from stirring or otherwise agitating warm milk.
8. Watch for cows that may be giving lipase milk. This means discarding questionable-quality milk, especially that from cows that have been milking a long time.
9. Cool the milk quickly and then keep it cool.
10. Avoid installing filters in the vacuum line.
11. Avoid operating milk pump continuously if the milk flow is below its capacity.
12. Avoid use of unnecessary fittings like tees, elbows, etc.
13. Eliminate risers as much as possible in pipeline installations. When lines are too long, a valve can be installed at the midpoint of the continuous pipe so the milk will be drawn only from the midpoint to the milk room.
14. Reduce the height of the risers if they must be used.
15. Reduce the slope of the line as much as possible.
16. Be sure that there are no air leaks in the pipeline.
17. Refrain from using air to clean out milker lines. If done, the milk removed should be discarded and fed to calves.
18. Be careful with disinfectants and udder ointments around the barn.
19. Keep hands and utensils clean at milking time.
20. Avoid foaming and churning in the milk tank as much as possible.

When Ring Tests are Positive

Not so long ago a dairyman told us that he had received notice of a positive ring test on his milk, thus requiring a blood test of his herd to identify the Bang's-infected animals. However, the blood test showed every animal in the herd to be completely negative! The owner then wanted to know how such a thing could happen, and hinted rather strongly that the ring test was worthless as a diagnostic measure. Since this sort of thing happens fairly often, it might be well to consider a few of the possible causes.

For a starter it is well to remember that the ring test is intentionally made extremely delicate to decrease the chances of any infected animals escaping detection. This is necessary because of the dilution factor involved when milk from an infected cow is mixed with that from numerous clean animals. This dilution factor is becoming increasingly important as more and more bulk milk tanks come into use throughout the country. Owners have always been warned that the ring test was so delicate that it might indicate infection where none existed.

For another, it is possible for ring test reactions to be caused by factors other than Bang's disease. As a group they're called "nonspecific" reactions, and we don't know too much about them. We do know, though, that various germs causing diarrhea and intestinal inflammation seem capable of causing ring test reactions, and cows in advanced stages of pregnancy appear capable of the same thing, even though they don't actually have Bang's disease. There are also various other possibilities along this line, including enzymes like lactase and reductase in the milk of certain cows, especially those that have been milking for long periods. Regardless of the exact cause, a single animal causing even a slight reaction may be enough to give a positive ring test.

Then it must be borne in mind that an owner usually receives his ring test report about a month after the milk has been tested. By the time a blood test is run, another month or so may have passed, and a lot of things can happen in two months time. Cows that were milking may have died or been sold so they aren't included in the blood test, even though they caused a ring test reaction. Temporary reactions due to something like an attack of winter dysentery or a diarrhea brought on by turning to pasture may have disappeared in the interval between the ring test and blood test. A calfhood vaccinated animal that was still showing a slight titer at the time of the ring test may have cleared up by the time she was blood tested. A heavily pregnant cow or one that was giving milk high in enzyme content may have freshened and be giving normal milk at the time of the blood test.

It is possible, of course, for records to be confused in a state office or milk plant so that one owner gets another's ring test report, but things like those we've mentioned are much more likely to be the cause of a negative blood test following a positive ring test. No test has ever been 100 per cent accurate, and the ring test isn't either. However, it's given a high rating in this respect, and it's had a thorough trial by this time. Authorities in several states are well satisfied with it as a part of an official Bang's-eradication program, so you're likely to be affected by it for years to come. In general, the ring test and blood test results have been demonstrated as highly correlated, and a blood test usually shows at least a suspect or two in a herd that has given a positive ring test. If it doesn't work out that way in your herd, you should first of all be thankful that none of your cows are diseased. Then you should be fair to the ring test by remembering that it has certain limitations and isn't completely dependable under all conditions any more than the average human being.

When Ring Tests are Negative

The other day we drew blood samples from a couple of cows to see if they could pass the Bang's test for sale. The owner was sure they were all right, for the last ring test of the milk had been negative. However, the blood test showed one of the animals as a strong suspect, automatically cancelling the sale. The owner demanded an explanation, claiming that either the ring test or blood test was wrong, and stating that neither could be depended on as a diagnostic measure. Since some of our readers may also be interested in this matter, we will repeat part of our explanation here.

First of all we'd like to point out that differences between the blood test and ring test are to be expected, and that's why the various states won't accept a negative ring test as proof that all animals in a herd are free of Bang's disease. The blood test is considered more accurate because it is a test of an individual animal, while the ring test is a test of an entire milking herd. Even though the ring test is made extremely delicate, it is still possible for an infected cow to escape detection when her milk is diluted many times with milk from a number of clean cows. This dilution factor is becoming more of a problem as the number of bulk tanks increases throughout the country. A couple of other facts regarding milk also add to the uncertainty connected with the dilution problem.

For one thing, the ring test is dependent on a distinct cream line, with a blue color appearing at the junction of the milk and cream. As most dairymen know, occasional cows produce milk that is naturally homogenized to the extent that the milk and cream don't separate on standing to show a distinct cream line. Such milk can't show a positive ring test, even if tested alone. In case the milk should happen to show a faint cream line, diluting it with milk from other cows might easily keep it from rising to the top in a herd sample so the cow producing it could be missed.

For another thing, the size of butterfat globules has a great deal to do with the accuracy of the ring test. An English study of cows known to be affected with Bang's disease that sometimes gave a negative ring test revealed an interesting fact. The ring test was invariably positive on these cows when their butterfat globules differed considerably in size, and was just as constantly negative when the fat globules were small and uniform in size. Accordingly, butterfat globules from an infected cow might be of uniform size so the ring test would be negative under all conditions. On the other hand, butterfat globules that varied in size might be kept from giving a positive ring test reaction if the milk was extremely diluted with that from clean cows.

Then it's possible for blood test reactions to be caused by factors other than Bang's disease, just as in the case of positive ring test reactions. The same non-specific reactions mentioned in regard to positive ring tests may also affect the blood test. These include hormones produced by cows in advanced pregnancy, and various germs causing diarrhea and intestinal inflammation. It seems possible that such reactions might affect the blood test without having any effect whatever on the ring test.

Finally, it must again be remembered that an owner usually receives his ring test report about a month after the milk has been tested. By the time a blood test is run, the milk may not be able to pass a ring test any more, even though it was negative a month earlier. Infected cows that weren't milking at the time of the ring test may have freshened, or diseased new cows may have been purchased. Some vaccinated first-calf heifers that are still carrying a slight titer may have freshened since the time of the ring test. It may also be that one or two slight blood reactions are only temporary and due to something like recent vaccination against shipping fever or an attack of diarrhea.

The Commonest Cause of Teat Injuries

Dairymen are often told that keeping cows in roomy stalls fitted with dividers will prevent most cases of teat injuries occurring in barns. We do not question this statement in regard to teat injuries that are caused by the feet of other cows. However, we contend that they won't affect the total very much, because few of these injuries are caused by other cows. This statement is supported by the fact that a great many teat injuries occur on cows that have been kept alone in box stalls at calving time. Owners seldom believe us at first when we tell them that a cow has injured one of her own teats, and point out that it would be practically impossible for a cow to step on herself in this manner.

We readily agree with them, but point out that the teat hasn't been hurt in this way. Reasoning will prove that this is true, for a teat that has been stepped on will probably be badly smashed and swollen. In contrast, practically all of the injured teats we see are either cleanly slashed lengthwise, or have the end sliced off so it hangs by a shred of skin without the slightest sign of bruising. Injuries of this type have been inflicted by a dew claw on the hind foot of the affected cow. We personally believe that at least 90% of all teat injuries are caused by dew claws.

A little observation in your own barn will show how easy it is for them to cause trouble. First of all, they are hard and have sharp edges that are quite capable of cutting soft flesh. Unfortunately, whenever a cow lies down she naturally exposes her teats in a way that invites injury by dew claws, and the larger the teats, the more likely they are to be cut.

When a cow is in a reclining position, a hind foot usually lies under the udder, often with the dew claws close to a teat, and the other hind foot is extended away from the body. When she rises to her feet, she gets up hind end first, of course. The extended hind foot is drawn up under the body as the first move, often bringing the inside dew claw against one of the teats. Sometimes a teat is caught between dew claws on opposite hind feet. In either case the next move to a standing position brings the udder upward at the same time that the dew claws are turned with the movement of the feet. If a teat is in contact with the sharp edge of a dew claw at that precise moment, it is cut. The injury is made worse if the teat happens to be caught between opposite dew claws when the cow lurches to her feet. Some cows are particularly susceptible to teat injuries, either through having large udders and teats, or because of some particularly bad position that they assume when lying down. Such animals are likely to injure teats year after year at freshening time.

Many teat injuries on these problem cows can be prevented by harnessing them with an udder support that completely covers the udder. Another method consists of trimming the dew claws and then using sand paper to remove sharp edges and round them off like buttons. As an alternative, owners may feel inclined to try out a device that has been used in Holland for many years with excellent results. Many Dutch dairymen use it routinely on all cows with large teats and pendulous udders, regardless of whether or not they have ever injured themselves.

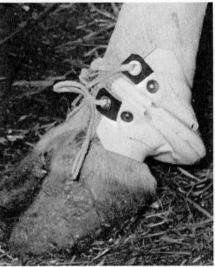

Special bandage, which covers the dew claws, helps prevent teat injuries.

It consists of an oilcloth-covered chrome leather bandage that circles the fetlock to cover the dew claws. It was originally fastened at the front of the foot with straps and buckles, but these caused sores, so they were replaced with leather strings. The device has a partition that fits between the dew claws to keep it from turning, and it is perforated to provide ventilation in case it has to be left on for long periods of time. It is made of chrome leather because this material will remain soft and pliable even after repeated soaking with mud and manure. The device can be secured through your local veterinarian.

6.

RESPIRATORY TROUBLES

Anatomy of the Cow's Respiratory System

The respiratory system begins with the nostrils. These are divided by a cartilage properly known as the nasal septum, and connect with the pharynx through two openings in the roof of the mouth which are called the choanae or posterior nares. As mentioned earlier, the pharynx is used for both breathing and swallowing. Leading from it is the larynx, and this upper end of the respiratory tract is always open except when swallowing is being done. At such times the soft palate raises to close off the pharynx above the esophagus, while a cartilage called the epiglottis shuts down over the larynx like a trapdoor to keep food and water from going into the lungs.

The larynx connects directly with the trachea or "windpipe" which can be felt from the outside as a tube composed of stiff rings. These rings are of cartilage and the trachea continues for about two feet before it starts dividing into so-called bronchi that go to different lobes of the lungs. These bronchi divide into progressively smaller branches known as bronchioles which eventually end as alveoli or air cells of the lungs.

The lungs are separated from the digestive organs by the diaphragm and with the heart occupy the space that is known as the thoracic cavity. They are unequal in size, with the right lung being about half again as big as the left one. This is largely due to the fact that the heart takes up a great deal of room on the left side of the thoracic cavity. Both lungs are covered with a thin membrane called the pleura which in the healthy state prevents attachment to adjoining structures.

The pulmonary arteries carry blood to the lungs from the right side of the heart after it is returned by veins from all over the body and is loaded with carbon dioxide and other waste products of living. These waste products are given up in the lungs and breathed out while the blood takes on a new load of oxygen. It is then returned to the left side of the heart, from where it is pumped

298

out through the body in various arteries. Eventually it replaces its oxygen with waste products and is again returned by veins to the right side of the heart.

Nasal Obstructions

CAUSE. Usually something like a stick or weed, although small boards and oil cups have also been reported. In addition, tumors of various types sometimes occur in the nostrils of cattle, and actinobacillosis has been known to close the posterior nares.

SYMPTOMS. Snoring sounds and noisy breathing are the commonest. Sometimes there is a gray or bloody discharge from the nose, as well as swelling or a bad odor. Occasionally an examination will show that no air is passing through one of the nostrils.

DIAGNOSIS. Sometimes the obstruction can be felt with fingers inserted in the nostril or seen in the posterior nares when the mouth is opened. Passing a small rubber tube through the nostril and down through the posterior nare will sometimes help in showing whether or not the passage is blocked.

TREATMENT. Surgery is needed for the removal of tumors and growths. Foreign bodies can sometimes be pulled out with the fingers, hooks, snares, or other improvised instruments. If deeply imbedded, surgery is often needed to free them.

Catarrh or Bronchitis

CAUSE. Almost anything that will result in "catching cold." Exposure to cold, storms, confinement in damp stables, overcrowding, poor ventilation, standing in drafts from open doors, etc., are often involved. This trouble is frequently associated with shipping fever and pneumonia, but may also be due to irritation by breathing dust or smoke.

SYMPTOMS. In mild cases coughing may be the only one. At other times lowering of the head, open-mouth breathing with frothing and protrusion of the tongue may be seen. Animals may appear dull or be "picky" about eating; they frequently lose weight and decrease considerably in milk production. Listening over the lungs may or may not reveal abnormal breathing sounds, although the temperature is apt to be raised a degree or two. The average animal recovers in a week or less, but sometimes persists in a chronic form as shown by a faster breathing rate under all conditions.

DIAGNOSIS. Usually through the mild symptoms and rapid recovery. However, it must be watched carefully, for the early stages of pneumonia show the same symptoms. Catarrh may also be confused with lungworm disease and mild forms of shipping fever.

TREATMENT. Largely a matter of complete rest in a dry warm stable that is well ventilated and free from drafts. Coughing is sometimes helped by a level teaspoonful of ammonium chloride given twice a day as needed. A half ounce of eucalyptus oil in a pail of boiling water will furnish a helpful medicated steam. Animals can be forced to breathe it by cutting the bottom out of a grain sack and fitting it over the pail while the other end is fitted around the animal's nose. Affected animals are best isolated as completely as possible in order to prevent possible spread of the trouble. Cases should be carefully watched and a change for the worse or appearance of a high fever should be taken as a sign of approaching pneumonia.

PREVENTION. Largely a matter of good management to avoid the causes listed earlier. Cattle are especially subject to catarrh during the wet cold nights of early fall when they have not yet been brought to the barns at night from pastures. Keeping them in at such times may easily mean the difference between sickness and health for certain animals.

Pneumonia (Bronchopneumonia)

CAUSE. Usually some predisposing factor which lowers the natural resistance of animals so that ordinarily harmless germs can cause serious trouble. Such factors include exhaustion from shipping, stress like thirst and hunger, or stabling in cold, damp, filthy, drafty, and poorly ventilated quarters. The virus of para-influenza-3 has been discovered to be a predisposing factor, and dairy calves housed in closed, over-warm buildings where the humidity is high often develop pneumonia. In addition, practically any ailment of cattle is capable of lowering the natural resistance so that pneumonia can develop. A list of the commoner ones includes mastitis, metritis, hardware disease, and kidney infection. Pneumonia that is directly due to infectious organisms is generally classed as shipping fever which is discussed in this book as a contagious disease.

SYMPTOMS. When cases are followed closely, a fever will generally be found to precede all others. However, the average owner notices fast breathing and coughing as the earliest signs of sickness. These are usually accompanied by dullness, refusal of feed, and greatly decreased milk production. There may be no abnormal breathing sounds at all or there may be rasping and wheezing noises that can be heard all over the barn. Thumping of the ribs usually produces signs of pain in affected animals. Often there are distinct differences in the breathing sounds of the two lungs which indicate involvement of different degrees. In the more serious cases it is not uncommon to see open-mouth breathing accompanied by frothing and occasional bleeding at the nose.

DIAGNOSIS. A combination of fast breathing, high fever, and coughing is usually enough to warrant a tentative diagnosis of pneumonia. The season of the year, the involvement of predisposing factors, difficult breathing, and abnormal sounds in the lungs will help to establish a definite diagnosis. Since secondary pneumonia is always a possibility, animals should be carefully examined for evidence of a possible primary cause. Sometimes a history of previous sickness will be of value in identifying these primary diseases. Under farm conditions pneumonia might be confused with lungworm infestation, gangrene of the lungs, emphysema, and such contagious diseases as shipping fever and mucosal disease.

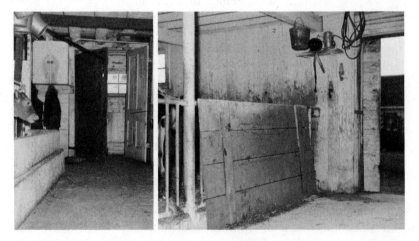

Left: Double doors to avoid drafts are helpful in the prevention of catarrh or bronchitis.

Right: Panel of boards set against calf pen cuts off drafts from open door for prevention of pneumonia.

TREATMENT. Good nursing is probably more important than anything else. Complete rest in warm dry quarters that are free from drafts is highly desirable, and removal from a damp stable to a dry one is often followed by immediate improvement. Blanketing may be desirable at times, for fresh air is more important than warm quarters if a choice must be made. In mild weather animals may be better off if left out-doors. Fresh water should be available at all times for fever is likely to encourage thirst. Grain rations should be light and slightly laxative, with bran being an old favorite. Root crops and leafy green feeds are also recommended. In cases of extreme weakness it may be advisable to give blood transfusions or sugar solutions intravenously.

Sulfamerazine and sulfamethazine have been demonstrated as highly effective in the treatment of pneumonia, either alone or in combination. The recommended first dose of 1 to 1½ grains per pound of body weight is best given intravenously, and then followed by daily doses of ½ to ¾ grains per pound given by mouth. Range or feed lot animals can be treated by putting sulfa in the drinking water at the rate of 1 pound to 100 gallons of water for every 20 animals.

Antibiotics are often effective in speeding up recovery and preventing complications. Penicillin alone may not give very satisfactory results, but in combination with sulfas may prove very helpful. It often appears that when streptomycin, dihydrostreptomycin, or penicillin and sulfas are given in combination, the results are better than when any of them are given alone. Recommended dosage for antibiotics includes: penicillin—3000 units per pound of body weight every 48 hours; streptomycin and dihydrostreptomycin—1 gram daily for calves and 5 to 10 grams daily for adult animals; oxytetracycline or chlortetracycline—2 milligrams per pound of body weight every 8 to 10 hours. Supportive treatment with atropine (¼ grain given subcutaneously), or strychnine sulfate (1 grain by mouth 3 times daily) may prove helpful too.

PREVENTION. Chiefly a matter of good management to avoid all possible causes of chilling and other predisposing factors. Stabling in well ventilated quarters is particularly important. Recommended practices should be followed before, during, and after shipment of cattle, and good care provided for all cattle that are sick with any kind of disease.

Coccidioidomycosis

CAUSE. A fungus called *Coccidioides immitis*. In the U.S. this disease seems to be confined to California and the southwestern areas along the Mexican border. Until a few years ago it was not considered to be a common disease of cattle, but recent surveys indicate that most of the animals in southwestern U.S. eventually become infected with coccidioidomycosis. In addition to cattle, the disease has been detected in man, dog, horse, burro, sheep, swine, cat, monkey, coyote, and several species of wild rodents. The disease is also known in certain dry areas of Mexico, Central America, and South America.

MEANS OF SPREAD. The fungus grows in the soil, and the spores are usually inhaled to cause infection of the lungs. Infection can also follow entrance of the fungus into a skin wound, but this seldom occurs. It is not believed that infected animals transmit the disease directly to people or other animals, and people are not believed capable of transmitting the disease to animals. There are probably several million infected cattle in the southwestern U.S. at all times, and 5 to 20% or more of cattle from this area are regularly found to have lesions of coccidioidomycosis when given postmortem examination in packing plants.

SYMPTOMS. None have been detected, even in experimental work in which cattle have been deliberately infected and kept under close observation for periods of three or four months afterward. Opening a dead animal will usually show tumor-like masses of varying sizes in either or both the lungs and lymph nodes of these organs. The growths are grayish-yellow to pale yellow in color, and have yellow pus in the center that is sometimes gritty like sand or even completely calcified.

DIAGNOSIS. Most practical in the field through the coccidioidin skin test that is run much like the tuberculin test for tuberculosis, with the side of the neck being the usual injection site. Tests involving blood samples have not been too successful for this disease. An accurate diagnosis is most important in packing plants, where coccidioidomycosis can easily be confused with diseases like tuberculosis, actinomycosis, actinobacillosis, lung abscesses, and the larval form of different parasites. A definite diagnosis can be made only in the laboratory through demonstration of the causative organism.

TREATMENT. Not considered as necessary for cattle.

PREVENTION. Entirely a matter of dust control and reduction of exposure to contaminated soil. Dust can be controlled by oiling or paving of feed lots. Removal of semi-barren land as pasture may help, and irrigation of pastures is a possible preventive measure. This is indicated by sampling studies carried on in Arizona which showed that *C. immitis* can be isolated only from non-irrigated soil. The eating of infected meat is not known to cause coccidioidomycosis, and cooking procedures usually destroy the fungus anyway. No vaccine is available at this time.

Lungworm Disease (Parasitic Bronchitis)

CAUSE. A worm two or three inches long called *Dictyocaulus viviparous* is the common lungworm of cattle, although animals may also become infested with *Dictyocaulus filaria* from goats, sheep, or deer. The condition may appear alone, but it is usually seen in association with malnutrition and infestation with stomach and intestinal worms. The adult worms seldom live long in the lungs, and unless they are being constantly reinfested, animals

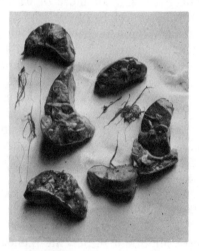

Lung worms and pieces of a cow's lung.

soon become free of the parasites. The worms suck blood and do the most damage through destruction of lung tissue.

They are usually spread through carrier animals that harbor a few of the worms without showing any signs of their presence. Spread is further encouraged by the use of permanent pastures, especially when they are wet and located in areas where the winters are mild. As previously noted, cattle may become infested with a different type of lungworm from pastures used by sheep, goats, and deer.

LIFE CYCLE. The mature worms live in the trachea and bronchi where they lay eggs. These are brought to the pharynx and swallowed with mucus, later hatching into larvae in the upper part of the digestive tract. The larvae pass out with manure and reach the infective stage in about a week. They thrive on moisture and may live in water or climb on forage when it is wet with dew or rain. At this stage they are resistant to drying but are killed by disinfectants and freezing. Under the most favorable conditions they seldom live longer than about six months when outside animals. The life cycle is continued when the larvae are swallowed with food or water and enter the digestive tract. They then burrow through the walls of the intestines, enter the blood stream, and eventually return to the lungs where they grow to maturity and start laying eggs of their own. An entire cycle may be completed in about a month under favorable conditions.

SYMPTOMS. Violent coughing is an early one, and pneumonia may follow within two or three days. In advanced cases there is apt to be extreme loss of weight, rough coat, sunken eyes, lack of appetite, weakness, and diarrhea. Frequently there is a nasal discharge and open-mouth breathing with lowered head and protruding tongue. Panting and coughing are likely to follow almost any kind of moderate exercise. Wheezing and labored breathing may resemble that of a horse with "heaves." Occasionally there is bleeding from the nose. The severity of symptoms will depend largely on the degree of infection and the immunity of the infested animals.

In recent years a different form of lungworm disease has been reported from England and Canada. In this atypical form, adult cattle show most of the characteristic symptoms, including coughing. However, they do not harbor mature worms in the lungs and, accordingly, no larvae are passed in the manure. An immunity on the part of the animals is apparently the reason why adult worms do not develop.

DIAGNOSIS. Definite through opening the trachea and bronchi of a dead animal and finding the worms, sometimes in masses large enough to block the air passages. Microscopic examination of manure may also show larvae. However, there is also a possibility that animals may be afflicted with the atypical form of the disease, and are not passing larvae with the manure. Under field conditions this trouble might be confused with almost any of the diseases causing respiratory symptoms.

TREATMENT. None was recognized until May, 1957. Then research workers in England announced that an old drug called cyanacethydrizide had been found effective against lungworms. It has the tradename of Dictycide, and is given subcutaneously. Since that time it has been thoroughly tested and shown to be effective against adult worms but not migrating larvae. Cyanacethydrazide can be given either by mouth (17.5 milligrams per kilogram of body weight), or subcutaneously (15 milligrams per kilogram of body weight), but it seems to be a little more effective when given subcutaneously. A single treatment will remove most of the adult worms, but severely infested animals should be treated each day for three successive days.

PREVENTION. Most practical through a vaccine made by using x-radiation on *Dictyocaulus* larvae. These larvae are then unable to develop to maturity, but they do migrate to the lungs where they produce a great deal of resistance to the parasites. Extensive trials have demonstrated that this vaccine is both effective and safe. In areas of severe infestation, monthly treatment with cyanacethydrazide is also recommended as part of a preventive program. However, a lungworm control program should not be completely dependent on the use of an effective vaccine and treatment.

Carrier animals are the most important source of infestation. Most of the adult worms are eliminated in two to four months, and most of the larvae die in less than six weeks on well-drained pastures, so good management practices based on these facts will also do a great deal to control lungworms. Since the larvae of lungworms usually remain in the manure, the contamination of feed and water with manure represents the most important way in which these parasites spread. Control will then naturally include means of preventing diarrhea from various causes, including infestation with other parasites like stomach and intestinal worms. Preventive measures as given for coccidiosis will also prove effective in a lungworm control program.

Gangrenous Pneumonia (Gangrene of the Lungs)

CAUSE. Usually through breathing liquids into the lungs while animals are being drenched. This may occur through improper drenching or forcing liquids down the throats of animals that are unable to swallow because of choke, milk fever, or other ailments that have paralyzed the throat muscles. Cows that are down with troubles like milk fever, botulism, or bloat often vomit and then inhale material that has been brought up from the rumen. In diseases like red nose and diphtheria, rotten tissues that have been sloughed from the back of the mouth may trickle down the trachea into the lungs. Gangrene of the lungs may also follow the breathing of smoke, fire, or chemical fumes.

SYMPTOMS. Usually those of early pneumonia, with coughing, dullness, loss of appetite, and labored breathing. Bubbling sounds can sometimes be heard in the lungs, and in late stages the breath may smell badly because of rotting lung tissues. Most cases end in death after a few days, but recoveries sometimes occur following a long period of sickness.

DIAGNOSIS. Difficult to distinguish from pneumonia, although the bubbling sounds and bad odor of the breath will sometimes indicate the nature of trouble. A history of recent drenching for some other ailment may also furnish a clue.

TREATMENT. The same as given for pneumonia.

PREVENTION. Chiefly a matter of using extreme care when drenching animals, with oils being particularly dangerous because they won't evaporate from the lungs like water. In all cases it is best to try animals on water to be sure they can swallow. If they can do this, drenching may be done as described in another section of this book. A stomach tube may be used on animals that are unable to swallow medicine.

Abscesses of the Lungs

CAUSE. Generally started by germs that have been carried by blood from infected areas in various parts of the body. Abscesses have been known to follow cases of metritis, mastitis, navel-ill, and other troubles. They may also be due to lungworm injuries or punctures caused by hardware in the stomach.

SYMPTOMS. Dullness and progressive loss of weight without apparent cause are common ones. The appetite may be poor for a long period or it may remain fairly good until almost the end. The general symptoms greatly resemble those of hardware trouble, with stiffness, slow movements, and arching of the back being frequently seen. However, such symptoms are not dependable, for the abscesses may show no signs of being present at all until perfectly healthy-looking animals suddenly drop dead. Bleeding or pus discharges from the nostrils may be seen in combination with labored breathing and foaming at the mouth. Tapping over the ribs may reveal areas of dullness and there may be bubbling breathing sounds that indicate fluid in the lungs.

DIAGNOSIS. Usually on the basis of symptoms and progressive loss of weight without evidence of serious general sickness. May be confused with lungworm disease, gangrene of the lungs, tuberculosis, hardware trouble, and others.

TREATMENT. Usually impractical. If attempted, the drugs most likely to help are streptomycin and neomycin. The streptomycin can be given at the rate of 1 gram per 100 pounds of body weight for a week or ten days, and the neomycin at the rate of 1 to 2 milligrams per pound of body weight for the same length of time.

Summer Snuffles (Hay Fever)

CAUSE. Unknown, but some kind of plant dust or pollen that promotes an allergy is suspected. Difficult breathing is due to swelling of the membrane lining the nasal passages and upper throat. It usually occurs during the pasture season, and disappears after a frost. Some kind of individual susceptibility is suspected because the same animals are often affected every summer.

SYMPTOMS. Snoring sounds and difficult breathing are the most noticeable. There may be watering of the eyes, yellow or bloody nasal discharges, and open-mouth breathing with frothing. The nose is sometimes rubbed viciously on objects and stubs or plant stalks may be forced far up in the nostrils. Occasionally there is considerable swelling around the eyes and the anus. The appetite usually remains good, but milk production may be greatly reduced. Cases are generally seen on pasture, but they sometimes appear when roughage is being fed during the winter. In either case the trouble is evidently due to a certain type of dust or pollen. There is seldom more than one affected animal in a herd, but the same one may be affected year after year while on pasture.

DIAGNOSIS. Usually on the basis of noisy breathing and other symptoms without a high body temperature and other evidence of general sickness as might be expected in diseases like pneumonia and malignant catarrhal fever. Under field conditions it might be confused with troubles like pulmonary emphysema and various other kinds of allergies. Occurrence during the pasture season and the involvement of animals with a past history of such attacks may help in making a diagnosis.

TREATMENT. Removal from the offending pasture and confinement in a stable on dry feed is probably the most practical. Medical treatments include injections of adrenalin (10 cc. of a 1:1000 solution); atropine (¼ grain), or antihistamines. Suggested antihistamines include chlorpheniramine maleate (7½ milligrams per 100 lbs. body weight) and mepyramine maleate (½ milligram per lb. body weight) given every 6 to 8 hours. Injections of a corticosteroid either alone or with an antibiotic may be tried. Flushing the nostrils with 40 to 100 cc. of a 50% glucose solution containing oxytetracycline, Furacin, and a corticosteroid has been reported as helpful. Such a solution is made by adding 55 cc. of Terramycin, 40 cc. of Furacin solution, and 5 cc. of dexamethasone to the glucose solution.

Inflammation of the Pharynx

CAUSE. Several that may be listed as: (1) Burning with medicines like creolin. (2) Unskilled use of instruments in treating choke. (3) Improper passage of hose to relieve bloat. (4) Foreign bodies like wire, tin, etc. (5) Tumors of various kinds. (6) Actinobacillosis. (7) Abscesses due to infection from injuries. (8) Damp stables and other causes of catarrh.

SYMPTOMS. Usually a partial or complete refusal of food and water because of the sore throat. Liquids that are swallowed may be returned through the nostrils, and coughing is a common symptom. There may be nasal discharges and the head is often carried in a peculiar manner with the nose raised. Difficult breathing and snoring sounds are likely to be noticed. Trouble due to injuries usually clears up in a week or less, while those due to infection may persist for long periods.

DIAGNOSIS. Usually through the symptoms and evidence of soreness in the throat. May be confused with "summer snuffles," catarrh, or the early stages of pneumonia.

TREATMENT. Dependent on cause, with removal being most important when foreign bodies are involved. Swollen mucous membranes are often reduced by steaming with eucalyptol or various of the creolin preparations. These are used at the rate of an ounce or two to a pail of hot water and animals forced to breathe the vapor as described under the treatment of catarrh. Ice packs over the throat may also help to make breathing easier. Million unit doses of penicillin in oil and wax injected intramuscularly are often found to be beneficial when infection is present. Water should be readily available at all times, and the early opening of abscesses is desirable. Food may be supplied as a thin gruel to make swallowing easier.

Inflammation of the Larynx

CAUSE. The same as given for inflammation of the pharynx.

SYMPTOMS. Much the same as for catarrh, since the two diseases often appear together. Common ones are open-mouth breathing and protrusion of the tongue in combination with snoring sounds and frothing at the mouth. Coughing is pretty sure to be seen in all cases, and may persist for weeks after apparently complete recovery.

TREATMENT. The same as given for inflammation of the pharynx.

Pulmonary Emphysema (Panting Disease)

CAUSE. Not always known whether started by an infectious or allergic or poisonous agent or merely the result of expulsion of air from the lungs with great force. Many cases are of unknown origin. However, the trouble often occurs when cattle are placed on lush pastures in the fall. This frequently happens in Canada where animals are pastured on kale or rape, and has been reported in our western states when cattle have been moved from mountain ranges to better lowland pastures. Under such conditions the disease is believed to be caused by some kind of allergic or toxic factor in the plants. This belief is supported by the fact that the number of cases often decreases after the first frost.

It has also been reported to occur after abrupt changes in rations, the feeding of moldy material or turnip tops, sudden increases in grain amounts, and after bringing cattle into feedlots. Irrigated pastures and those of alfalfa, grain stubble, and meadow grasses have been involved, and spoiled forage has been an apparent cause in some cases. In addition, this condition often appears as a symptom and is secondary to troubles like pneumonia, smoke inhalation, shipping fever, lungworms, hardware trouble, poisonings, and practically any other trouble that causes prolonged difficult breathing.

SYMPTOMS. The most prominent one is labored breathing which has a sudden onset, and is associated with the appearance of foam in the mouth and nostrils. Affected animals usually stand with the head lowered and neck extended, drooling saliva with the mouth open and tongue protruding. Breathing is of a fast, gasping type, and exhalations are often accompanied by grunts of pain. If the animal lives for 24 hours, air can often be felt under the skin of the neck, and sometimes along the back to the root of the tail. If not treated, most affected animals die within a matter of a few hours to a couple of days. When pulmonary emphysema is secondary to some other disease, there will also be symptoms of the primary trouble, of course. Although usually seen in an acute form, old animals may develop the disease in a chronic form resembling heaves in horses.

DIAGNOSIS. Usually on the basis of sudden appearance in cattle that have recently been moved from poor to good pastures in the fall of the year. However, this ailment must always be considered as possibly being caused by, or secondary to, some of the various troubles already referred to under CAUSE.

TREATMENT. When symptoms are due to moldy feed, treatment is not likely to be very satisfactory, although mildly affected animals usually recover without any treatment, anyway. Best results have been obtained through intramuscular injections of 10 to 15 cc. adrenalin and 25 to 50 cc. of antihistamine solutions in combination. These drugs may also be given alone. Other treatments reported as of value include subcutaneous injections of atropine in doses of ¼ to ½ grain, and intramuscular injections of an antihistamine with penicillin. In secondary emphysema, the primary trouble should also be treated, although it is unlikely to do much good. Affected animals should be kept as quiet as possible so their oxygen needs are not increased by body exertion.

PREVENTION. Since the cause of this disease is unknown, no preventive measures can be given.

Malignant Catarrhal Fever (Malignant Head Catarrh)

CAUSE. A virus that appears to be closely attached to white blood cells and lymph glands when it attacks cattle. The disease was recognized in the United States in 1913 and first reported in Canada in 1924. It also exists in Europe and Africa. Although not usually considered as a contagious disease, disastrous outbreaks have occurred in both Canada and the United States. Cattle of all ages, breeds, and both sexes are susceptible. Although sheep do not show typical symptoms of the disease, they apparently can carry the virus and several outbreaks have been coupled with direct and indirect contact with sheep. Recovered animals may carry the virus for several months, suggesting that they may act as reservoirs of infection. Certain kinds of deer are also susceptible, and in Africa the wildebeest is believed to play a part in transmitting the disease.

MEANS OF SPREAD. Not definitely known, but probably by the swallowing of contaminated material. In some cases the virus seems to be airborne, with the respiratory system being affected first. Sheep seem able to transmit the disease, and it has been experimentally passed from cattle to sheep and from sheep back to cattle. The possibility of insect spreaders must be considered, even though cases have occurred during the winter months. A wide variation in the incubation period (14 to 150 or more days) and the possibility of recovered carriers may serve to explain such cases.

SYMPTOMS. Somewhat dependent on the form taken, for the peracute, intestinal, head and eye, and the mild forms are all recognized. In general, though, the most outstanding is a sudden sickness that is accompanied by a fever of 105 to 108° F. Animals go off feed, milk production drops off to almost nothing, and weight is lost at a rapid rate. The head is often extended because of a sore throat, there may be swelling and watering of the eyes, and a reddish or yellow discharge from the nostrils. Eating and drinking are slow, and the upper throat may appear swollen. Within a day or two a white film may form over the eyeballs, and various types of nervous symptoms may be shown. These range all the way from trembling and twitching of muscles to staggering, convulsions, and attacks on people. In the early stages the muzzle has a fiery red color, but it is soon covered with a yellowish scab which is a very characteristic lesion of this disease. A diarrhea develops early, and there may be considerable decay of tissues in the mouth. Animals weaken rapidly, often become lame, and the nostrils may become almost completely clogged with a thick discharge.

The course is variable, but most cattle with the head and eye form will die within about a week. In some cases only a single animal is affected, and it may die within 24 hours with no evidence of spread. In others, an outbreak may assume epidemic proportions, and sick animals may either die suddenly or linger for two or three weeks before finally dying. In rare cases animals may make an uneventful recovery in three or four days but, as a rule, most affected cattle will die. Experimental work indicates that immunity in recovered animals lasts for only a few months.

Opening a dead animal will usually show a fibrous membrane covering the lining of the pharynx, larynx, nostrils, and upper air passages. The lining of the mouth is apt to be brick red or purplish colored, and ulcers may be found on the lips, tongue, and hard palate. The upper part of the esophagus often bears ulcers, and the lining of the true stomach may also be thickened and ulcerated. Ulceration and thickening may be seen the full length of the small intestine, and to some extent in the large intestine. The lymph nodes of the head and neck are enlarged and sometimes crimson, and the lining of the urinary bladder, vulva, and vagina is often bloody and ulcerated.

DIAGNOSIS. Usually on the basis of typical symptoms, evidence of a non-contagious nature as shown by involvement of only a few animals, and the high death rate. Under farm conditions this trouble might be confused with shipping fever, red nose, BVD, rinderpest, and stomatitis. The diseases can sometimes be differentiated by these facts:

1. Shipping fever. Nervous symptoms are lacking and evidence of pneumonia is more pronounced.
2. Red nose or IBR. More animals are sick, but with fewer deaths. The disease spreads readily, lesions are restricted to the upper respiratory tract, and recovery is rapid.
3. Bovine virus diarrhea or BVD. Nervous symptoms are lacking, as are eye lesions and enlargement of the lymph glands.
4. Rinderpest. Shows no eye involvement, enlargement of the lymph glands, or nervous symptoms. In addition, it spreads rapidly, is primarily confined to the digestive tract, and has a high death rate.
5. Stomatitis. Largely limited to the upper digestive tract, and without eye lesions, nervous symptoms, and enlargement of the lymph glands.

TREATMENT. None can be recommended for the viral infection, but secondary bacterial infections may be helped by sulfas. When animals are showing nervous symptoms it is usually best to do nothing more than move them into quarters where they can be kept free of disturbances, and have access to feed and water. Glucose and vitamin A may be administered, and if animals will not drink, water may be given through a stomach tube. Eyes should be cleaned daily, and given appropriate treatment with ointments or ocular powders. Regardless of what is done, the chances of recovery are very poor for affected animals.

PREVENTION. Due to a lack of knowledge concerning the means of spread and reservoirs of the causative virus, it is difficult to prescribe effective measures. Experience has indicated that sheep are important in spreading this disease, so it is recommended that sheep and cattle be separated, particularly at lambing time. In experiments, the disease was apparently eliminated by separating sheep from the diseased cattle. Similarly, in Africa the native herdsmen believe that wildebeest are a source of infection for cattle only when the wildebeest calve, and move their herds away from them during this season. Experiments have indicated that available vaccines have little or no value in preventing this disease. Owners will do well not to purchase animals through community sales or auction barns because of the danger of buying recovered carriers of malignant catarrhal fever.

Pulmonary Adenomatosis

CAUSE. Not definitely known, although when first reported from Texas in 1953,* it was associated with the feeding of moldy sweet potatoes, corn stalks, higari, and milo. At various times the condition has been blamed on moldy feeds, bacteria, viruses, and allergies, but none of these causes have been involved in all cases. It has been suggested that lungworm larvae may sometimes be a contributing factor to this condition.

The similarity between lung lesions of this disease and those found in human beings with "silo-fillers disease" has caused authorities to suspect that the cattle disease was also caused by the inhalation of nitrogen dioxide. A recent experiment at Iowa State College** using this gas reproduced both the symptoms and lesions of pulmonary adenomatosis. Such a cause is possible, for

* North American Veterinarian, April 1957, page 109.
** Southwestern Veterinarian, 6, 1953, page 267.

the fermentation of silage in a silo with the resultant production of nitrogen dioxide may be duplicated in the rumen of a bovine. Nitrates and nitrites are known to be increased in young plants, drouth-stricken plants, and plants grown on soils heavily fertilized with nitrogen. As additional evidence, the Iowa workers point out that both of these diseases occur in rural areas of that state where both animals and human beings have a chance to come in contact with nitrogen dioxide. However, at this time nitrogen dioxide has not been definitely established as a cause of pulmonary adenomatosis.

SYMPTOMS. Much like those of pulmonary emphysema, and beginning with labored breathing that is accompanied by a slight grunt on exhalation. The respiratory symptoms gradually become more severe, with the rate and grunting both increasing until animals finally go down in a stupor and die. Most affected animals show a thick mucus discharge from the nostrils. Opening a dead animal is likely to show the lungs as being greatly enlarged. Unlike rubbery, air-filled normal lungs, these can be cut quite easily because of their thick and meaty structure. Examination of the lungs will show the presence of small tumor-like growths in the cells lining the alveoli to account for the name "adenomatosis." In this respect the lungs will be different from those of animals affected with pulmonary emphysema where the alveolar walls are stretched, thinned, and often ruptured. The nasal passages are apt to be badly inflamed, and tiny blood spots may be found on the lining of the trachea and bronchi. As a rule, only a few animals are affected in a herd, but practically all of those showing symptoms die within two to four days.

DIAGNOSIS. Usually on the basis of a post mortem examination that reveals the characteristic structure of the lungs and shows both of these organs uniformly abnormal. Under farm conditions this disease might be confused with troubles like pneumonia, shipping fever, pulmonary emphysema, allergies, and red nose. The high death rate and evidence of being non-contagious may also help in making a diagnosis.

TREATMENT. None have been very successful. However, recoveries have resulted following massive doses of atropine (1 to 2 grams) given subcutaneously in combination with complete rest and a change of ration.

Nasal Granuloma (Rhinosporidiosis, Maduromycosis)

CAUSE. The single-type found in feedlots of the northern U.S. appears due to infection with *Spherophorus necrophorus,* the same germ that causes foot rot in cattle. The multiple-type found in the southern states was originally described in Africa as a disease of horses, and was believed to be caused by a parasite called *Rhinosporidium equi.* The first occurrence in cattle in the U.S. was reported in 1933. A case in a cow was then reported from Colorado in 1936, and two cases in cattle from Texas in 1951. All of these were believed to be caused by *Rhinosporidium.* However, three ·new cases were reported from central Texas in 1960, and together with the four cases reported earlier, the condition was called a maduromycosis caused by a fungus. Infection of both types is believed to start with an injury to the lining of the nasal passages or turbinates.

SYMPTOMS. Labored breathing and a smelly grayish nasal discharge are the first ones noticed. Breathing becomes progressively more difficult as the growth becomes larger, snoring sounds are made, and open-mouth breathing develops. Breathing has a tendency to become more difficult during the summer months, and easier during the winter. However, the breathing never becomes completely normal again.

The growths may or may not be visible, depending on their location. The single-type appears as one mass of granulated tissue resembling "proud flesh." The multiple-type associated with *Rhinosporidium* usually appears as a number of nodules of varying sizes. The symptoms may last for two or three years, but the difficulty in breathing eventually prevents eating, and animals may starve to death unless slaughtered. During the summer growths may become fly-blown to make a bad condition even worse.

TREATMENT. Streptomycin or dihydrostreptomycin injected at the rate of 1 gram per 100 pounds of body weight for a week or so will sometimes ease symptoms and reduce the size of a single-type growth, but surgical removal represents the only complete cure. Even then, the injection of streptomycin or dihydrostreptomycin may have to be repeated every two or three months to prevent recurrence. No treatment has been demonstrated as effective against the multiple-type of granuloma. Accordingly, affected animals are best slaughtered as soon as they are discovered before they have a chance to lose a great deal of weight.

When Cattle Cough

Whenever an owner hears some of his cattle coughing quite a bit, he is apt to start worrying. This is because such a symptom may be an early sign of extremely serious trouble. On the other hand, a fit of coughing may mean nothing more than one of those that suddenly affect human beings for no good reason at all. Only the appearance of other symptoms will indicate whether or not the coughing is a sign that warrants concern. Even then, it may be quite a job to decide exactly what is the matter, for there are at least 19 possible causes of coughing by cattle. The list looks like this:

1. AIR STARVATION. Caused by poor ventilation in barns. Animals are usually noticed as coughing in the morning after being compelled to breathe foul air all night. The coughing is likely to be cured in a few minutes after the cattle are turned outdoors. Installation of a window fan may be the only treatment needed for this condition.

2. IRRITATING SUBSTANCES. Air may contain smoke, dust from hay, or nitrogen dioxide from fresh silage. Applying hydrated lime to barn floors may cause coughing by many of the cattle that are inside.

3. GANGRENE OF THE LUNGS.

4. CHOKE.

5. ALLERGIES.

6. INFLAMMATION OF THE PHARYNX.

7. LUNG ABSCESSES.

8. RED NOSE, or IBR.

9. VIRUS DIARRHEA.

10. MUCOSAL DISEASE.

11. SHIPPING FEVER.

12. PNEUMONIA.

13. MALIGNANT CATARRHAL FEVER.

14. WOODEN TONGUE.

15. DIPHTHERIA.

16. WINTER DYSENTERY.

17. LUNGWORMS.

18. TUBERCULOSIS.

19. BRONCHITIS.

With these various possibilities in mind, owners shouldn't be too sure that they know the exact cause of trouble when cattle begin to cough. This is particularly true any time there's danger that a contagious disease is involved. In such cases a veterinarian should be called at once for the sake of obtaining a definite diagnosis. Owners will save money by doing this in the event that something like shipping fever is getting started.

7.

SKIN TROUBLES

Anatomy of the Cow's Skin

The skin covers all parts of the cow's body and at the natural openings is continued by the mucous membranes lining the digestive and respiratory and reproductive tracts. It consists of two distinct layers, the outer one called the epidermis and the deeper one known as the corium. The cow has a thicker skin than any of the other farm animals, and it is subject to considerable variation in different body areas. It is generally thickest across the back and grows progressively thinner over the sides and belly. However, at the brisket or point of the hock it may be twice as thick as at other points. The skin is attached to the body by so-called subcutaneous tissue. This contains quite a bit of muscle which in many areas has fibers attached to the skin to permit twitching or wrinkling of the epidermis. Both the arteries and veins form networks in the corium and send off branches to the hair follicles and glands. The color of the skin varies greatly in cattle, but it is generally concealed by the hair which is really a specialized part of the epidermis.

The hoofs are also considered as a specialized form of the epidermis, and are made up of three parts known as the periople, sole, and wall. These are naturally doubled on each foot because of the cloven hoof. The periople surrounds the top of each hoof as a flat band. It is about a half inch wide except at the back where it widens considerably to cover the heels. The sole covers the bottom of the hoof and merges with the periople at the heel. The wall covers the sides of the hoof and is joined to the other two parts. The corium underlies all of these harder structures just as the case of ordinary epidermis.

The horns represent another specialized form of the epidermis which covers the bony horn processes given off by the skull. It is thin except near the tips of the horns where it may be practically a solid mass. The corium lies beneath this outer covering and is attached to the bone by so-called periosteum.

Eczema

CAUSE. Usually an accumulation of dirt which first leads to inflammation of the epidermis and then to the formation of vesicles and pustules. These rupture to make the skin moist and covered with dry crusts matted in the hair. Decomposition and infection are likely to occur under these crusts to make the inflammation progressively worse. When destruction has worked deep enough to involve the corium the condition is more properly known as dermatitis. An example is furnished by the suppurative dermatitis described under mammary troubles. Wading through mud or manure is often to blame for eczema, while overfeeding seems to be concerned with certain cases, too.

SYMPTOMS. Usually starts as a simple reddening of the skin which becomes progressively worse with the formation of vesicles and pustules. The skin becomes covered with scabs and crusts and itching is intense. Constant rubbing and scratching serves to thicken it and cause wrinkling and loss of hair. Often there is bleeding and involvement of the corium. Healing may occur only to allow the trouble time to break out all over again.

DIAGNOSIS. Usually through the elimination of other possible causes. May be confused with ringworm, mange, lousiness, vitamin deficiencies, and various kinds of allergies.

TREATMENT. Begins with clipping hair from around affected areas and scrubbing them with mild soap and warm water. After that the application of mild sulfurized oil or the lime-sulfur dip recommended for mange treatment will help to promote healing. A suitable remedy can be made at home by mixing one part of sulfur iodide in ten parts of olive oil. When itching is severe the mixture can be improved by adding five parts of alcohol. A five per cent mixture of either tannic acid or salicylic acid in alcohol may also prove helpful.

PREVENTION. Usually a matter of keeping animals clean and feeding them properly. However, eczema can sometimes start in areas between the legs and body under the best of conditions, so a watch must be kept on such places.

Light Sensitization (Photosensitization)

CAUSE. The eating of certain plants and drugs that results in sensitization to sunlight. It is sometimes caused by buckwheat, trefoil, and alsike clover, while poisoning from lantana in the southeast and lechuguilla in the southwest is also considered a form of light sensitization. In addition, trouble has followed the grazing of crimson clover, Ladino clover, Dutch white clover, coastal Bermuda, common Bermuda, or fescue. Sensitization is commonest when grasses die because of drouth, become moldy when it rains, and then are eaten with new growth which comes up through the old. Symptoms may also appear following grazing on frozen grass like Bermuda. The grass dries after freezing, then becomes moldy, and when new growth starts, animals are forced to eat a mixture of new and old grass. Since trouble may appear following the use of phenothiazine for worming calves, this drug must be considered as a sensitizing agent in young calttle, although older animals show much more resistance to it.

SYMPTOMS. The commonest type of sensitization causes little more than a reddening and peeling that affects only white areas of the skin. A much more serious form occurs when a so-called "icterogenic" substance is eaten with plants. This damages the liver so that bile pigments accumulate to produce severe jaundice. In addition, the liver is unable to eliminate a substance called phylloerythrin which is made in the intestines from chlorophyll and is released into the blood to sensitize tender skin areas.

In the early stages affected cattle slobber, water at the eyes, act sick, and often have a diarrhea. They may appear nervous, shaking their heads, switching their tails, and moving restlessly. The eyes often become yellow-colored, and skin areas appear "sunburned" especially on the shoulders, flanks, and around the eyes. Evidence of burning may also appear on the udder and teats to make them so painful that cows kick at milking time or refuse to let their calves suck. Skin lesions develop first as slight swellings over small areas, and within a few days the affected skin areas crack open and serum escapes to cause matting of the hair. Crusts form and the cracks widen until large sections of the skin become dried out and slough away to reveal raw sores. In some cases animals die before severe skin lesions have a chance to show up. The severe form may also cause lesions in the mouth, crusting of the muzzle, and evidence of lameness. Although usually not considered very serious, the death rate sometimes ranges between 2 and 10 per cent of an affected herd. Attacks are most likely to occur on hot days following a heavy rain.

DIAGNOSIS. Usually on the basis of typical symptoms and a history of recent worming with phenothiazine or feeding on suspicious pasture or forage. In some cases the fact that only white areas of the skin are affected will help to indicate the trouble.

TREATMENT. Begins with getting animals in out of the sun and taking them off causative pasture or removing moldy roughage from the ration. A veterinarian should be called for seriously affected animals, since they may die if not treated immediately. In an emergency they may be given a 30% solution of sodium thiosulfate intravenously at the rate of 1 ounce per 100 pounds of body weight. Sodium thiosulfate may also be given by mouth at the rate of 2 ounces per 100 pounds of body weight. However, it is often difficult to drench affected animals, and when given this way the drug will not act as fast as when given intravenously. The intravenous treatment can be repeated or supplemented by giving an ounce per 100 pounds of body weight by mouth. The itching and pain can often be relieved by the intramuscular injection of a corticosteroid. Skin lesions can be treated with an oily preparation like carron oil or zinc oxide ointment, and those of the udder with something like a mastitis ointment containing a corticosteroid.

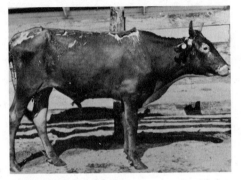

A steer suffering from light sensitization following exposure to mouldy Bermuda grass. (Picture, courtesy Dr. W. J. Gibbons, A.P.I., Auburn, Ala.)

PREVENTION. Do some or all of these things:
1. Keep calves inside for at least a week after treatment with phenothiazine.
2. Mow, rake off, or burn pastures after drouths or frost to get old growth out of the way.
3. Let new grass get at least six inches high in pastures before turning in animals.
4. Avoid overgrazing that encourages animals to eat down into dead or moldy old plant growth.
5. Change animals to other pastures or a dry lot at the first sign of light sensitization.
6. Avoid the feeding of moldy or mildewed forage.
7. Supply extra feed to avoid the danger of overgrazing.

Allergies (Hives, Urticaria)

CAUSE. Not always known, but at one time or another this trouble has been traced back to certain plants, frozen feed, dusty hay, spoiled silage, and various types of pollen, molds, and yeasts. Reactions have occurred when milk was left in the udders of cows being dried off or exhibited. They have also occurred when vaccination was done, or following the injection of drugs or serums, or when "grubs" were crushed under the skin while being squeezed from the backs of cattle. Calves have been affected by milk substitutes, and cows may show symptoms when they fail to "clean" after calving. Impairment of breathing is due to swelling of the membranes lining the nostrils and the rest of the respiratory system.

SYMPTOMS. A large number of swellings usually appear on various parts of the body. These are most likely to be seen around the eyes, ears, anus, vulva, teats, and udder, but they may show up anywhere, either as small scattered wheals or so close together that they may merge to cover large areas of the body. The skin often becomes pink in color, and may appear to be wrinkled.

Animals sometimes show signs of intense itching, run high fevers, and shiver violently. Swelling of the lining of the nostrils and upper throat frequently causes slobbering, panting for breath, and snoring sounds. There may be watering of the eyes, yellow or bloody discharges from the nostrils, and frothing at the mouth. The nose is sometimes rubbed viciously against anything handy so that pieces of wood or stalks of plants are forced far up the nostrils. Although symptoms are frightening when seen for the first time, they are seldom serious and usually disappear in an hour or so, even when nothing is done to relieve the condition. Affected cattle soon start eating again after an attack, but milk production may be greatly reduced for two or three days.

Cases may appear at any time of the year, either when cattle are on pasture or being kept inside on dry feed. When roughage or pasture is to blame, trouble is almost always due to dust, pollen, yeasts, molds, or some type of plant substance. Although it is seldom that more than one or two animals are affected in a herd, the same ones may suffer attacks every few days over a considerable period of time. In some cases a certain animal will be affected year after year, but only during a specific part of a single season. At the other extreme, an animal may have a single attack and then never have another one as long as it lives.

DIAGNOSIS. Usually made on the basis of typical symptoms that disappear in a short time without animals showing symptoms of general sickness. In some cases a history of recent vaccination, treatment with drugs and serums, or manual removal of warbles will help to indicate the nature of trouble. In the beginning of an attack this trouble might be confused with pulmonary emphysema, shipping fever, pneumonia, the nervous form of acetonemia, or red nose.

TREATMENT. Largely a matter of correcting the primary cause in order to prevent a recurrence of attacks. When cases occur on pasture, it is generally best to take the affected animals off pasture and to keep them on dry feed for a few days. If symptoms reappear when they go back on pasture, the animals can be returned to dry feed for a couple of weeks and again tried on pasture.

Cases that occur during the fall and winter call for an attempt to find the cause through one-by-one elimination of various feeds from the diet. Since frozen and moldy silage or dusty hay is often involved in these cold weather cases, it will be a good idea to start with the removal of such feeds from the ration. If cows are being dried off, it may help to milk them out a few more times before forgetting about them.

When symptoms are known to be due to something like vaccination, retention of afterbirth, injection of serum, or crushing of warbles under the skin, it will be advisable to call a veterinarian to administer drugs like adrenalin or antihistamine compounds.

In an emergency, treatments listed under Summer Snuffles can be tried. An owner can sometimes relieve intense itching by applying snow or ice packs to affected areas. An alternative is the use of a thin paste made by mixing ordinary baking soda with water. This is applied to the itching area, rubbed in well, and allowed to dry on the animal.

Stings by Insects

CAUSE. Stings by insects like bees, wasps, hornets, and occasionally massive attacks by mosquitoes. Bites by spiders have also been reported as causing trouble at times.

SYMPTOMS. Pretty much as described for hives, although the swellings are apt to be more painful and limited to a smaller area. They also tend to persist for a longer period of time.

DIAGNOSIS. Generally through the appearance of symptoms after known or suspected attacks by insects. The confinement of swellings to certain areas may also help to indicate the true nature of trouble.

TREATMENT. The same as given for hives.

Grubs in the Back (Cattle Warbles)

CAUSE. The larvae of two different flies. *Hypoderma lineatum* (heel flies, warble flies, cattle warbles) are found in the southern and southwestern parts of the United States; *Hypoderma bovis* (bomb flies, cattle grubs) are confined to the northern part of this country.

H. bovis is active through most of the summer and is generally to blame for the frenzied running of cattle on pasture since they terrify animals by their bullet-like attacks when laying eggs. *H. lineatum* is active for only about six weeks during the early spring and works so quietly that it seldom excites cattle. Both flies lay eggs on the hairs of the legs and lower parts of the body, and their life cycles are practically identical.

The most obvious damage is generally produced by the larvae cutting holes in the skin and spoiling it for leather. However, additional damage results from absorption of poisons excreted by the larvae and destruction of normal tissue to make it "jelly beef" that has to be trimmed away at slaughter time. At times the larvae get into the brain and spinal canal to cause serious nervous symptoms and all kinds of crazy actions. Everything considered, the losses due to cattle warbles are estimated at 50 million dollars every year.

LIFE CYCLE. Larvae hatch from the eggs in about a week after they are laid on hairs, and immediately penetrate the skin through hair follicles. The larvae of *H. lineatum* make their way into the body cavities, and require about two months to reach the esophagus, where they remain for another two or three months. Finally, they move backward and upward, often through the spinal canal, and lodge under the skin of the back. This journey requires about 30 days. They then pierce the skin again, but this time they back up to the hole so that it serves both as a breathing place and an outlet for wastes during the period that the larvae are developing. In 40 to 80 days the larvae emerge through the skin opening, drop to the ground, and go into the pupal stage. This stage may last from one to three months, depending on weather conditions. Adult flies eventually emerge from the pupal case, mate, and lay eggs to start the cycle all over again. Most of the larvae found in the spinal canal are those of *H. bovis*. This is taken to indicate that these larvae rarely migrate to the region of the esophagus as those of *H. lineatum* almost always do.

SYMPTOMS. Chiefly through the typical swellings on backs during the early spring. Many of the early cases of hives are believed due to allergic reactions caused by the larvae. Cases have been reported where the larvae entered the backbone and caused crazy actions through serious damage to the brain or spinal cord. During the egg-laying season running of animals and interrupted feeding may cause loss of weight and decreased milk production in addition to body injuries due to running through fences and into objects of various kinds. Younger animals seem most severely affected by these parasites, but the reason is not definitely known.

DIAGNOSIS. Based on demonstration of larvae in the swellings along the back. Eggs can sometimes be found on the hair of animals during the summer.

TREATMENT. Rotenone is the old standby for killing grubs and several ready-mixed liquid and powder preparations are available through veterinarians. The powders are apt to be more practical during cold weather when wetting of animals may be undesirable. Instead of the commercial preparations your druggist can make up either of the following mixtures:

1. One part of derris powder containing 5% rotenone and one part of double ground tripoli earth.
2. One part of derris powder containing 5% rotenone and two parts of prophyllite.

The powder is dusted on liberally and thoroughly worked into the skin with a stiff brush. The initial application should be made about six weeks after the swellings first appear, with a second one being made about three days later. A third treatment is recommended about two weeks after the second one.

A liquid solution can be made by putting twelve ounces of derris powder containing 5% rotenone in every gallon of warm water and then adding two ounces of granulated soap. This can be applied either with a brush or power sprayer at the same intervals suggested for the powder. The only treatment approved for warble control in dairy cattle is rotenone used as a spray or 1.5% dust. Removal of grubs by squeezing them out is dangerous, since abortions and even deaths have been caused by allergic reactions when parasites were crushed under the skin.

Although helpful, the rotenone treatments have the disadvantage of killing grubs only after they have already done a great deal of damage. Aware of this, for years USDA scientists tried injecting or feeding various drugs in search of one that would kill the grubs earlier. Dieldrin, lindane, aldrin, diazinon, and other drugs were used with considerable success. However, none of the tested chemicals were any better than rotenone because they didn't prevent emergence of the grubs from the back after they had seriously damaged both the hide and meat of an infested animal.

Then in 1955 the Dow Chemical Company announced the discovery of a drug that kept grubs from developing in cattle. This was an organic phosphate chemical known as ET-57, and later sold under various trade names, like Trolene and Viozene. It was given to cattle either as a drench or in bolus form, and was carried by the blood to destroy grubs wherever they were located in the body at the time of treatment. Eventually other organic phosphates were developed which gave almost 100% control of grubs when given to animals either as a drench, bolus, or mixed with feed. Other compounds like Co-Ral were equally effective when applied to animals as a spray or dip, or even poured on along the back, as in the case of Ruelene or Rid-Ezy. In South Dakota tests, excellent results were secured when a long-handled dipper was used to pour the insecticide evenly along the animals' backs. This method has the advantage of being faster than spraying, and does not require special equipment. Animals that are sprayed should be treated with a sprayer that gives at least 250 pounds of pressure per square inch, and the skins should be thoroughly wetted. For best results movements should be restricted to permit working at close range, and the spray should be directed at right angles as nearly as possible.

The best time for application will depend on the area where cattle are kept, but to get complete control treatment should be delayed until the adult "warble fly" season is over, and preferably at least four weeks before grubs normally appear as lumps in the back. With this in mind, the following treatment times are suggested: Southern areas—May through October; Northern areas—July through November. In far Northern areas, treatment into mid-December has been found to be effective. Regardless of the compound used, directions should be followed exactly. Do not treat dairy animals, animals less than three months old, animals that are sick, or within ten days of shipping, weaning, or vaccination, animals that are to be slaughtered in less than the time limit afterward.

PREVENTION.   Entirely a matter of destroying the larvae before they can develop into flies to lay eggs. An eradication program is successful only when owners cooperate on a township or county-wide basis because the flies travel for long distances. Consequently, control on a single farm isn't very effective when the neighbors persist in raising flies.

Lousiness (Pediculosis)

CAUSE. Five different species of lice occur on cattle in the United States. One of these, *Bovicola bovis,* the red louse, is a biting louse. The other four are sucking lice: *Linognathus vituli,* the long-nosed blue louse; *Haematopinus eurysternus,* the short-nosed blue louse; *Solonopotes capillatus,* the hairy cattle louse, and *Haematopinus quadripertusus,* the tail louse. The first four are widely distributed throughout the United States, but the tail louse, first reported from Florida in 1948, is pretty much limited to the southern states. This is probably because it is unable to stand low temperatures, being almost completely wiped out by extremely cold spells during the winter.

LIFE CYCLE. About the same for all species. Eggs are laid and fastened to hairs close to the skin, and hatch into nymphs in about two weeks. These nymphs look much like adults except for their smaller size. After going through three nymphal stages, they become mature lice in two or three weeks after hatching, and shortly start laying eggs on their own to start a new cycle.

With the exception of the tail louse, all species tend to grow best and do the most damage during cold weather. This is generally believed due to the fact that only lice that find protected areas such as between the legs, in the brush of the tail, or inside the ears, can survive the heat of summer.

SYMPTOMS. Itching shown by restlessness, rubbing, and licking is common. Continued irritation often results in loss of hair, thickening of the skin, and scab formation as seen in mange or ringworm. Heavy infestations commonly cause severe loss of weight and decreased milk production. Young and poorly fed animals are apt to be most seriously affected. Lice are commonest and most numerous during the winter season when hair coats are longest and dirtiest. With the arrival of spring, shedding of hair, and turning of animals out in the sunshine, the parasites seem to disappear.

DIAGNOSIS. Made by finding the lice or their eggs on the animals. Sucking lice prefer the poll, backbone, or inside surfaces of the hind legs while the red biters favor the area around the base of the tail. However, they may be found almost anywhere on affected animals. Several different kinds can sometimes be found on the same animal, and may even appear in company with mange mites, ringworm, and other forms of skin infection. As a result, the finding of lice should not be taken as proof that they are the sole cause of trouble.

TREATMENT. Several effective products are available in either liquid or powder form for ridding cattle of lice. Powders are usually preferred in cold weather, although liquids can be used to advantage in the early fall when days are still warm and there are only a few lice to be removed. The rotenone preparations recommended for grubs in the back will also kill lice, but are ineffective against the eggs or nits. The same thing is true of 5% coal tar dips and the lime-sulfur mix used against mange mites. Consequently, follow-up treatments at two-week intervals are needed when such preparations are used.

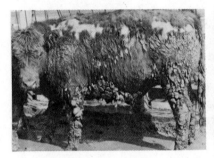

Continued irritation by lice often results in loss of hair and thickening of skin.

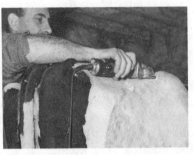

Lice can be controlled by close clipping of animals at six-week intervals.

Dairy cattle can be sprayed with solutions of 0.25% ciodrin, 0.25% pyrethrins plus 0.25% synergist, 5.0% rotenone, or treated with a 0.5 to 1.0% rotenone dust. Any of these can be repeated after two weeks if needed, and may also be used on beef cattle.

Beef cattle can either be sprayed or dipped with solutions of 0.06% coumaphos, 0.15% dioxathion, 0.03% lindane, 0.25% ronnel, 0.5% toxaphene, or sprayed with solutions of 0.5% malathion, 0.5% methoxychlor, 0.59% carbaryl, or 0.375% ruelene. The only dusts recommended for use on beef cattle are 5.0% malathion, 10.0% methoxychlor, 5.0% toxaphene, or 1.0% lindane. Automatic treatments like oilers and backrubbers are not completely satisfactory for lice control, since the entire body must be treated for best results.

Tail lice can be controlled by a 1.0 to 1.5% methoxychlor spray.

Recent experiments at the University of Wisconsin have indicated that cattle lice can be controlled without any kind of dipping, dusting, or spraying. The method simply calls for close clipping of animals at six-week intervals. It appears effective because the lice evidently need the protection of long hair if they are to remain on cattle during the winter months. When animals are clipped the beasts will need to be protected against cold and bad weather.

PREVENTION. Pretty much a matter of good feeding and keeping animals clean in well-lighted and properly ventilated quarters. The disinfection of stables before animals are brought in for the winter will also help, while the "delousing" of newly purchased animals may keep parasites from being brought into a herd.

Stephanofilariasis

CAUSE. A tiny worm called *Stephanofilaria stilesi* which burrows in the skin. The life cycle is unknown but it is suspected that the parasites are spread by blood-sucking insects.

SYMPTOMS. Much like those of ringworm, but the lesions are usually found on the bellies of animals instead of the sites preferred by the fungus. Infection is usually shown by bald areas of thickened skin which are covered with dry crusts. Itching frequently causes rubbing which leads to bleeding and swelling of the infested skin areas.

DIAGNOSIS. Made through microscopic examination of skin scrapings taken from beneath the crusts and demonstration of the threadlike worms.

TREATMENT. None is known, although recoveries sometimes occur without anything being done.

Myiasis (Screwworm Infestation, "Blowing" by Flies)

CAUSE. The laying of eggs by certain varieties of flies in dead or living animals. These then hatch into larvae or maggots that burrow around in the area while feeding. The filth-smeared buttocks of animals afflicted with diarrhea, wounds of various kinds, or the raw navels of new-born calves are common sites of egg-laying, and affected animals are commonly said to be "struck" or "fly-blown." The so-called "screwworm flies" are often blamed for such trouble, but various of the ordinary blowflies are sometimes involved, too.

LIFE CYCLE. The screwworm fly lays eggs in batches of 200 to 300 at the edges of raw areas. These hatch within 24 hours, and the larvae move into the wounds where they live for about a week and then drop to the ground and pupate. Flies must emerge from the pupae within 60 days, and the temperature must be at least 54° F. for their development. The flies can complete their development within 3 weeks, but they cannot survive more than 4 months without at least one generation being produced. This means that the screwworm flies can survive the winter only in Texas, Florida, and California. Then they migrate north each year until they are stopped by temperatures too cold for their development. In nature the screwworm larvae develop only in the wounds of living animals.

The ordinary blowflies have a slightly different life cycle. A single female will lay about a thousand eggs in either dead or living animals, and in filthy areas as well as wounds. The eggs hatch into larvae in 8 hours to several days, depending on the weather. The larvae immediately start to feed on their surroundings and become full grown in 2 to 19 days according to the food available. They then leave the animal to enter the ground where they pass through the pupal stage. Adult flies usually emerge in 3 to 7 days, although hibernation through the winter may occur in the pupal stage. In either case the flies start laying eggs soon after emerging from the pupal stage, and a complete life cycle has been known to be completed in 7 days. As a result, there may be several generations of the pests in a single summer. The adult flies live about a month and are also capable of hibernation through the winter.

SYMPTOMS. Uneasiness due to pain caused by the burrowing maggots is usually the first one noted. Dullness, refusal of food, reluctance to move and other evidence of general sickness is sometimes seen in bad cases. A peculiar sweetish odor due to the rotting of flesh is always present and may indicate trouble before any other symptoms are noticed. Infested wounds are always inflamed and badly swollen and are likely to give off a foul-smelling bloody fluid. Examination will show the maggots, sometimes so deeply buried that only their tapered rear ends can be seen sticking up out of the flesh.

DIAGNOSIS. Through demonstration of the larvae or maggots in the bad-smelling "struck" areas.

TREATMENT. Starts with clipping hair from around "struck" areas. Such material is best burned immediately, for it may contain maggots or unhatched eggs. Larvae that have burrowed deeply can be killed with applications of chloroform, benzene, Smear 62, or EQ335. In addition to these compounds, beef animals can be treated with others, like Co-Ral and ronnel compounds. Dead maggots should be removed with tweezers or forceps. Treatment is concluded by applying an agent that will help healing at the same time that it repels flies and keeps them from laying eggs in the area to start trouble all over again. Ordinary pine tar is an old favorite for this purpose, and the compounds mentioned for treatment are also effective.

PREVENTION. Consists of a five-point program:

1. Prompt disposal of all dead animals through burning or chemical treatment recommended by your state livestock officials. This is desirable because flies often lay eggs on dead animals as well as living ones, and covering carcasses with earth does not prevent the hatching of eggs and later development of larvae into flies that find their way to the surface of the ground.

2. Trapping of flies with carcasses used for bait. Your county county agent or state livestock officials will be able to advise you on the construction and use of such traps. Fewer flies mean fewer eggs and maggots, so their large-scale destruction is important.

3. Good management practices that have things like dehorning, branding, castration, ear-marking, etc., being done before or after fly season. When such jobs can't wait, resultant wounds are best treated regularly until healing is complete. All new-born calves should have their navels treated as soon as possible when there is danger of "blowing" by flies.

4. Proper feeding and methods of parasite control to decrease the danger of diarrhea will also lessen the danger of animals being "struck" around the rump region where soiling is likely to occur.

5. Frequent inspection of all pastured animals will make it possible to treat wounds before serious myiasis occurs. A well-organized program of carcass disposal must be followed over a large area, since blowflies are capable of traveling for long distances.

Screwworm flies have been largely eradicated from the southeastern United States, and encouraging progress is being made along the same line in the southwestern states by making use of a natural trait of these flies. That is the fact that the female flies mate only once, while the male flies mate several times. Large numbers of screwworm flies have been raised and then sterilized before release into screwworm areas so as to flood such areas with sterile male flies. It has been shown that the sterilization does not affect the mating behavior or life span of the treated flies.

Gangrene of the Skin

CAUSE. Usually a lack of bedding or impaired circulation of blood in animals that have been "down" for long periods. The condition may also follow injuries by chemicals or freezing, while cases resembling apthous stomatitis but without lesions in the mouth have been described and are probably due to some type of fungous infection. Trouble is often made worse by the use of chaff or sawdust for bedding which has a tendency to stick to moist and injured areas.

SYMPTOMS. Areas that become swollen, dark-colored, and free of hair in any body area. At first the swellings may ooze yellowish or bloody serum, but within a short time the entire thickness of the skin becomes hard, leathery, and apparently without feeling. General symptoms of sickness may be shown through dullness and impaired appetite when large skin areas are involved. The final stage consists of sloughing the affected skin, with the depth of trouble being determined by the severity of injury.

DIAGNOSIS. Through the appearance of affected areas and the lack of feeling in them. A history of freezing, dipping, spraying, or long confinement in a certain position may help to indicate the nature of trouble, too.

TREATMENT. Packs made by dipping gauze in solutions of 1 part corrosive sublimate to 2000 parts of alcohol are often helpful when applied to gangrenous areas. The packs must be covered with bandages to keep animals from eating them and must not be continued for more than two or three days at a time because the sublimate is a highly poisonous mercury compound. Protectives like zinc oxide ointment or carbolized vaseline are in order and will help to soften the hardened areas. On moist surfaces it may be desirable to use antiseptic powders like mixed sulfas for their drying action. Thuja and penicillin ointments are recommended for healing purposes. The wounds are best kept lightly covered at all times to prevent contamination and infection.

PREVENTION. All animals should be furnished with a deep bed of clean straw at all times, and those that are "down" for any reason should be turned at least six times daily. Areas like legs that are exposed to constant friction should be wrapped in cotton and then bandaged for protection whenever possible. Other preventive measures consist of avoiding the various causes given earlier.

Injury by Chemicals

CAUSE. Usually by application of dips that have been improperly mixed and made too strong. Occasionally some of the home-made fly and insects sprays contain harmful oils. At other times cows lie down in puddles of lye water or similarly strong solutions that have been used for scrubbing stalls.

SYMPTOMS. Pretty much as described for gangrene of the skin, with severity of injury dependent on the amount and strength of the offending chemical involved.

DIAGNOSIS. Usually on the basis of symptoms that follow dipping, spraying, or disinfecting of barn floors.

TREATMENT. Animals should be protected from sunlight while the remedies suggested for gangrene of the skin are also useful for this type of injury. Immediate washing of affected areas with mild soap and warm water may help to remove some of the harmful chemicals before they can do additional damage.

PREVENTION. Largely a matter of carefully following directions when dips and sprays are being compounded. Mixtures of crankcase oil, kerosene, etc., should be used carefully, for they often cause skin damage. Animals should be kept out of the sun for a few hours following the application of all types of oily mixtures.

Vitamin A Deficiency

CAUSE. Once believed to be entirely a lack of carotene in the ration. However, in recent years vitamin A deficiency has been identified in herds fed adequate rations to indicate that the conversion of carotene to vitamin A is blocked in some cases. Studies at the University of Missouri have shown that cattle, eating feeds containing high levels of nitrate, are apt to develop a serious vitamin A deficiency when carotene in forage is the only source. Access to water containing a high level of nitrate will have the same effect. Although the exact mechanics of interference with conversion are not known, it has been suggested that nitrate may modify enzymes that do the actual converting, or it may impair processes involved in the metabolism of vitamin A. Farming methods may be partly to blame for the increased incidence of vitamin A deficiency cases, and in some cases the weather may be a contributing factor. Thick planting and heavy nitrogen fertilization will increase the nitrate content of corn, and so will periods of drought. Until continued research makes more definite information available on the relationship of nitrate and vitamin A, owners should consider the possibility of vitamin A deficiency as a cause of trouble, even when rations appear to contain adequate amounts of carotene.

SYMPTOMS. Roughened hair coat, scaly skin over the neck, withers, and tail head, staggering, spasms, a dropsy-like condition of the brisket, watering and clouding of the eyes, blindness, premature births, weak or still-born calves, breeding troubles, enlarged joints, lameness, and swelling of the feet. Bulls may become temporarily sterile, and fattening cattle may suddenly collapse or go off feed.

DIAGNOSIS. On the basis of suspicious symptoms, especially when they occur in connection with a ration which is obviously deficient in carotene, or during hot weather when conditions favor the destruction of carotene in forage. Under farm conditions this trouble may be confused with others like pinkeye, foot rot, hardware trouble, mange or lousiness.

TREATMENT. Often only a matter of adding vitamin A to the ration. This can sometimes be done by supplying leafy green hay. Even though a great deal of the carotene is destroyed by field-curing, forage that retains its green color will still be an excellent source of vitamin A. Yellow corn is an important source of this vitamin, but it contains only about a tenth as much carotene as good hay. Corn gluten feed, gluten meal, and hominy feed made from yellow corn are higher in carotene than the corn itself. Ripe peas of green varieties equal yellow corn in vitamin A content. When nitrate is believed to be a causative factor, vitamin A supplements can be supplied. For range cattle, a protein pellet fortified with vitamin A is easiest to feed. A highly concentrated form of vitamin A can be added to water, but this requires a tank or attachment on a self-waterer to insure a fixed amount of vitamin A in the water. Another method consists of mixing the vitamin A with water and molasses, and then sprinkling it on the roughage. Adding vitamin A to salt is a convenient way to supply it, but it does not insure an adequate amount for all animals, since some will eat more than others when it is supplied on a free-choice basis. The vitamin A may also be given in the form of capsules. High energy feeds like molasses and corn have been successfully used in reducing nitrate levels in rations.

PREVENTION. Through supplying carotene in the ration either by feeds or vitamin A concentrates. Dairy cows should receive at least 15,000 units of vitamin A daily for a couple of weeks before calving, and 4,000 units daily afterward. Feeder cattle should go on high-level vitamin A for a few weeks as soon as they enter lots to make up for any shortage that may already exist, and be fed the vitamin at a lower level all through the feeding period.

Melanomas

CAUSE. Unknown, since these are types of cancers.

SYMPTOMS. Usually start as small black mole-like structures

that increase in size until they reach considerable proportions. There are believed to be two kinds: a slow-growing type that appears singly and evidently does little harm, and a fast-growing one that appears in clusters and may spread all through the body, both inside and out. This latter type may cause death when it has spread

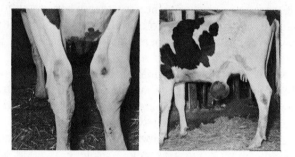

Left: Hygroma of hock or big hock.
Right: Slow-growing type of melanoma on a Holstein heifer.

to the liver, lungs, and other important organs. The growths have the appearance of black warts and are commonest along the back in cattle.

DIAGNOSIS. Usually on the basis of their color and appearance which has sometimes caused the growths to be called "black cancers." It may be confused with warts.

TREATMENT. Best left alone, since tampering with the growth may cause it to become suddenly dangerous and malignant. There is no satisfactory treatment for the fast-growing type, but the less dangerous variety may be removed surgically if the owner wishes to take chances on possible spread.

Big Hock

CAUSE. Generally continuous bruising over a long period that leads to an accumulation of fluid under the skin. Most frequently seen in older animals or those in short, poorly-bedded stalls which have a chance to strike the sides of the hocks on the gutter edge when they lie down.

SYMPTOMS. A gradual enlargement of the hock, usually most pronounced on the outer side. The swelling is almost entirely due to fluid in the early stages, but later on there is increased size of tissues in the area, too. Continued bruising may cause enlargement to the extent where it interferes with walking and is extremely unsightly. The growths seldom become sore, although they may reach the size of a half-bushel basket. In the later stages the growth may become infected through the breaking of skin, and an abscess may develop which oozes pus at various times.

DIAGNOSIS. Based on the typical appearance and location of the swelling.

TREATMENT. None is satisfactory unless the animal is turned to pasture or placed in a deeply bedded stall where continued bruising of the hock is impossible. Under such conditions the swelling may be reduced by daily painting with iodine when it is caught in the early stages. Larger growths will require surgery to drain them. This is best done by making an opening at both the top and bottom, being careful not to injure the joint capsule. The entire sac of fluid may also be dissected out by a skilled surgeon. When the swelling is opened the entire area should be bandaged to prevent contamination of the wound and resultant infection. Healing is likely to require several weeks because of the constant movement of skin around the joint.

PREVENTION. Entirely a matter of providing plenty of bedding and stalls that are long enough so that hocks aren't bruised over gutter edges when animals lie down.

Big Knee

CAUSE. Constant bruising of the knees that leads to an accumulation of fluid under the skin as in the case of big hock. Most frequently due to bumping against the manger curbing while getting up and lying down or through eating in a kneeling position while reaching for food.

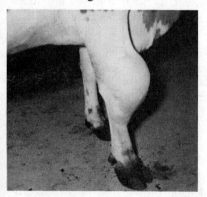

Big knee

SYMPTOMS. The same as given for big hock except that the swelling appears on the front part of the knee.

DIAGNOSIS. Based on the gradual growth and location of the swelling.

TREATMENT. The same as given for big hock.

PREVENTION. Placing a sack of hay or straw against the manger curb may pad it so injuries aren't likely to occur. Setting the stanchion back an inch or so may also prove helpful.

Big Brisket

CAUSE. The same as given for big knees and hocks except that bruising occurs to the lower part of the brisket, usually through bumping on the lower edges of mangers, feed racks, or stanchions.

SYMPTOMS. A large swelling that appears at the brisket. No other signs of sickness are shown.

TREATMENT. The same as given for big knees and hocks.

DIAGNOSIS. Usually through the location of the swelling, although it may easily be confused with hematomas discussed a little later. Hardware trouble in the latter stages will also sometimes cause swelling in the brisket area.

PREVENTION. As already given in regard to preventing bruises of the involved area.

Big Pin Bones

CAUSE. As given for the three preceding troubles except that bruising occurs on the back part of the pin bones on each side of the tail. Such injuries are often called "car bruises" because of their appearance in cattle that have stood with their rumps braced against walls during shipment in trucks or stock cars.

SYMPTOMS. Swelling in the region mentioned, with either one or both of the pin bones being affected. Such injuries are more likely to be seen in thin cattle than in fat ones because of a lack of protective fat in the area.

TREATMENT. The same as already given for the three preceding troubles.

PREVENTION. Entirely a matter of preventing bruising. Injuries may be due to bumping on gutter edges when cattle lie down or on joists that cows repeatedly back into.

Hematomas

CAUSE. Any kind of an injury that breaks a blood vessel and causes it to release blood under the skin instead of letting it escape to the outside through a wound. Kicks, blows, and falls are commonly involved, as are accidents occurring in jumping over doors and gates.

SYMPTOMS. A swelling that suddenly appears in areas that were perfectly normal a short time before. In cattle it is most common along the belly wall where some of the milk veins have been damaged. They are also frequently seen along the sides of the neck due to stanchion injuries or behind the ears where they have been caused by "pulling back" on restraining devices. The enlargements are usually cold to the touch and cause the animal no pain. They seldom cause any indications of general sickness.

DIAGNOSIS. Usually on the basis of sudden appearance, although those along the belly wall may be confused with ruptures mentioned a little later in this section. When animals have not been closely watched for long periods, a hematoma might also be mistaken for an abscess. Sometimes it is well to insert a hypodermic needle in the swelling and draw out a sample of material in a syringe before making a definite decision as to the nature of trouble.

TREATMENT. Nothing should be done in less than a week, since such a delay will give the broken blood vessel a chance to be repaired. After that time the swelling can be opened and clotted

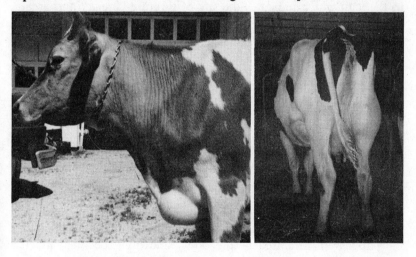

Left: Hematoma brisket.
Right: Abscess of thigh started by bruising against stall divider.

blood removed so the skin can settle back and healing occur in a normal manner. Dusting the interior of the cavity with sulfas or antiseptic powders will help to prevent possible infection. Smaller hematomas will sometimes be resorbed by the body without any treatment whatever.

Abscesses

CAUSE. Usually a bruise that has become infected or some sort of penetrating wound that has been contaminated with pus-forming bacteria. Hematomas may also become infected and develop into abscesses.

SYMPTOMS. Pretty much the same as given for hematomas, although swellings usually take longer to develop and are thicker-walled. In the early stages they are also apt to feel hot and appear painful to the animal. Large ones may cause evidence of general sickness in the form of increased body temperature and loss of appetite.

DIAGNOSIS. Usually through the slower growth. although those along the belly may be confused with ruptures that permit increasing amounts of the intestines to escape under the skin. In fact, both abscesses and ruptures sometimes exist at the same time, particularly when the navel region is involved. Using a syringe to draw out some of the contents may help to establish the true nature of trouble. In the latter stages a "soft" spot can sometimes be felt in the wall which indicates the site of a future "break" and escape of pus.

TREATMENT. Hot packs or poulticing will often help to bring abscesses to a "head" so they will rupture by themselves; otherwise, as soon as ready, the abscess may be opened and drained of pus. The cavity can then be packed daily with gauze soaked in Lugol's solution. The packs are decreased in size as the cavity closes.

Bruises

CAUSE. Any kind of a blow that injures tissues without breaking the overlying skin. When large blood vessels are broken a hematoma results, and when nerves are destroyed gangrene may result in the area.

SYMPTOMS. Much like those given for a hematoma, but with swelling due to inflammation and serum instead of blood. They may appear in any area of the body, and often become infected to develop into abscesses.

DIAGNOSIS. Usually through elimination of other troubles like hematomas, abscesses, or ruptures. When appearing around the jaws, bruises may be confused with lumpjaw or wooden tongue.

TREATMENT. The application of ice packs and bandages often helps resorption of serum with decrease of swelling, while daily painting with iodine is also recommended.

Ruptures or Hernias

CAUSE. Usually a blow or sudden strain that has produced a tear in the belly muscles without breaking the skin. As a result the intestines escape under the skin instead of being confined within the body in a normal manner. Ruptures are sometimes inherited and calves may be born with the defect.

SYMPTOMS. A swelling that either appears suddenly or is present at birth at some point along the lower sides or belly wall. In calves the condition is commonest at the navel where an abnormally large opening persists. Ruptures in bulls sometimes permit the intestines to come down inside the scrotum with the testicles. The swellings are not apt to be painful, but loops of intestine may become pinched off or "strangulated" to cause symptoms as described under intussusception of the intestines in an earlier section of this book.

DIAGNOSIS. Usually through the symptoms and location of the swelling. Sometimes a break or ring in the muscle wall can be felt with the fingers, or the swelling can be completely reduced by re-

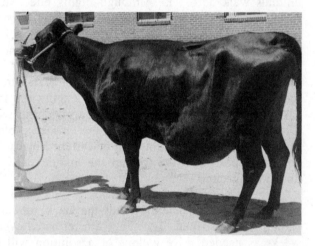

Rupture of lower flank muscles in cow.

placing the contents inside the body where they belong. Sometimes intestinal contents can be withdrawn by use of a syringe and hypodermic needle. Ruptures may be confused with hematomas, abscesses, or rupture of the prepubic tendon. In the bull a swelling of the scrotum caused by hernia may be thought due to infection or a tumor of the testicles.

TREATMENT. Surgery is usually the only practical treatment and this may not be advisable in the case of older animals with extensive tears in the muscles. The practice usually consists of opening the skin over the swelling, replacing the intestines or other organs, and then sewing up the tear with catgut. The skin is generally sewed separately with different material that has to be removed in about a week. Calves with small ruptures that are only an inch or so across may outgrow the condition by the time they are three months old if they are kept on a concentrated diet of milk and grain that doesn't put too much weight in the digestive tract. Unimproved animals are best operated on at that age, since growth of the digestive organs has a tendency to make existing openings even larger.

Controlling Flies on Cattle

Spraying or dipping at fairly regular intervals are probably the commonest methods of controlling flies, and while effective, they take considerable time and labor. Accordingly, many owners will be interested in one system or another that lets the cattle protect themselves.

Many owners are using the treadle sprayer that works whenever animals walk across it. Although highly effective, these sprayers need frequent servicing to keep the nozzles open. Another automatic device is represented by the cable-type back-rubber. Several different kinds are on the market, but a good one can be built at home for little or nothing.

It is made of three or four strands of barb wire, each 15 to 20 feet long which are twisted together lengthwise. Twelve or fifteen old gunny sacks are then wrapped around the wires and tied at intervals with binder twine so that the finished cable has a diameter of 4 or 5 inches. This cable can be fastened by the ends between a couple of posts or trees so that the middle sags about 18 inches above the ground.

When the first application is made, one gallon of a solution is poured slowly and evenly along the back rubber, for the sacks should not be soaked. The sacks are retreated every three or four weeks as needed. Five gallons of a solution will just about take care of a back-rubber for the season, and one back-rubber should be supplied for every 75 to 100 animals.

The most important point in using a back-rubber is to see that it is set up in a shady place where the cattle loaf, or near a watering place. The vicinity of a salt box is also good, and some owners fasten the cable between a couple of gate posts where the cattle pass every day. A modification of the back-rubber idea can be used in pastures where there is underbrush, with treated sacks being tied to trunks or low branches.

The repellent that is used will depend somewhat on the type of herd, for pesticide residues in milk have been causing the Food and Drug Administration considerable concern in recent years. Because most of the chlorinated hydrocarbon insecticides can be excreted in milk, they are no longer recommended for insect control on dairy cows. Either malathion or methoxychlor powder can be dusted on dairy cows, but not within five hours before milking or oftener than once every three weeks. Compounds like lindane, DDT, chlordane, toxaphene, and others cannot be used on lactating animals.

Continued research work will probably reveal new safe treatments, but at this time only pyrethrins plus synergist, dichlorvos, malathion, methoxychlor, coumaphos, ciodrin, lethane, or thanite are approved for direct application to milking cows for the control of flies and mosquitoes. These may be mixed with either oil or water but the oil solutions are generally preferable for use because of their slower evaporation rate. Official recommendations for dairy cow sprays are as follows:

Pyrethrins (0.05-0.1%) plus synergist (0.5-1.0%) for daily spraying by hand sprayer, treadle sprayer, or electric eye sprayer at the rate of about 2 ounces per animal.

DDVP (1.0%) for daily spraying with all kinds of sprayers, but at a rate of not over 2 ounces per cow. This is not a repellent, but will kill flies on sprayed animals for about 10 hours.

Organic thiocyanates (3.0-5.0%) as oil solution at the rate of 1 to 2 ounces per animal daily as a mist spray.

For beef cattle, dry cows, and young stock, all of the insecticides approved for use on dairy cattle can also be used. In addition, carbaryl, dioxathion, DDT, toxaphene, ronnel, and ruelene can be used for either spraying or backrubber application. Directions on the label should be closely followed in regard to mixing and application, and also in regard to use of the compound a certain number of days before slaughter.

Face Flies

The face fly (Musca autumnalis) is a comparatively new pest in the United States. It originated in either Asia or Europe and was first reported in North America from Nova Scotia in 1952. From then until 1959 it was recognized as existing in the U.S. only in New York, Vermont, Ohio, and Illinois. In that year it was reported from 11 other states east of the Mississippi. These were in an area north of, and including, Tennessee and South Carolina. Since that time it has crossed the Mississippi and appeared in Iowa, Missouri, Minnesota, both Dakotas, Nebraska, and Kansas. In 1961 it was recognized in 25 states as far west as Colorado, and is eventually expected to reach the Pacific coast. Authorities believe that face flies exist in other states but have not been reported, only because they do so little damage in small numbers that they have not been noticed.

The face fly gets its name from the fact that it is usually found on the faces of cattle. The flies swarm about the head, concentrating around the eyes, nostrils, and lips. Here they form tight clusters, dabbing at the mucous membranes for liquid food. In addition, they sometimes congregate on the shoulders, neck, brisket, and legs, feeding on saliva smears left when cattle lick themselves, or on blood coming from wounds left by injuries or biting flies. Irritation by the flies is apt to cause severe watering of the eyes, and scientists believe they may be potential spreaders of pinkeye, eye worm, and navel ill in newborn calves. When not on animals, the flies can be found on the sunny side of trees, fence posts, and buildings, especially during early morning and evening hours.

This pest closely resembles the ordinary housefly, but is much larger than either the horn fly or stable fly. If the size difference is not enough, the face fly can be identified by an outstanding characteristic, for it does not like the shade. Face flies quickly leave animals when they enter barns or shady areas, and will then wait outside in the sun until the cattle come out again. The female lays eggs in fresh manure, and the eggs hatch in 24 hours. The larvae become adult flies in 22-30 days, when the females begin laying eggs of their own to start another life cycle.

Although face flies are not biting flies, a heavy infestation will annoy cattle so that they will stop grazing and bunch together for protection. Dairy cows will then decrease in milk production and beef animals will lose weight. Concentrations of 75 flies per cow in a New Jersey herd caused a 20% drop in milk production. Their preference for sunlight naturally causes face flies to be chiefly an annoyance of pastured cattle in the day time. A spray program that is effective against other flies will provide only limited protection against face flies, and additional control measures are necessary. Dairymen can:

1. Pasture cows only at night. Green crops can be cut and fed during the day.
2. Spray cows daily with permissible materials approved by the USDA which have been listed earlier in this book.
3. Use an organic phosphate insecticide, called DDVP, which has been USDA approved for use in baits. This product is now marketed as a prepared sweetened liquid under various trade names, and it can also be mixed by the user at the rate of 75% corn syrup, 25% water, and 0.2% DDVP. Flies

feeding on it die and drop off in 40 seconds. It is best applied daily in the form of a six-inch X on the animal's forehead with a narrow brush or cellulose sponge. Treatment is continued daily for two or three weeks and afterward if needed.

4. Apply a 0.5% solution of dichlorvos across the forehead in the same manner as described for DDVP.

5. Spray with solutions containing ciodrin, dichlorvos, pyrethrins plus synergist, or coumaphos.

The control of face flies in beef animals is more difficult, since the DDVP can't be applied by hand every day. The most efficient method probably consists of providing back rubbers loaded with a 5% toxaphene oil mixture. Other products approved for backrubber use on beef animals include methoxychlor, DDT, coumaphos, ronnel, and the newer Anti-Resistant DDT, all of which should be used as a 5.0% solution with an oil base. Be sure to follow label directions when using them. insecticides, and set up a regular schedule for reloading the back rubbers. The back rubbers should be set up with one end near the ground so that cattle can rub their faces and heads. Since underbrush and trees will offer competition for fly removal, the back rubbers should not be placed near them. The best locations for back rubbers have already been listed under CONTROLLING FLIES ON CATTLE in this book. Treated sacks can also be hung low on bushes and underbrush to supplement back rubber control.

In addition to being troublesome cattle pests, face flies may become a household annoyance for human beings in the fall of the year, when they often invade farm homes looking for a place to hibernate through the winter. Once inside, they continually swarm around windows and travel throughout the house. It may be possible to get rid of them by using dieldrin, chlordane, DDT, or malathion in the attic, but owners should be sure to follow label instructions and observe safety precautions when such products are used inside buildings, for they are all poisonous to some degree.

Controlling Ticks on Cattle

The control of ticks is primarily important because of the fact that many species have been proven as transmitters and vectors of various diseases. A few of them are piroplasmosis, anaplasmosis, and Q fever. However, even if they did not help to spread diseases, they do enough damage in other ways to justify control measures.

All ticks that prey on cattle are blood-suckers, and with the exception of the spinose ear tick, require a feeding of blood between molts. Assuming the average female tick will require 1 cc. of blood to complete its development, this could result in the loss of considerable blood to affect milk production and weight gains, while lowering resistance to various diseases. In addition, the feeding ticks of certain species may inject a salivary secretion which is capable of causing paralysis and even death. Finally, the feeding ticks do considerable skin damage, and the wounds caused by their bites provide a starting place for bacterial infections and attract flies to cause "strikes." It was once estimated that 90% of the screwworm strikes in the Gulf Coast area are started by tick bites.

Either spraying or dipping at regular intervals can be used to control ticks, but many cattlemen prefer to use a back rubber that lets the cattle protect themselves. An applicator of this type that can be made at home is described on page 289 of this book under CONTROLLING FLIES ON CATTLE. The type of insecticide that is to be used will depend largely on whether a beef or dairy herd is being treated.

Ticks on dairy cattle can be controlled through spraying with a 0.3% ciodrin, 0.1% pyrethrin plus 1.0% synergist, or 5.0% rotenone solution. Malathion or methoxychlor powder can also be dusted on them under the same restrictions that apply when these compounds are used for controlling flies on dairy animals. These chemicals can also be used on beef cattle. In addition, ticks on beef cattle can be controlled by 0.5% carbaryl spray, 0.125% coumaphos spray or dip, 0.15% dioxathion dip or spray, 0.5% malathion spray, 0.75% ronnel spray, or 0.5% toxaphene dip or spray. Since only the adult stage of any three-host tick is found on cattle, dipping and spraying will help control ticks, but will never completely eradicate them. Accordingly, the cattle will have to be treated year after year. When animals are sprayed, solutions should be applied to the "run-off" stage, and particular care should be used to soak the belly, ears, and tail-head area. When water is highly acid or alkaline, certain emulsions may "break," so a preliminary testing of the emulsions with water may be desirable. Wettable powders are usually safe under almost all conditions.

Controlling Flies in Dairy Barns

In addition to controlling flies on their animals, dairymen are also likely to be faced with the problem of controlling flies in their barns and milk houses during the summer months. After they have studied the matter thoroughly, they will probably conclude that selection is a matter of choosing from a group of different chemicals, each with certain advantages and disadvantages. Continued research will probably reveal others, but at the time of this writing there are seven approved chemicals that can be used either as space or residual sprays. When used as a space spray the insecticide is discharged into the air as a fine floating mist or fog. When used as a residual spray, the insecticide is sprayed directly onto walls, ceilings, fixtures, etc. When used in either way, it is recommended that:

1. Feeds, feed troughs, drinking cups, and other sources of water be covered before spraying is started.
2. Animals and human beings stay out of sprayed buildings for at least four hours after application.
3. The breathing of spray mist be avoided by wearing a respirator while spraying is being done.
4. Goggles be worn to keep spray mist out of the eyes.
5. Gloves and waterproof clothing be worn to prevent contact of spray with the skin.
6. Operators wash thoroughly after spraying.
7. Special attention be paid to the operation so that the contamination of milk and other human foodstuffs is avoided.
8. Oil emulsions be used inside buildings only as a last resort because of possible danger when such mixtures are inhaled. Water will evaporate from lungs, but oil will not.
9. Manufacturer's directions be carefully read and even more carefully followed in regard to mixing, application, and unapproved places for use. For example, diazinon is not generally approved for use in milk houses, but it may be used in barns as a residual spray.

One of the seven chemicals is methoxychlor, the first of the so-called residual sprays to be approved for use in dairy barns. Although an excellent fly-killer in some cases, it has the disadvantage of having been used long enough so that flies in certain areas have become resistant to it. However, it will prove highly effective in sections where there is no problem of fly resistance to the chlorinated hydrocarbon insecticides.

A second is malathion, first generally used in 1955. Another is ronnel, also known as Korlan and Trolene. The fourth is DDVP, sometimes called Vapona, and the fifth is diazinon. The sixth is dimethoate, and the seventh is dibrom. They are generally recommended for mixing as 1% solutions, with the exception of malathion, which is suggested as best when mixed as a 2% solution.

The frequency of spraying will depend on the chemical used. Dimethoate is the longest-lasting, and will remain effective for six to nine weeks. Ronnel and diazinon are good for three to six weeks, while DDVP and malathion are only effective for about a week. Dibrom is really not a residual spray at all, since it kills flies for only a few hours. Adding syrup to a spray of any kind may lengthen effectiveness by about 10%. All of these approved chemicals are still poisonous to some extent, so directions and precautions on the label should be carefully followed.

Whatever is used, early-season sprayings seem to last longer than those made later. Tests in New Jersey have shown that sprayings made in mid-May when flies were first appearing in numbers have outlasted applications made in mid-June by two or three weeks. It is possible that earlier spraying would have given still better results.

Methoxychlor is the only approved barn spray that cannot be used in milk houses, too, and several of these chemicals are also approved for bait use. Most of these baits contain the chemicals as a base, with something like sugar or hominy grits serving as a lure, but such baits run a poor second when competing with barn odors for fly interest. When failures occur, they are probably due to the fact that baits have been placed in areas seldom visited by flies. They may also have failed because of rapid deterioration resulting from contact with lime or direct sunlight. Although dry baits are effective as fly-killers, there are very few locations where they can be placed in dairy barns that are washed or swept daily. Accordingly, frequent spot applications of sprays in warm sunny areas frequented by flies are generally preferred to the flake or granular baits. As an alternative, wet baits or sprays may be applied to gunny sacks which are easily moved out of the way when required and replaced later.

Painted-on baits have also been tried. Mixed with syrup, the bait was then applied to gathering places of flies. In exposed areas the painted-on bait would kill flies for two or three weeks, but soon became covered with dirt so it was ineffective. When applied to the underside of light fixtures, the bait remained effective for about a month. The disadvantage of baits lies in the fact that they must be put out frequently and with discretion for best results. Even then, they cannot be expected to prove as satisfactory as a cheaper residual spray that can be applied to any surface.

The effectiveness of treated cords suspended from barn ceilings is largely dependent on the weather when they are used. They may not do much good during hot, dry summer days when flies avoid the ceiling area in favor of relatively cool, moist floors and lower walls. On the other hand, these cords may account for a heavy fly kill during the cool nights of late summer when the barn ceiling has become an attractively warm roosting place.

Effective though these fly-killers are in various forms, it must be remembered that chemicals alone cannot be depended on for the control of flies. You will have to help them out by eliminating the places where flies breed. This means cleaning up strawpiles and removing rotting hay from around feed racks. It also means hauling away manure piles, cleaning out loafing sheds, and keeping milking barns clean. If you clean your barn at least twice-weekly and keep your barnyard as dry as possible all summer, you will be doing a great deal to cut down the number of flies that require killing. When a space spray must be used every day, something is wrong with control methods. Poor sanitation is usually the basic reason, and flies are then being hatched as fast as they are killed.

Since changes are being constantly made in recommended insecticides for cattle, the list should be checked before using any of those listed in this book. An authoritative reference is represented by the USDA Handbook 331, "Suggested Guide For The Use of Insecticides To Control Insects Affecting Crops, Livestock, Households, Stored Products, Forests, and Forest Products." In addition, lists of currently recommended insecticides can usually be obtained from the Agricultural Experiment Stations in most states.

Skin Tuberculosis, Ulcerative Lymphangitis

CAUSE. Acid-fast, rod-like organisms resembling those of tuberculosis, but lesions are definitely not caused by tubercle bacilli. This disease was first reported in the U.S. in 1916, and it or a very similar disease was described in France as early as 1913. It has also been recognized in England, Denmark, and Sweden.

SYMPTOMS. Nodules usually occur on the legs. Although they seem to be in the skin, they are really located just beneath the skin. As time goes on, these nodules generally soften and eventually break through the skin to form ulcers. Additional nodules appear along the course of the lymphatic vessels, and animals in advanced stages of skin tuberculosis may show twenty or more of these nodules, usually arranged in fairly distinct rows. After breaking and discharging, the nodules usually heal. However, in some cases the nodules merge together instead of breaking open one by one. They then form large hard masses with several openings dis-

charging pus. Affected animals may or may not react to the tuberculin test or they may react at one time but not at another. The
disease is not serious, but it causes unsightly blemishes. From an
owner's standpoint, the worst thing about it is the fact that this
disease may confuse the status of a herd that is being tested for
tuberculosis. Reactions to the tuberculin test cannot be safely
blamed on this condition unless herd history makes the occurrence
of tuberculosis highly improbable in the animals.

DIAGNOSIS. Usually on the basis of typical lesions appearing in
characteristic lines on the legs without the neighboring lymph
nodes becoming involved. It might be confused with skin infection
caused by a germ called *Corynebacterium pseudotuberculosis*
(Preisz-Nocard Bacillus), but this germ is not acid-fast, and can
be detected as such in the laboratory.

TREATMENT. None recognized.

8.

NERVOUS TROUBLES

Anatomy of the Cow's Nervous System

For all practical purposes the nervous system can be thought of as consisting of the brain, spinal cord, and nerves which branch off them and go to various parts of the body. Movements and sensations of all kinds are first of all due to the nerves. These are of two kinds: either carrying messages to the brain or away from the brain, and are known as either sensory or motor nerves. For example, a sensory nerve carries a message that a certain part of the body is being hurt by an electric fence. The brain responds by sending a message to appropriate motor nerves that put muscles in action and move the animal out of danger. Another example is furnished by the optic nerves that send messages of sight to the brain. A different set of nerves close the eyelids against insects and move the body so animals don't run into obstacles. These various nerves are given off by the brain and along the full length of the spinal cord. In turn they branch and combine in a complicated communication system which reaches all parts of the body and makes possible the five senses and the most intricate patterns of movement.

The brain is essentially an enlargement of the spinal cord which consists of three major parts. The front part is the cerebrum composed of two equal parts called the cerebral hemispheres. Just back of it is the cerebellum, and still further back is the medulla oblongata. Beyond this point the brain is continued as the spinal cord in the middle of the backbone. The brain proper is divided into several other parts, one of the more important being the hollow interior of the medulla oblongata which is known as the fourth ventricle. Another is the pituitary gland which manufactures many of the hormones important in growth, reproduction, and milk secretion. The brain and spinal cord together are frequently referred to as the central nervous system. Nerves are given off in pairs from opposite sides throughout its full length.

351

Twelve pairs known as the cranial nerves are given off by the brain proper. These go chiefly to the head and throat region, including the eyes, ears, and nose, but the vagus nerves also send branches to the stomach and other internal organs.

Thirty-seven pairs commonly come off the spinal cord and are therefore known as spinal nerves. They are further classified according to the point where they leave the cord. For example, there are usually eight pairs in the neck region between the poll and shoulders which are known as cervical nerves. These largely serve the skin and muscles of the region, although some of the branches combine to form the phrenic nerve which goes to the diaphragm. Some of the branches also combine with certain of the thoracic nerves to form the so-called brachial plexus or network of nerves which lies deep under the inner muscles of the shoulder. This plexus gives off many nerves, with some of the more important being the suprascapular, median, ulnar, radial, and volar. Most of them are important in regard to movement of the front legs.

Thirteen pairs, which are known as the thoracic nerves, leave the spinal cord between the shoulders and last rib. These are pretty much devoted to the skin and muscles of the abdomen, although some of them combine with cervical nerves to form the brachial plexus as mentioned earlier.

Another six pairs, called lumbar nerves, are given off between the last ribs and the hip bones. These go largely to the skin and muscles of the region, although some of them combine with two of the sacral nerves to form the lumbo-sacral plexus. This is another network, with some of the more important nerves coming from it being the femoral, obturator, sciatic, tibial, and plantar.

The sacral nerves are the five pairs that are given off between the hip bones and the root of the tail. They supply branches to the skin and some of the adjacent structures as well as the lumbo-sacral plexus just mentioned. There are usually five pairs of so-called coccygeal nerves that are given off from the tail.

In addition to the nervous system already described there is another one which is known as the sympathetic nervous system. In general it is concerned with the various internal organs and is of little practical interest to cattlemen, so it will not be discussed here.

Injuries to any of the nerves or parts of the central nervous system are shown by various kinds of symptoms. Generally they are concerned with some degree of paralysis, abnormal position, or crazy actions of some kind.

Rabies or Hydrophobia

CAUSE. A virus that causes inflammation of the brain and is present in the saliva of affected animals from one or two days before symptoms are shown until the time of death. Infection usually occurs through bites, but may take place when saliva gets into cracks or wounds of the hands when the mouths of rabid animals are invaded for examination. It affects all animals, but is most common in dogs, foxes, skunks, and other animals which may bite cattle and cause the disease in them. Bites are most dangerous when they are deep or close to the brain as in the case of face and neck injuries. This is because there are many nerves in this area and the virus follows them to the brain where the real damage is done.

SYMPTOMS. Usually appear in two stages, the first being that of excitement commonly known as "furious" rabies. At this time arching of the back and straining as though trying to pass manure is common in cattle. Occasionally they bellow in a peculiarly hoarse tone, paw the ground, and attack people or other animals. Extreme nervousness may be shown by restlessness, constant switching of the tail, jerking of the legs, boring in the ground with horns or head, and sometimes signs of being in heat. Food and water is refused because of the paralysis of throat muscles which makes swallowing impossible. Grinding of the teeth, slobbering, and bloating are also common symptoms. This first stage lasts for two or three days and is gradually replaced by the second, which is often called "dumb" rabies.

Animals become more and more completely paralyzed, finally going down in a helpless condition and even unable to pass urine or manure because of nerve involvement. Death usually occurs about a week after the first symptoms are noted and recoveries are unknown. These symptoms are not to be taken as infallible, for the disease frequently appears as a paralytic condition without any signs of a "furious" or excitement stage. In these cases the animal usually dies within two or three days after being noticed as sick.

DIAGNOSIS. Made definitely only in the laboratory. The quickest way consists of finding Negri bodies in the brain cells under a microscope. However, this method isn't too accurate since they may be absent in the early stages of the disease. On the other hand, they may appear because of other troubles and not be due to rabies at all. Consequently, mice are usually inoculated with some of the suspected brain as a more precise diagnostic measure. Death of the mice in six to ten days with typical symptoms is taken as positive proof of rabies.

It is recommended that suspected animals be permitted to die a natural death whenever possible in order to give the Negri bodies a better chance to appear in the brain cells. If they must be killed, it should be done in a manner that spares the head, for it's practically impossible to examine a brain that has been blown to bits by a shotgun blast or pounded to pulp with a club. Entire heads are best sent to laboratories packed in ice to prevent decomposition that will interfere with microscopic examination. Two waterproof containers are recommended, with one fitting inside the other and the head being packed in the inner one and ice around it in the outer one.

From an owner's standpoint diagnosis is usually based on the typical symptoms that often cause him to suspect choking on something or other. When the early symptoms gradually develop into paralysis the suspicion of rabies should be more pronounced than ever. Animals that don't present the "furious" stage are more of a problem, but paralysis and symptoms of choke should always cause an owner to be a little hesitant about putting his bare hands in a mouth that is dripping saliva. A history of animals that have been bitten some time earlier is often helpful in suggesting the cause of trouble, although the incubation stage varies between 2 to 10 weeks and may be as long as three months. Animals that live longer than two weeks after symptoms are first noted don't have rabies.

TREATMENT. None known after symptoms have developed. It is customary to vaccinate animals that have been bitten by rabid beasts, but the vaccine will not save all treated animals. However, it is recommended that exposed animals be given 100 cc. of vaccine immediately after they are bitten, and two more 50 cc. doses later at two day intervals.

PREVENTION. Preventive measures are difficult to prescribe, since practically all cases of rabies in the United States are transmitted by wild animals like skunks and foxes. In some areas bats are a dangerous source of infection, particularly because apparently normal animals may carry the causative virus in their saliva. Dogs have decreased in importance as spreaders of the disease because of improved vaccines used on them. Aside from vaccination, a practical rabies control program for dogs consists of:

1. Confinement or destruction of all stray and ownerless dogs.
2. Keeping farm dogs home and tied up at night.
3. Quarantining all rabies-infected areas for at least 30 days.

Although people often object to tying up their dogs when they are harmless, confinement is designed for the animals' own protection, not that of others. While running loose, pets may be bitten by rabid dogs or wild animals. Once bitten, they have a good chance of developing rabies themselves, and then biting people or cattle on the home farm.

Pseudo-Rabies or Mad Itch

CAUSE. A virus that causes inflammation of the brain. In swine the disease is mild, contagious, and causes few deaths, while in cattle it is non-contagious but generally fatal. The virus evidently gets started in cattle through invasion of cuts or wounds, and is generally seen in animals that have been running with swine. However, outbreaks of the disease are common in rats, and it often appears that the trouble is spread through bites of these rodents. A single attack gives life-long immunity if the animal survives.

SYMPTOMS. Usually signs of intense itching with continuous licking of the hind quarters that soon removes all the hair from large areas. The condition seems to become progressively worse.

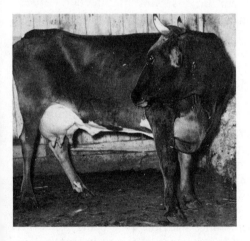

Cattle affected with mad itch are apt to lick themselves a great deal.

and animals often end up by rubbing against barbed wire or anything else in sight. Some of the beasts bite and gnaw at themselves, and itching may become so intolerable that animals go crazy and attack people. Within a short time the entire hind quarters are dark, leather-like, and smeared with blood. In about twenty-four hours affected animals go down in a paralyzed condition, slobbering profusely and often grinding the teeth. Paralysis is likely to be accompanied by bellowing, fast breathing, and convulsions, with death usually occurring within a couple of days after the first symptoms are noted.

DIAGNOSIS. Largely on the basis of the extreme itching and other typical symptoms. It has often been mistaken for the so-called "skin form" of shipping fever, and may also be confused with rabies, acetonemia, and other troubles showing derangement of the nervous system.

TREATMENT. No satisfactory medical remedies are known, but cattle should be separated from swine in the event an outbreak occurs. If cases appear when cattle aren't running with hogs, a program of rat eradication may be needed to stop the trouble.

Circling Disease (Listerellosis, Listeriosis Silage Disease)

CAUSE. A germ called *Listeria monocytogenes* that produces inflammation of the brain. How the germs get into the body is not known. However, carrier animals have been identified, and *Listeria* are common in wild animals. Research work indicates that the soil may be an important reservoir of infection. Since outbreaks are commonest in the winter and early spring, and in the northern states, it has been suggested that germs may be transmitted to cattle through contaminated feed when carriers or infected animals come closer to farm buildings for food. In addition, *Listeria* have been isolated from silage, although the means of entry is not known. It is possibly through soil, carrier birds or animals, or infected rodents like rats and mice. Undernourished animals or calves with scours appear to be highly susceptible.

SYMPTOMS. Usually a tendency to move in circles or stand with the head pressed against something like a building or fence post. At other times affected animals may wander aimlessly or show difficulty in walking. Food and water are completely refused, and milk cows drop off to nothing in production. The head is often carried low and to one side, sometimes with the eyes being rolled far back in the head. If the head is straightened out, it promptly flies back to its former position when released. Paralysis of one side of the face may be shown by a drooping ear or corner of the lower lip. Slobbering is common and animals often appear completely blind. The pulse rate and temperature are variable according to the severity of attacks, but both have a tendency to remain about normal. The urine test for acetonemia may be positive in the later stages of circling disease. All animals older than six weeks are susceptible, but it is seldom that more than one or two are affected in a herd. The disease is generally fatal, with death resulting in two days to a week.

DIAGNOSIS. Definite only through laboratory tests. Under farm conditions it might be confused with lead poisoning or rabies. In dairy cows it might be confused with acetonemia, particularly in the latter stages of the disease when the urine test may show a positive reaction. When specimens are sent to the laboratory, an examination for both rabies and listerellosis should be requested.

TREATMENT. None definite, although favorable results have been reported following the intramuscular injection of penicillin in massive doses. Various of the sulfa solutions have also been claimed as beneficial when given intravenously in the early stages of an attack. Since most of these cases were not confirmed by laboratory diagnosis, there is a possibility that some of them were other ailments instead of circling disease.

PREVENTION. Vaccination with a bacterin has given poor results thus far. It is likely that a live-culture vaccine would give immunity against the disease. However, the disease can affect human beings, and the resulting public health hazard serves to make the procedure very questionable.

Sporadic Bovine Encephalomyelitis (SBE), Buss Disease

CAUSE. A virus of the psittacosis group which is responsible for the disease of this name that affects many wild birds, domestic fowls, pet birds, and even human beings. It is sometimes called Buss disease because the first reported outbreak occurred in cattle owned by a man of that name. There is no way of telling how extensive the disease really is, but at the present time it has been recognized only in Iowa, Texas, Minnesota, South Dakota, Missouri, California, and Idaho. The disease is usually seen in cattle under three years of age, and as a rule only a few cattle are affected in a herd. The disease generally does not appear again in herds after the first attack has subsided, but it is possible for cases to appear year after year on a farm. Infection is rarely spread from sick to healthy animals, but calves being nursed by an affected cow have been known to contract the disease. In spite of extensive work done on this angle, the actual means of spread is still not known. The incubation period is four to twenty-seven days after exposure. Experimental work indicates that sheep, goats, swine, horses, and turkeys are not susceptible to SBE.

SYMPTOMS. The first is a fever of 104 to 107° F., and in some cases this is the only sign of trouble. Such mild cases might escape notice entirely. Most severely affected animals go off feed, lose weight, show evidence of a diarrhea, and have discharges from the nose and eyes. Many will slobber and breathe with effort. Some cattle will recover at this stage, but most of them will get worse and show trouble in moving. They become stiff, stagger, circle, and have a tendency to stumble over small objects. There are a few recoveries, but the majority of affected cattle become progressively weaker, finally become paralyzed, and die.

Opening a dead animal will usually show a considerable amount of yellowish fluid in both the abdonimal and pleural cavities, and the lungs may show signs of pneumonia. In addition, a yellowish fibrinous network may be found covering the lungs, heart, and digestive organs. The disease generally runs its course in one to three weeks. The death rate will vary between 40% and 70%, with calves being most likely to die.

DIAGNOSIS. Definitely made only in the laboratory through isolation of the causative agent from the brain. When suggestive symptoms are shown before death, a tentative diagnosis can sometimes be made on the basis of typical postmortem findings. Under farm conditions SBE might be confused with IBR, BVD, listerellosis, rabies, malignant catarrhal fever, lead poisoning, and various other troubles.

TREATMENT. None recognized at this time.

PREVENTION. No preventive measures can be recommended.

Corn Stalk Disease (Corn Stalk Poisoning)

CAUSE. An unknown poisonous substance that is evidently dependent on drouth conditions for its production. It is usually considered as being largely confined to the stalks, and is apparently destroyed when the stalks are run through a shredder or ensilage cutter. However, there is a possibility that mold and smut on corn ears may also carry the dangerous element. Reports from Illinois in 1954 indicated that losses were reduced or completely eliminated when fungus growths were removed and the corn fed by hand. There were fewer reports of deaths when corn fodder was picked over and fed by hand in this area, too. Trouble usually occurs where cattle are grazing drouth-stricken corn stalks, but several cases have been reported where deaths followed feeding of hand-cut stalks, stalks cured in the shock, or even the grain itself. No

causative bacteria have ever been demonstrated; there are no patho-
logical changes like those produced by nitrate poisoning; and
treatment that is effective in cases of prussic acid poisoning does
not help cases of corn stalk disease. Accordingly, it is considered
as a distinct and entirely different type of poisoning.

SYMPTOMS. An unsteady, staggering gait is apt to be the first
one noticed, with most animals panting and many of them acting
crazy or appearing to be blind. Inability to swallow causes considerable slobbering. Cattle may show signs of colic, tremble
violently, grind their teeth, keel over, and go into frightening
convulsions. They usually die a few minutes after going down.
Some cows will lie quietly with the head extended on the ground
like a resting dog, only to jump up and unexpectedly attack anyone
who comes near them. These crazy brutes may crash headlong
into almost anything, and most of them die shortly after making
such a charge. Some owners have reported that the groaning of
"downer" cattle caused them to investigate. In other cases owners
have not suspected anything was wrong until they found dead
cattle in the corn fields. Affected animals usually live only a few
hours after first showing symptoms, and in practically all cases
death occurs within twenty-four hours. The temperature, heart,
and breathing rates are likely to remain well within the normal
range throughout an attack. Trouble usually starts about five days
after corn has been picked and animals are turned into the stalks.
Losses in various areas have ranged all the way from a few animals
per farm up to entire herds. Although sheep and horses are also
susceptible to corn stalk disease, losses aren't so high in these
animals as when either beef or dairy cattle are involved.

DIAGNOSIS. Usually through a history of feeding on uncut corn
stalks that grew during a season of drouth, but symptoms may
cause corn stalk disease to be confused with various other troubles.
The appearance of convulsions may cause strychnine to be suspected, while crazy actions of different kinds are much the same
as those sometimes due to lead poisoning. Panting and gasping
for breath can be caused by nitrate or prussic acid poisoning. It
is possible for blindness, a dazed appearance, and sudden deaths
to be blamed on lightning stroke. A practical diagnostic procedure
calls for comparing a sample of blood from the jugular vein of a
normal animal with that taken from one suspected of being affected
with corn stalk disease. Blood from a poisoned cow has a cherry
red color resembling oxygen-carrying blood from an artery instead

of the much darker blood normally carried by a vein. Blood from a poisoned animal also shows an abnormal pink color when it is placed in a glass tube and clotted by mild heat.

TREATMENT. None generally recognized, although the intravenous injection of dextrose solutions has been reported as effective in some cases. However, cases invariably result in death once severe symptoms have been shown, and affected animals have little chance of living more than 24 hours. It will probably be best to sell for slaughter any animals that seem to recover because many of them will develop degeneration of the brain within 30 days.

PREVENTION. Largely a matter of keeping animals out of corn fields as soon as the first suspicious case is reported in a neighborhood. The breaking of stalks with a picker, disc, or stalk-cutter before turning cattle into them does not seem to have any value as a preventive measure. Owners may be able to feed dangerous fodder and corn without killing any of their cattle if they will also supply the animals with plenty of good legume hay along with a good grain ration. Even then, though, at least a few deaths must be expected if animals are left in poisonous stalks for more than a couple of hours at a time. To be on the safe side, owners will do well to consider their corn stalks as dangerous just as soon as they hear that first story of something that might be corn stalk disease in their area. Dr. A. A. Case of Missouri reports that dangerous corn stalks can be revealed by using the test for nitrites as described under nitrate poisoning in this book.

Lockjaw (Tetanus)

CAUSE. A germ known as *Clostridium tetani* which is found almost everywhere in soil and manure. Infection probably always occurs through wounds or at calving time when the genital tract is contaminated. Punctures of the flesh are bad, with the deeper ones being the most dangerous. Strangely enough, the germs do no direct damage, since this is due to the poisons they give off while growing and multiplying in the body. These poisons act on the various nerves, particularly those of the motor type, to account for the stiffening and paralysis that characterizes the disease. The toxin of lockjaw is one of the most powerful known, and is believed to be over one hundred times stronger than strychnine.

SYMPTOMS. Usually starts as a stiffness which may affect all or only certain parts of the animal's body. This is seldom in the region of the original wound, which may be completely healed before symptoms appear. Instead, the muscles of the throat, jaws, or hind quarters are more likely to be affected. As time goes on the head and neck are apt to be stiffly extended and the legs spraddled in a characteristic "saw-horse" attitude of rigidity. Movements become increasingly difficult, the belly is tucked-up, and trembling is common. Sudden noises may cause convulsions or protrusion of the third eyelid in the corner of the eye. Feed and water are commonly refused because of inability to swallow, and bloating is a frequent symptom. Inability to eat in combination with paralysis of the digestive tract is likely to cause evidence of constipation. The temperature, pulse, and breathing is apt to remain close to normal throughout an attack. There are a few recoveries, although most affected animals die within two to ten days' time. Animals that live past the first four days have a chance of recovery, especially if they are able to drink and eat a little food. However, complete recovery may take several weeks, with recurrent attacks after a few days of apparent improvement being common. The incubation stage is generally from one to three weeks, but may be as long as several months.

DIAGNOSIS. Usually on the basis of typical symptoms, although a history of recent calving, castration, dehorning, or injuries may help to indicate the nature of trouble. This is particularly true on farms where lockjaw has appeared previously.

TREATMENT. Although antitoxin probably has no value once the toxin has become fixed to the nervous tissues, it can be given in 100,000 to 300,000 unit doses in the hope of doing some good. This is because some of the toxin may still exist in the blood, or is still being produced so that the antitoxin will be able to counteract it. Massive doses of penicillin appear to be helpful, and are probably the best bet in regard to treatment. The earlier treatment is given, the better are the chances of beneficial results.

In addition, managment practices will often prove helpful. Animals can sometimes be helped by placing feed and water at shoulder level, since the head cannot ordinarily be lowered without considerable difficulty. Grain is best furnished as a thin gruel so it will bypass the first stomach, and chewing movements are usually impossible anyway. Animals should never be drenched, because they may be unable to swallow, and liquid will then go into the lungs to cause pneumonia. In such cases feed and water should be given by means of a stomach tube. It will also help to keep affected animals in a cool dark place where they can be kept quiet and free from flies.

PREVENTION. Usually not necessary to give tetanus antitoxin or toxoid at the time of exposure because cattle are so highly resistant to the disease. In areas where lockjaw is a serious problem in cattle, 1,500 units of tetanus antitoxin given at the time of surgery or exposure through wounds will give immunity which lasts about two weeks. When permanent immunity is desirable, it can be secured by giving three injections of tetanus toxoid at three-week intervals followed by once-a-year vaccination with the same product.

Sun Stroke or Heat Stroke

CAUSE. Overheating either through direct exposure to the sun or confinement in hot, poorly-ventilated quarters. Animals in closed trucks, railroad cars, or pavilions at sales and fairs are often affected. A lack of salt and water are predisposing factors.

SYMPTOMS. Dullness, staggering, panting, and open-mouth breathing are usually seen, with paralysis likely to occur in the latter stages. Slobbering is profuse, with convulsions and evidence of delirium also being common. An extremely fast pulse and high body temperature are nearly always present, with thermometer readings sometimes approaching 110 degrees. Animals may die within a few minutes or several days later, although mild cases usually respond to treatment within a short time.

DIAGNOSIS. Usually on the basis of typical symptoms that appear suddenly in hot weather. It may be confused with any of the troubles listed as causing inflammation of the brain.

TREATMENT. Almost entirely a matter of cooling the body as quickly as possible in order to prevent permanent damage to the brain. Ice packs applied above the eyes and injections of cold water in the rectum are recommended. Sometimes animals may be sprayed with water from a hose or garden sprinkler, while confinement in a shady place where there is plenty of fresh air is always desirable. An electric fan may prove helpful for cooling purposes, while placing a tub of ice under the muzzle may supply cold air for breathing by affected beasts. An ounce or more of chloral hydrate well-diluted with water can be given orally to quiet animals showing signs of delirium. A pint or more of 4% salt solution may be given intravenously to good advantage.

PREVENTION. Largely concerned with good management that provides free circulation of air in shaded quarters. Constant access to salt and cool fresh water is also important in avoiding this trouble.

Lightning Stroke

CAUSE. Usually lightning that has struck animals at pasture. They need not be struck directly, since lightning frequently "jumps" after hitting something else first. Under proper conditions it will travel down fences for long distances until grounded by some poor beast that happens to be touching the wire. When animals are jammed together and touching each other, several may be killed at once. This frequently happens when stock is bunched under a tree during a storm.

SYMPTOMS. Animals may be found dead after being killed instantly, but they often remain alive while showing signs of being deaf, blind, dazed, or partly paralyzed. Paralysis due to lightning seldom lasts for long, but when the brain or important nerves are seriously injured, animals may be permanently crippled. Instant death is shown by a lack of evidence indicating dying struggles, and dead animals are sometimes found with a last bite of grass still clutched in their teeth. Carcasses usually stiffen in an unexpectedly short time after being killed by lightning, while bloody foam is apt to be present in the mouth and nostrils. There may or may not be burned areas or singed streaks down the legs to show where lightning struck and traveled to the ground.

DIAGNOSIS. The finding of singed hair, skin burns, or dark, branch-like patterns of lines on the skin is enough to warrant a diagnosis of lightning stroke. Opening a dead animal and finding the branch-like pattern on the flesh side of the skin in combination with veins distended by dark fluid blood will support such a diagnosis. Symptoms involving the nervous system like staggering, blindness, and paralysis that appear suddenly in connection with an electrical storm are sufficient for a tentative diagnosis.

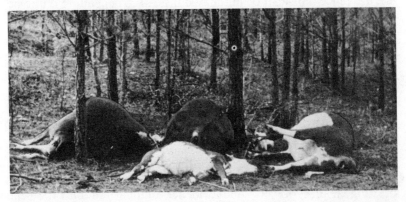

When animals are close together several may be killed at once by lightning. (Picture, courtesy Dr. W. J. Gibbons, A.P.I., Auburn, Ala.)

TREATMENT. Seldom needed. However, if animals remain unconscious for very long, they should be propped up on their breastbones with sacks, bales of hay, etc., to prevent bloating. Stimulants like caffeine or sodium benzoate can be given subcutaneously at the rate of 4 to 8 cc. to hasten recovery. Animals showing aftereffects like blindness or partial paralysis should be protected against injuring themselves.

PREVENTION. Chiefly a matter of good management. Animals should be kept out of wooded pastures and fields where they have a chance to bunch up under isolated trees during electric storms. Steel fence posts will assure regular grounding of wires at short intervals, and the same results can be secured by placing ground wires on each wooden fence post. Under such a system lightning is then dangerous only between any two consecutive posts.

Electric Shock

CAUSE. Usually some kind of a short circuit in milking machines, feed grinders, and other machines. Sometimes cows are injured while chewing on extension cords running to lights or warmers for calves. Homemade electric fence units have also been reported as causing trouble along this line.

SYMPTOMS. Pretty much as just given for lightning stroke, with animals either being found dead or showing evidence of shock. One or several animals may be involved at the same time.

DIAGNOSIS. Pretty much dependent on finding the short circuit, although symptoms furnish a clue to the trouble.

TREATMENT. The same as for lightning stroke.

PREVENTION. Accidents can't be entirely prevented, but reliable electric fence units can be purchased instead of depending on homemade devices of questionable safety.

Inflammation of the Brain (Encephalitis)

CAUSE. Usually some specific disease like rabies, pseudo-rabies, sporadic bovine encephalomyelitis, red nose, listerellosis, or malignant catarrhal fever. It may also follow selenium poisoning, corn stalk disease, toxoplasmosis, and various other bacterial and mycotic infections that happen to localize in the brain.

SYMPTOMS. Twitching of various muscles with occasional spasms and convulsions are more common ones. Walking in circles, pressing against objects, and evidence of delirium may be seen, while alternate periods of dullness and excitement are likely. Refusal of feed, grinding of the teeth, labored breathing, groaning, staggering, and partial or complete paralysis are also common symptoms. Weight is often lost rapidly, and apparent blindness may sometimes be noted.

DIAGNOSIS. Largely through an elimination of other troubles that cause similar symptoms. Paralysis of varying degrees in combination with evidence of delirium can usually be taken as definite proof of brain involvement. It may be confused with any of the diseases already described in this section as well as others like shipping fever and tuberculosis affecting the brain.

TREATMENT. None is known, although symptoms may disappear by themselves within a short time if the brain is not permanently damaged. Determining the primary cause may permit appropriate remedial measures.

Abscess of the Brain

CAUSE. Usually pus-forming germs that have been carried by the blood from diseased areas of the body. Often from infection following dehorning and head injuries, but sometimes reported as originating from infection as far away as the uterus or udder.

SYMPTOMS. Any or all of those already described under inflammation of the brain.

DIAGNOSIS. Usually made only after the abscess is found in the brain of a dead animal, although symptoms may cause suspicion of its existence.

TREATMENT. None known.

Tumor of the Brain

CAUSE. Unknown, since these growths are forms of cancer. They evidently are sometimes started by cells that are carried by the blood from tumors in other areas of the body.

SYMPTOMS. The same as given for inflammation of the brain. They usually occur over long periods, becoming worse and worse as the tumor grows.

DIAGNOSIS. Made only after they are found in the brains of dead animals.

TREATMENT. None is known.

Pressure on the Brain or Spinal Cord

CAUSE. Usually an abscess as already discussed, with troubles like tuberculosis, navel ill, metritis, and liver infection having been reported as starters. Tumors, parasites, bony growths, and injuries to the skull and backbone may also cause pressure on the central nervous system.

SYMPTOMS. Usually a weakness and progressive paralysis that appears back of the point where pressure is being exerted on the spinal cord. Pressure in the brain is shown by affliction of body areas furnished with nerves from that particular part of the brain. When the spinal cord is involved, functions are apt to be normal between the brain and the point of pressure. For example, pressure in the small of the back will probably cause paralysis of the hind quarters, while pressure in the shoulders would probably cause general paralysis except for the head and neck. Symptoms usually develop gradually except in the case of bone injuries, when they appear suddenly. Pressure may affect sensory as well as motor nerves so that neither sensation nor movement is possible in certain body areas. Passage of urine and manure may even be stopped.

DIAGNOSIS. Usually through evidence of paralysis beyond a certain point along the spine. Sometimes a painful area can be located. Pressure on any part of the brain will give the symptoms of inflammation already noted and so indicate the seat of trouble. Examination of the central nervous system after death will probably be needed to show the exact nature of the agent causing pressure.

TREATMENT. None is known except in cases where surgery may serve to remove the cause of pressure.

Parasites in the Brain

CAUSE. Usually the larvae of warble flies that have entered the backbone at some point and followed the spinal cord to the brain. Larvae of the tapeworm *Multiceps multiceps* have also been reported as invading the brains of cattle.

SYMPTOMS. The same as given for inflammation of the brain.

DIAGNOSIS. Usually made only by finding the parasites in the brain of a dead animal. It may be confused with any of the other troubles showing similar symptoms.

TREATMENT. Usually none is practical. An exception must be made when pressure causes softening and bulging of the skull to indicate the location of trouble. Under such a condition surgical removal of the parasites may be possible, and followed by recovery of the animal.

Epileptic Fits

CAUSE. Unknown, but generally believed to be an inherited characteristic.

SYMPTOMS. Twitching of muscles, excitement, tongue-chewing, and foaming at the mouth with animals usually going down in convulsions. In a short time the affected animal gets up and seems perfectly all right again. In some cases symptoms simply consist of sudden dropping to the ground as if shot, accompanied by brief periods of convulsions with frothing at the mouth. In any case the attacks recur at irregular intervals to indicate the chronic nature of the trouble.

DIAGNOSIS. Chiefly on the basis of recurrent attacks showing typical symptoms. The fact that only certain blood lines are involved may further help to single out the disease. May be confused with any of the other ailments causing similar symptoms.

TREATMENT. None is likely to help. Animals subject to such attacks are dangerous, anyway, and may pass the undesirable characteristic on to offspring besides.

"Sweeney"

CAUSE. An injury to the suprascapular nerve that originates from the brachial plexus and passes over the front edge of the scapula or shoulder blade. Although usually thought of as affecting horses wearing poor-fitting collars which injure the nerve, the condition sometimes appears in cattle that have bruised the nerve against doorways, stanchions, and other objects as well as through injuries received while fighting.

SYMPTOMS. At first a severe lameness and difficulty in lifting the affected front leg more than an inch or so off the ground. With the passage of time the muscles covering the shoulder blade are likely to shrivel away to leave a depression in the area. In minor injuries no lameness may be shown, and only a limited shriveling of the shoulder muscles may be evident.

DIAGNOSIS. Usually on the basis of the shriveled shoulder muscles, either with or without lameness of the corresponding leg. It may be confused with other types of front leg lameness, since a lack of use from any cause is likely to cause shriveling of the shoulder muscles.

TREATMENT. Cases that show severe or complete paralysis are not likely to be helped by any measures. Shriveled muscles can sometimes be helped by subcutaneous injection of Lugol's solution. The injections should be made in several areas over the depression, with 2 cc. being used at a time. Such treatment must be followed by complete rest, for the Lugol's solution causes severe inflammation and swelling.

Radial Paralysis

CAUSE. An injury to the radial nerve that originates from the brachial plexus and helps to straighten the various joints of the front leg when movements are made. Damage usually occurs through kicks and blows, but it has been known to follow stepping into holes in the ground when animals were running.

SYMPTOMS. Lameness and dragging of the toes when an affected animal walks. All joints of the affected leg are doubled back and can't be straightened in a normal manner. However, some animals can walk satisfactorily if the leg is pulled forward with a rope fastened around the pastern when they attempt to walk. Most animals can stand normally if the leg is placed under them and pulled back at the knee to prevent buckling.

DIAGNOSIS. Usually on the basis of typical symptoms and the ability to stand and walk when functions of the disabled radial nerve are performed by human beings.

TREATMENT. Complete rest with the leg joints held in correct position. A special shoe can sometimes be made with an iron brace extending from the heel up the back part of the leg past the knee The entire leg is then bandaged fast to the brace so it is held in a stiff position. Mild injuries showing little evidence of paralysis will sometimes require no treatment save rest in a box stall. Most cases usually recover, but the process may take all the way from a few days to several months, depending on the severity of injury.

Sciatic Paralysis

CAUSE. An injury to the sciatic nerve that comes off the lumbrosacral plexus and goes to many of the big muscles of the buttock on each hind leg.

SYMPTOMS. The affected leg hangs limply, with even the hamstring relaxed. Attempted movement causes the limb to be jerked ahead and upward so the foot is dragged on the toes. If the foot is placed under the body in a normal position the leg will usually support the animal until movement is attempted. Backing is extremely difficult, and the fetlock will ordinarily be forced into the ground when it is tried. There is no feeling in the lower part of the leg.

DIAGNOSIS. Made on the basis of typical symptoms and the ability of the leg to support weight when placed in proper position.

TREATMENT None known. Recovery may occur if the animal is rested and given good care, but the chances are against it.

Calf Paralysis or Obturator Paralysis

CAUSE. Injury to one or both the obturator nerves which originate from the lumbo-sacral plexus and help to hold the hind legs under the body in a normal position. Injury occurs most frequently at calving time, particularly in the case of first-calf heifers with a small birth canal. This is because the nerves lie in an exposed position against the pelvic bones on each side where they are easily bruised by the passage of a large calf.

SYMPTOMS. The leg has a tendency to be turned out from the body because muscles that hold it in place are paralyzed. If both nerves are affected the legs are likely to stick out on both sides while the cow rests on the udder in a spraddled position. Animals are unable to get up by themselves, but can stand if helped up and the hocks held together in a normal position. However, the cow goes down again as soon as movement is attempted. Struggling to get on the feet may break some of the pelvic bones or throw the hip out of joint.

DIAGNOSIS. Based on the typical symptoms that show the paralysis of muscles that ordinarily hold the hind legs under the body.

TREATMENT. The hocks are best strapped or tied together to prevent further injuries due to extreme spraddling. Barring complications from infected wounds of the genital tract and broken bones, most cows will recover. However, the recovery period varies all the way from a couple of days to several weeks, depending on the severity of nerve injury.

Brachial Paralysis

CAUSE. An injury to the brachial plexus of nerves that controls movements of the front leg on that side. It probably occurs oftenest when cattle are cast, or when the front feet are tied to encourage struggling that results in bruising of the plexus. It may also be injured by foreign bodies being forced under the shoulder blade, hematomas or abscesses on the inside of the shoulder blade, and growths on the inside of the shoulder blade or the outside of the ribs.

SYMPTOMS. Complete paralysis of the foreleg on the affected side. The foot is dragged on the ground, the fetlock is doubled back, and the leg is usually held away from the body. As in the case of radial paralysis, most animals can stand normally if the foot is placed in a normal position, and the leg is pulled back at the knee to prevent buckling.

DIAGNOSIS. On the basis of typical symptoms after dislocation of joints and broken bones have been eliminated as possibilities.

TREATMENT. Dependent on the extent of injury, with none being recognized for severe cases. In mild cases the entire leg can be placed in a cast and the animal rested until recovery occurs. Even under the best of conditions, this is likely to take several weeks.

Femoral Paralysis

CAUSE. An injury to the femoral nerve which helps to straighten the various joints of the hind leg when movements are made. This trouble is most likely to be seen in pastured calves when the leg is stretched by roping or after the foot has been caught in a fence.

SYMPTOMS. Lameness and dragging of the foot. All joints of the leg are doubled back and cannot be straightened in a normal manner when walking is attempted.

DIAGNOSIS. Through typical symptoms after stifle injuries have been eliminated as a possibility.

TREATMENT. Complete rest in a stall where food and water is easily reached with a minimum of movement being required. It will usually be advisable to place a cast on the entire leg below the hock to provide support and prevent injury to the top of the hoof when it is dragged. A fair share of these cases will eventually recover under such treatment.

Peroneal Paralysis

CAUSE. An injury to the peroneal nerve which controls extensor muscles of the hind leg. This nerve lies close under the skin on the outside of the hock where it is unprotected and easily injured when cattle are thrown, slip, fall, run into objects, or are down and struggling to get up. In this latter case, peroneal nerve injuries often occur when cows have milk fever. Treatment for milk fever may then prove successful, but still leave the cow in a partly paralyzed condition.

SYMPTOMS. An affected animal will stagger, totter about, and try desperately to stand squarely on the hind feet, but one of the hoofs turns under. The animal will stand and even try to walk on the ankle and front of the knuckled-under foot. If the fetlock doesn't straighten out after a few steps, the animal may go down and be unable to get up again by itself. Walking can be accomplished if a rope is fastened around the fetlock and the leg and foot is pulled forward whenever the animal steps.

DIAGNOSIS. Through typical symptoms and knuckling under of the hoof.

TREATMENT. A plaster cast around the fetlock will help to keep the hoof from turning under. Another treatment consists of a device that substitutes for the lost action of the extensor muscles. A strap is fastened above the hock joint, and a piece of wire is fitted through both toes of the affected foot. These two points are connected with a strip of an old inner tube. When the foot is lifted, the toes are pulled up by the rubber band, making it possible for the sole of the foot to contact the ground when the step is completed. Untreated animals may recover by themselves, but should be kept confined, since walking on a turned-under hoof reduces chances of recovery.

PREVENTION. Largely a matter of keeping cows in well-bedded box stalls at calving time. Following this single recommendation will eliminate most of the cases of peroneal paralysis that occur on dairy farms.

Spastic Syndrome, "Stretches," "Crampiness"

CAUSE. An inherited characteristic that is believed to affect some part of the central nervous system, probably located in the upper brain stem. Ailments like arthritis and foot rot appear to be contributing factors in some cases.

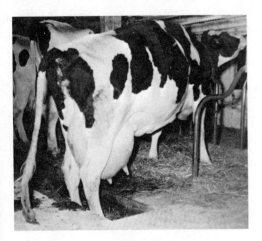

Spastic syndrome cow during a seizure.

SYMPTOMS. Spasms cause the animal to stand with the hind feet extended backward, and the head raised and thrust forward in a stretching attitude. Certain muscles become rigid, and there is evidence of considerable pain. One or both hind legs may be affected, together with muscles of the back. In advanced cases practically all muscles of the body may be involved. An attack comes on suddenly, and may last a few seconds to a few minutes. It stops just as suddenly, but spasms recur. Attacks may become increasingly frequent, or animals may become progressively worse until slaughter is advisable. Spasms do not occur when animals are lying down, but often begin immediately after they get up. Animals of either sex are susceptible, and the syndrome is consistently found in cattle with excessively straight hind legs and weak hocks. Many animals carrying the same blood lines may be affected on a single farm. Animals are usually around five years old when symptoms first appear, although cases have been reported in cattle two and three years old.

DIAGNOSIS. Usually on the basis of sporadic attacks that occur only in standing animals. These intermittent attacks will help to distinguish the spastic syndrome from troubles like arthritis, foot rot, tetanus, and various kinds of nerve injuries.

TREATMENT. None recommended, chiefly because the condition is inherited and it would seem unwise to perpetuate it by keeping affected animals in a herd. It is generally regarded as incurable, but when animals are in agony and suffering a severe attack, temporary relief can usually be afforded by the use of spinal cord depressants. One reported as particularly effective is mephenesin, "Tolserol" (Squibb) given in doses of 8 to 10 grams in a 2% solution intravenously or in 8 gram doses orally. Treatment is discontinued when the condition improves.

PREVENTION. Entirely a matter of keeping affected animals out of a breeding program as well as their close relatives. It will also be a good idea to eliminate animals with weak hocks and abnormally straight hind legs from consideration as breeding stock in a herd.

9.

URINARY TROUBLES

Anatomy of the Cow's Urinary System

The urinary system of cattle can be considered as beginning with the kidneys. The right one usually lies near the small of the back and partly under the last rib on that side. The other one usually lies a little to the left of the backbone in the same general area, but when the rumen is full it may be crowded over so it lies behind and below the right kidney. The organs consist largely of so-called renal or uriniferous tubules which connect with blood vessels and remove waste products while secreting urine. The tubules drain urine into collecting ducts, which in turn empty it into the pelvis of the kidney. This is nothing more than the funnel-like beginning of a tube called the ureter which runs from each kidney and empties into the upper side of the bladder near its neck.

The bladder can be thought of as a pear-shaped sac which lies in the body with the enlarged blind end in front and the narrower neck behind just inside the pelvic cavity. In the bull it lies on the bony floor of the pelvic cavity below the rectum, seminal vesicles, prostate gland, and the ends of the deferential ducts leading from the testicles. In the cow it also lies on the floor of the pelvic cavity, but is beneath the vagina and body of the uterus. The neck of the bladder is continuous with the urethra.

In the bull this goes backward on the floor of the pelvic cavity for a short distance, then turns sharply downward and is continued inside the penis to its outlet in the end of the organ. In the cow the urethra goes straight back and opens on the floor of the vagina about four inches inside the vulvar opening and just above a blind pouch known as the suburethral diverticulum.

Bloody Urine

This condition is a symptom rather than a specific ailment, and may appear in connection with several different troubles. A list of the more common causes looks something like this:

1. Stones or calculi that cut delicate tissues while passing through various parts of the urinary system.

2. "Hardware trouble" that causes internal bleeding, with the blood being eliminated through the kidneys.

3. Indigestion that sometimes injures the lining of the digestive tract and also causes internal bleeding with elimination in the urine.

4. Infection of the uterus that causes bleeding of this organ and elimination of blood in the urine.

5. Mastitis attacks that may cause tissue damage and bleeding in the udder.

6. Sweet clover poisoning that may be responsible for severe internal bleeding when normal clotting fails to occur.

7. Poisoning by lead, mercury, etc., that may destroy tissues and cause serious internal bleeding.

8. Diseases like anthrax and shipping fever that may be accompanied by high fevers that destroy red blood cells in the body.

9. Prolonged use of sulfas that may lead to crystal formation in the kidneys and damage to the organs.

10. Phenothiazine that has been used to remove various internal parasites has been reported as capable of giving the urine a red color resembling blood.

11. Infection with *G. hemolyticum* to cause so-called "bacillary hemoglobinuria."

12. Infection with *C. renale* to cause so-called "pyelonephritis."

13. Infection with one or more types of leptospira organisms to cause leptospirosis.

14. Eating of feeds like beets, pokeberries, etc., may give the urine a red color as in the case of phenothiazine.

15. A lack of phosphorus in the ration and consequent destruction of red blood cells to cause so-called "parturient hemoglobinuria."

Pyelonephritis

CAUSE. Usually a germ called *Corynebacterium renale,* although other organisms could be to blame. Since *C. renale* lives only a short time outside the body, transmission is believed to take place through direct contact with infected animals, with the germs entering the urinary tract from the urethral opening in the vagina. Bulls are probably infected by invasion through the urethral opening in the end of the penis. Mechanical spread through tail switching, splashing of urine during urination, and the use of contaminated brushes and curry combs has been reported. Many cases seem to be the result of calfhood exposure that has taken a long time to develop, and spread is possible through the breeding act. It has also been suggested that high protein rations may be a predisposing factor, and outbreaks are apparently aided by exposure to cold wet weather. There may be other triggering factors like advanced pregnancy and bladder stones (urinary calculi) which encourage infection without actually blocking the flow of urine.

SYMPTOMS. Usually a gradual loss of weight and declining milk production while the appetite remains fairly good. However, symptoms may appear suddenly and include arching of the back, frequent urination, restless treading, kicking at the belly, and gen-

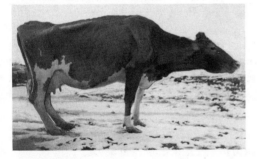

Cow in the final stages of pyelonephritis.

eral evidence of colic. The urine is apt to be bloody, and sometimes contains clots of blood or bits of pus and mucus. It is frequently positive to the test for acetonemia, and may have a bad odor suggestive of retained afterbirth. The pulse, respiration, and temperature generally remain about normal, but loss of blood may cause pallor of the mucous membranes in the latter stages of an attack. Pain may be shown in the kidney areas and manual examination may reveal greatly enlarged ureters or kidneys. These symptoms aren't constant, for sometimes there is no enlargement of these organs. Attacks may end in death within a few days or become chronic and last for months. At times there are periods of improvement followed by recurrence of symptoms. It may affect animals of either sex of any age, even including suckling calves.

DIAGNOSIS. Positive when *C. renale* is found under the microscope in connection with typical symptoms of the disease. It may be confused with hardware trouble, bacillary hemoglobinuria, liver disease, acetonemia, leptospirosis, parturient hemoglobinuria, and metritis.

TREATMENT. The intramuscular injection of procaine penicillin G in a water solution is probably best. It should be given in large doses (3 million units) every day for at least a week or until the urine clears up and other symptoms disappear. Penicillin which is excreted by the kidneys through the urine will bathe infected tissues which also receive penicillin through the blood. The injection of enzymes has been reported as helpful, and can be given every other day at least three times. It is also advisable to cut the grain ration to almost nothing during attacks. The disease has a tendency to recur, epecially when animals are exposed to cold, wet weather, and are fed heavily on grain.

PREVENTION. Largely a matter of management, with these steps being recommended:

1. Isolate infected animals from the rest of the herd.
2. Remove all possibly infected bedding as soon as possible.
3. Disinfect stalls that have been occupied by infected animals.
4. Breed infected cows artificially, since there is always a chance of infecting bulls that may then spread the disease through an entire herd.
5. Do not use infected bulls for either natural or artificial service.

Bacillary Hemoglobinuria (Red Water Disease)

CAUSE. A germ known as *Clostridium hemolyticum*. When first recognized as a disease, it was believed to be confined to the western part of Nevada and nearby counties of California, but it is now known to exist in many other states west of the Mississippi as well as in Mexico and Chile. It probably exists in midwestern and eastern states, too.

The disease is most likely to appear in lowland pastures or on poorly drained irrigated lands. It seldom occurs on dry upland ranges or pastures where cattle do not have access to swampy land, although it can appear at any elevation. The organisms are somewhat like those of lockjaw because they produce a powerful poison which is the actual cause of death.

MEANS OF SPREAD. Not definitely known, although floods can carry infection, and outbreaks of red water disease have occurred in areas previously free of the disease following flooding. It is likely that carriers exist, for feeder cattle from infected areas can apparently carry the disease to clean premises. Reports indicate that possibly the disease may also be spread by carcasses and trucks used to haul infected cattle. Outbreaks have been known to occur when susceptible animals which had never been exposed to the disease were moved to a known infected area. Although the liver is primarily involved, the importance of liver flukes in this disease has not been established.

SYMPTOMS. Much like those of a sudden attack of hardware trouble, but dark red, foamy urine is one of the first. Animals stop eating, chewing their cuds, and drop off to nothing in milk production. They stand in a humped-up position, are reluctant to move, often grunt at each step, appear constipated, and run fevers between 104 and 106° F. Cases usually appear during the summer and early fall, and the death rate among unvaccinated cattle may run from 10 to 25% in a single season. In the late stages animals show difficulty in breathing, and a bloody diarrhea may develop. The average course of the disease is about 36 hours, and practically all untreated animals will die.

Opening a dead animal will usually show the nostrils and trachea to be filled with a bloody froth, and the lymph nodes bloody and swollen. Large amounts of bloody fluid are likely to be found in both the pleural and abdominal cavities. The liver is usually enlarged and yellowish in color, and almost invariably will show a characteristic light-colored area several inches across. This area is known as an infarct, and is slightly higher than the adjacent liver tissue. Carcasses give off a characteristic disagreeable odor.

DIAGNOSIS. Definitely made only in the laboratory through identification of *C. hemolyticum*. However, a tentative diagnosis can sometimes be made on the basis of the characteristic infarct appearing in the liver of a dead animal. Under farm conditions the disease might be confused with pyelonephritis, anaplasmosis, leptospirosis, hardware trouble, postparturient hemoglobinuria, and sometimes anthrax.

TREATMENT. Since the course of the disease is so short, treatment must be given early if it is to do any good. Massive doses of broad-spectrum antibiotics at 12-hour intervals may do some good, but unnecessary excitement should be avoided as sick animals may die before treatment can be given. Affected animals should be sheltered and given free access to fresh water and good quality feeds. Affected bulls should be held out of service for about a month after recovery because of possible rupture of the liver infarct as a result of use. Such a rupture could result in internal bleeding that would kill an animal.

PREVENTION. Most practical through semiannual vaccination of all cattle over six months old with a bacterin. One of the vaccinations should be performed about a month before cattle go out on infected ranges or pastures. Cattle coming into infected areas from disease-free sections should be vaccinated immediately. Animals dying of this disease should be burned or deeply buried in quicklime to prevent spread of the disease by water, wild animals, or human beings.

Postparturient Hemoglobinuria (PPH)

CAUSE. Essentially a low phosphate blood level in combination with a low intake of phosphorus. A ration low in phosphorus is particularly dangerous in lactating cows because of the drain of phosphorus in milk. Some authorities believe that the low phosphate blood level must be accompanied by saponins present in feeds like sugar-beet leaves and alfalfa hay or a hemolytic factor in plants like kale, cabbage, rape, and lush spring pastures, or beets and turnips. In Europe the disease is seen most often on old farms with poor soils, and attacks often follow a summer with long periods of drouth. The disease has been produced experimentally by feeding beet pulp and alfalfa. Beef cattle are seldom affected, and the condition does not appear in heifers or calves. Whatever the exact cause may be, it acts in some way to destroy the red blood cells.

SYMPTOMS. Usually appears in mature cows a week to a month after calving, and is more prevalent in stabled animals. The earliest sign of trouble is apt to be bloody urine. Within a few days the animal goes off feed and becomes weak because of loss of blood. Weight is lost at a terrific rate, and animals may go down in a paralyzed condition and die within three or four days. The urine is either red or almost black, and often reacts to the test for acetonemia. The mucous membranes are apt to be pale at first, but may soon become yellow and jaundiced. The death rate is not usually high, but recoveries may take several weeks, with recurrent attacks being common. Both the pulse and breathing rates are likely to be increased and temperatures often run between 104 and 107 degrees. Bloody urine may persist for several days and there are mild cases in which it is the only symptom shown.

If left untreated, affected animals will usually go down in a paralyzed condition and die within three or four days. However, this is not always true, for some severely affected animals will slowly recover. During this recovery period animals will often eat dirt and other indigestible material, probably in an instinctive attempt to replace the minerals lost through red blood cell destruction. Opening a dead animal will usually show an anemic and jaundiced carcass with an enlarged liver that is yellow with grayish-red pinpoint spots visible on the surface.

DIAGNOSIS. Usually on the basis of typical symptoms that appear a short time after calving and in combination with a history of feeding on roughage capable of causing this disease. Under field conditions it might be confused with red water disease, pyelonephritis, leptospirosis, hardware trouble, chemical poisoning, Texas fever, and liver diseases.

TREATMENT. Blood transfusions of a quart or more at a time are probably best in severe cases. A ration of leafy hay with no grain is recommended for affected animals, and turning to pasture may prove helpful. Free-choice availability of minerals is desirable, particularly a mix containing plenty of iron and copper.

The intravenous injection of either calcium hypophosphite (1 ounce in 100 cc. of distilled water) or sodium acid phosphate (2 ounces in 300 cc. of distilled water) has been recommended. Such treatment should be followed up by adding 4 ounces of bone meal to the feed daily, and providing bone meal and trace mineralized salt on a free choice basis.

PREVENTION. Largely a matter of providing plenty of phosphorus in the ration, particularly before and after calving. An average cow will require about 2 ounces of phosphorus daily if producing 50 pounds of milk, and a little over 3 ounces daily if producing 100 pounds of milk. In addition, it will be good insurance to hold the intake of plants like rape to less than 35 pounds daily, and to limit the feeding of root crops, alfalfa, and lush pastures.

Abscesses of the Kidneys

CAUSE. Usually pus-forming bacteria that reach the organs through blood that has carried them from infected body areas. They are commonly associated with hardware trouble and metritis, and often may represent the terminal stages of pyelonephritis. They may appear in calves because of infection through navel-ill.

SYMPTOMS. Variable, but usually include loss of weight and general failure to do well over a considerable period of time. Pain may be shown in the kidney area, sometimes there is bloating, and pus flakes may appear in the urine.

DIAGNOSIS. Usually through elimination of other troubles in combination with a rectal examination which reveals the enlarged kidney. It may easily be confused with pyelonephritis and various of the other diseases already mentioned.

TREATMENT. None is known.

Water Belly (Urethral Calculi, Bladder Stones)

CAUSE. Not definitely known, but generally believed to be a combination of several different factors. Hard or alkali water, a deficiency of vitamin A, an improper balance of calcium and phosphorus in the ration, lack of water, and infection of the urinary tract have all been believed responsible for certain cases. Large amounts of sorghum feeds in the ration have been reported as a contributing factor. Cattle with the smallest urethral opening, like steers under a year old, are most likely to be affected. The primary cause is an accumulation of gritty, stone-like material that prevents the normal passage of urine through the urethra. The doubling or sigmoid flexure of the penis in bulls and steers favors lodging of the stones.

SYMPTOMS. Most generally seen in bulls and steers, since the stones are usually passed without much trouble once they have reached the urethra of cows. Animals may act colicky and be constantly up and down. Kicking at the belly, backing up, treading, bawling, winding the tail, and general uneasiness are common. The animal is off feed, generally unable to pass urine, and sandy deposits may appear on the preputial tuft of hair. In the early stages a rectal examination is apt to show a greatly distended bladder and urethra. Within a day or two the pain is apt to be lessened enough so that beasts will eat and drink a little. This is usually because of rupture of the bladder that distends the abdomen and allows the accumulation of a barrel or more of urine in it which makes the meat unfit for use. Rupture of the urethra may occur instead of rupture of the bladder, usually occurring between the scrotum and end of the sheath, with the formation of a large swelling at the point of rupture. Sometimes there is an odor of urine on the breath.

DIAGNOSIS. Usually on the basis of typical symptoms and a rectal examination that reveals the greatly enlarged bladder. When the bladder has ruptured, drawing a sample of abdominal fluid with a syringe may show it to be urine. Heating it a little will confirm suspicions through the smell. The odor of urine on the breath may also serve to indicate the nature of trouble.

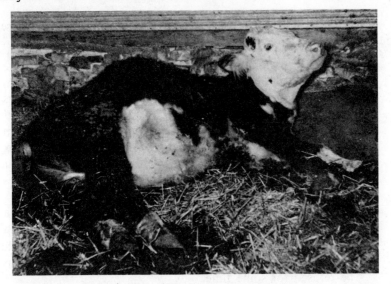

"Downer" steer with distended abdomen responsible for name "water belly."

TREATMENT. Depending on the severity of symptoms, value and number of affected animals, any one or more of six different procedures:

1. Immediate butchering of animal before the meat is ruined by absorption of urine.
2. Intramuscular injections of antibiotics to control infection so the swollen urethra will relax and permit passage of the stones.
3. When calculi can be palpated from the outside, they can sometimes be crushed with towel forceps.
4. Ammonium chloride given orally three times daily or pine oil given orally twice daily in half-ounce doses.
5. One to three intramuscular injections at daily intervals of an extract of mammalian pancreas with the trade name of Depropanex.* This product tends to produce a local, permanent, but prompt relaxation of muscles in the ureters and urethra so that calculi can be passed.

* Tonken, Canadian J. Comp. Med. & Vet. Science, February 1958.

6. Surgery to remove the stones and drain urine from the peritoneal cavity.

7. Surgery that opens the urethra above and to the rear of the scrotum so the urine can escape at this point.

PREVENTION. Despite all of the various possible causes, these measures are recommended for all areas:

1. Supplying vitamin A through feeds high in carotene, like dehydrated alfalfa. In some cases it may be more practical to feed vitamin A concentrates so that each animal gets 10,000—30,000 units daily.

2. Feeding a balanced ration, with an improper ratio of calcium and phosphorus being avoided by adjusting the mineral mix to the amount of concentrate fed. This means that the higher the amount of concentrate, the lower the amount of phosphorus and the higher the amount of calcium should be.

3. Encouraging animals to drink more water by furnishing a constant supply of fresh water in the summer, and warming it in the winter. The regular source of drinking water should never be used for mass medication, since treated water may be refused for some time.

4. Supplying loose salt on a free-choice basis.

5. Research and experience have shown that "water belly" can be largely prevented in both range animals and feed lot steers by the feeding of protein concentrate meal or pellets, containing from 10-20% salt. An alternative and equally effective method consists of adding an extra 3-5% salt to the regular grain ration. Using more than 5% salt in the ration may lead to smaller daily gains. The extra salt induces drinking of more water, and causes dilution of the urine so that fewer and smaller "stones" are formed. Since calves are often affected at weaning time when they are reluctant to drink water, it will be best to add extra salt to their creep rations some time before they are taken away from their dams. This practice will help to get them in the habit of drinking water even before they are weaned.

6. Castrating animals late (three to six months) instead of at an earlier age. This has the effect of producing a larger urethra that is less likely to become blocked by calculi. In 3,000 head of range steers observed by Montana State Experiment Station workers, there was an incidence of urethral

calculi in only 0.7% of late castrated calves as contrasted with an incidence of 4.7% in early castrates.

7. Adding ammonium chloride to the ration at the rate of 1¼ ounces per head daily. Animals which are treated surgically should receive the ammonium chloride to prevent recurrence and, whenever range animals are fed supplements, ammonium chloride should be included at the recommended dosage in the supplement.

8. Rotating or otherwise limiting the grazing on pastures associated with a great deal of water belly trouble in past years.

10.

REPRODUCTIVE TROUBLES

Anatomy of the Cow's Reproductive System

The reproductive system of the cow can be thought of as beginning with the ovaries. There are two of them which are located on opposite sides near the middle of the pelvic cavity and about a foot and a half inside the vulvar opening of a medium-sized cow. In mature animals the ovaries are about the size of a pigeon egg, with one usually being larger than the other because of alternate periods of activity in heat cycle. They may be perfectly smooth, enlarged with fluid-filled follicles, or marked with firm protuberances known as "yellow bodies" which are formed after follicles rupture to release eggs at the time of heat. Each ovary is pretty much surrounded by a membranous pouch which is known as the ovarian bursa. These pouches are formed by a folding over of the broad ligament which supports the uterus and is attached on each side to the upper part of the flank about four inches below the hip bone. The funnel-like top of a so-called uterine or fallopian tube is attached to the edge of each ovarian bursa and serves to catch eggs that are released by the ovary. These tubes are about the size of a large thread and follow a winding course over the sides of the bursae to eventually end in the uterus.

This organ is shaped like the letter "Y," with the forks usually being known as the cornua or "horns" of the uterus. These horns extend toward the front end of the cow, and a fallopian tube empties into the tip of each one. The horns separate at what is generally known as the bifurcation point of the uterus. The distance between this spot and the narrowed neck or cervix is called the body of the uterus. The cervix is the area which divides the uterus from the vagina. The vagina is the passageway which connects the cervix with the vulva or external genital organ. About four inches inside the vulva a blind pouch can be found on the floor of the vagina. This is about the size of a finger end and is known as the suburethral diverticulum. Just above it is a slit marking the open-

384

ing of the urethra which conducts urine from the bladder.

In non-pregnant animals the vagina is about a foot long, the cervix about four inches, and the body of the uterus a little over an inch long. The horns have an average length of around fifteen inches and taper off gradually to the junction with the fallopian tubes. Beginning at the bifurcation, the cornua commonly curve down, under, and then forward and outward like the coils of a sheep's horns. Most of the uterus lies in the abdominal cavity, and can be felt just below the rectum, where it partly covers the bladder. The inside of the uterus is studded with about one hundred oval elevations which are often called "buttons" but are more properly referred to as uterine caruncles or cotyledons. These are ordinarily about a half inch in diameter. The main blood supply is the middle uterine artery which is important in making rectal examinations for the determination of pregnancy. Changes in size and location occur gradually throughout the reproductive tract when cows are carrying calves.

Reproductive System of the Bull

The reproductive system of the bull can be assumed as beginning with the two testicles. They are carried in the scrotum between the hind legs and each terminates in the so-called "head" of a vessel which is known as the epididymis. This follows a winding course along the testicle until the "tail" of the epididymis joins the ductus deferens or deferential duct. Each of these ducts leaves the base of the corresponding testicle in company with nerves, blood vessels, and muscles which are grouped to form a spermatic cord. The two cords pass upward and enter the abdominal cavity through so-called inguinal canals, one on each side of the belly wall. Once inside the body, the deferential ducts leave the spermatic cord and turn backward into the pelvic cavity. Both cross the upper surface of the bladder and come close together at its neck where they empty into the urethra. These ducts are primarily concerned with furnishing a passageway for spermatazoa that originate in the testicles.

The seminal vesicles are two glands which lie on each side of the bladder near its neck. Each has a duct which empties into the urethra either with or near that of the deferens on that side. The prostate gland is made up of two connected parts which are located at the neck of the bladder just behind the seminal vesicles in a position so that they cover the ends of the deferential ducts. Several ducts lead from the prostate and empty into the urethra a little to the sides of the deferential openings. There are two bulbo-urethral glands, sometimes known as Cowper's glands. One lies on each side of the urethra behind the prostate, and each has several ducts which open into the urethra behind the openings of the deferential ducts. These different glands supply parts of the fluid collectively known as semen, and which is conducted through the urethra to the end of the penis at mating time.

The penis is about three feet long and is attached to the ischial bones high between the hind legs by two fibrous bands which are known as the suspensory ligaments of the penis. The organ follows the general slope of the body wall from this point to one behind and above the scrotum. Here it turns sharply backward and then forward again to form an S-shaped curve which is called the sigmoid flexure of the penis. A muscle known as the retractor penis is attached on each side near the under side of the organ at a point about six inches behind the glans and extends backward so that the other end is attached near the root of the penis. The organ is straightened out at the time of service, otherwise these two muscles serve to keep about a foot of it folded up in the flexure. The penis ends in a pointed and enlarged flattened head which is called the glans penis. In it is the opening of the urethra which serves as a common passageway for both semen and urine. The fold of skin surrounding the penis along the belly is called the sheath, and the patch of long hairs marking its end is known as the preputial tuft.

Failure to Come in Heat

There are several possible reasons why cows may fail to come in heat. A common one is pregnancy, even though there is no record of breeding. Although there are exceptions to the rule, conception generally suppresses heat periods in cattle. Heavy production of milk is another common cause of cows failing to come in heat. Production and reproduction are closely related, and a hormonal balance that permits heavy milk production may act at the same time to prevent heat periods. Poor feed or starvation rations may also cause trouble in this respect. After all, Mother Nature decrees that a cow has to live first and reproduce as a sort of secondary activity. When animals don't get enough feed to do both, there's a good chance that they won't come in heat until times get a little better. Aside from an actual shortage of certain minerals and vitamins, lack of enough food during the winter is often the reason why cows suddenly start coming in heat after being turned out to a good living on grass in the spring of the year. This fact is a reminder that cold weather is sometimes a factor in preventing heat, too. Cows are naturally supposed to come in heat during the spring months while remaining sexually dormant during the winter. Even though we've changed the animals so that they come in heat the year 'round nowadays, an occasional one still holds with old customs to the extent of refusing to come in heat during the cold months. Heavy infestation with parasites has also been noted as a cause of failure to come in heat. This is probably indirectly related to a shortage of food, for stomach worms and lice and mange mites live off the cows and so may rob them of badly needed nutrients. In addition, a heavy load of parasites can make animals really sick to cause cessation of heat periods. For that matter, any kind of serious sickness is usually effective in preventing heat periods. Cows may be a long time in "coming around" after an attack of milk fever or acetonemia, and the same thing is true in regard to a bout with some contagious disease like shipping fever. Even more serious effects are possible in some cases, for diseases like Bang's and vibriosis may injure or destroy parts of the ovaries so that normal heat periods are no longer possible. Similar results may follow unskilled manipulation of the ovaries when rectal examinations are being made. Then there's always the possibility of so-called persistent or retained "yellow bodies" being to blame for failure to come in heat. Although generally seen in connection with some of the causes already listed, the condition may appear independently and for no apparent good reason.

Persistent "Yellow Bodies"

Under normal conditions a cow comes in heat about every three weeks. Shortly after the end of the heat period a follicle ruptures on one of the ovaries, releasing an egg and leaving a bloody cavity. A lump of scar tissue soon appears at this site which is appropriately called a "yellow body" because of its characteristic color. If pregnancy occurs at the time of heat, the structure persists through most of the gestation period and apparently secretes a hormone which prevents heat. If conception doesn't occur, the yellow body grows larger for a time and then starts to decrease in size at the same time that another follicle is developing on one of the ovaries. The follicle also secretes a hormone, but this one encourages the appearance of heat. Thus we have a contest between two opposites, with one growing stronger while the other grows weaker. Eventually the time comes when the follicular hormone can overpower the one formed by the "yellow body." The cow then comes in heat, the follicle ruptures, and another yellow body is formed to start things all over again.

Although the basic reason isn't always definitely known, upsets frequently occur and the yellow bodies don't disappear. Follicles don't show up, either, and it's sometimes a question of whether the yellow bodies prevent follicle formation or failure of follicle formation prevents the absorption of the yellow bodies. Whatever the relationship, cows don't come in heat and the trouble is often said to be caused by retained or persistent "yellow bodies."

The structures can be removed by manipulation of the ovaries through the wall of the rectum, although unskilled removal may cause internal bleeding that will kill animals. The subcutaneous injection of hormones is probably more practical for farmers. Stilbestrol in 5-10 cc. doses may be used, with second or third treatments at weekly intervals sometimes being needed. Either method will usually start animals coming in heat again, but animals should be definitely known to be open before they are treated. This is important, for most pregnant cows also carry persistent "yellow bodies" and removal of the structures by any method is very likely to cause abortion.

Nymphomaniacs or Chronic Bullers

CAUSE. One or more blister-like cysts or fluid-filled structures which appear on the ovaries, although the actual reason for their appearance is unknown. At times the structures may approach the size of a hen egg. Like follicles, they evidently secrete a hormone that produces symptoms of heat.

SYMPTOMS. Cows first appear to be in heat for long periods or all the time, thus accounting for the name "chronic bullers." They "ride" other cows and stand while others "ride" them. However, in later stages they refuse to let other cows "ride" them although they continue to "ride" other animals. As time goes on they act more and more like males, "breeding" cows that come in heat and even fighting the bull away from such animals. They paw the ground while bellowing in a hoarse tone like a bull and even walk like a herd sire. The head becomes increasingly coarse in appearance, the shoulders thicken, and the tail head has a tendency to rise. Milk production drops off to nothing and the cow stops coming in heat even though she is definitely not with calf.

DIAGNOSIS. Usually on the basis of typical symptoms, and made definitely by a manual examination through the rectum that reveals cysts on the ovaries.

TREATMENT. Breaking the cysts in combination with intravenous injection of hormone preparations made expressly for the correction of this condition. Breaking the cysts without hormone injections gives temporary results, but the structures have a tendency to recur in a short time. Hormones used alone will correct the condition, but recovery is hastened when the cysts are broken in connection with such treatment. Effective hormone preparations can be obtained through veterinarians, but they are not generally available in places like feed mills and drug stores. A single treatment is usually enough to make a cow normal again, but a second or third one is sometimes needed. The chances of success are increased when animals are treated early, since ovaries may be hopelessly damaged in cases of long standing.

Irregular Heat Periods

Cows naturally vary a little in the length of cycles, so heats occurring every 18-23 days are usually considered within the normal range. However, individuals should be consistent so that one heat doesn't occur after 18 days, the next at 23, the next at 20, and so on. Such an occurrence is usually a sign of trouble. Heats at short intervals or extremely long ones after a period of normal cycles are also likely indications that something has gone wrong.

Cows that suddenly start coming in heat at 10-12 days or shorter intervals are usually afflicted with cystic ovaries, a condition that was just described under the heading of "Chronic Bullers." In fact, heats at extremely short intervals may be an early symptom of this particular trouble. Heats may occur at short intervals once in a while because of unknown factors that upset hormonal balance in the animal body. They may also appear in connection with various infections of the reproductive tract and certain diseases like rabies, but a series of heats at short intervals should cause suspicion of cysts on one or both ovaries. Diagnosis and treatment is the same as given for "chronic bullers."

It sometimes happens that cows come in heat weeks or even months after they were believed safely settled with calf. In most of these cases the animals were actually pregnant for a while, but lost their calves for some reason or other. Diseases like vibriosis, Bang's, and trichomoniasis are often involved, but there are other causes of abortions in cattle as listed in this book under that heading. There are other reasons why cows may fail to come in heat for long periods, and include such things as heavy milk production, poor feed, sickness, and others described in an earlier part of this section. Under such conditions cows may never have been pregnant

at all, but simply stopped coming in heat and resumed the cycles at
a later time when conditions were more favorable. Treatment is dependent on the cause, and identifying the right one may call for
considerable detective work on the part of an owner.

It must also be remembered that pregnant cows sometimes come
in heat and fool people into thinking they are open. They aren't
supposed to do such a thing, but an occasional animal will break
the accepted rules of proper behavior, anyway. Consequently, it's
usually a good idea to check cows for pregnancy when they suddenly show up in heat after a long period when they were believed
to be settled with calf.

Causes of Abortion

There are at least sixteen possible causes of bovine abortions:
1. Bang's disease is the commonest. This is true even on
   farms where calfhood vaccination is being done, for a
   large number of reactors may supply more exposure than
   vaccinates can resist.
2. Trichomoniasis. Although usually associated with early
   miscarriages, this disease can cause abortions in the latter
   stages of pregnancy, too.
3. Leptospirosis. Abortions may be the only symptom.
4. Vibriosis. Appearing in Bang's-free herds, it may be un-
   recognized as a cause of abortions so it leads to condemnation of the blood test for Bang's as being inaccurate.
5. Mucosal disease. Recently named as a possible cause of
   bovine abortions in a report from the North Dakota Station. The entire calf crop was lost or born dead in some
   of the Dakota cases.
6. Nitrates in weeds, crops, or water supplies. Dangerous
   weeds include certain species of goldenrod, broomweed,
   pigweed, and nettles. Crops that are sometimes high in
   nitrates include oat hay, cornstalks, wheat straw, and
   frosted beet tops.
7. Body injuries. Being carried in a sac of liquid, an unborn
   calf is pretty hard to injure. Nevertheless, kicks by horses,
   jamming in narrow doorways, etc., may still cause abortions.
8. Various types of yeasts and molds that sometimes invade
   the uterus. Once started in a herd, this type of infection
   can be spread from cow to cow by diseased bulls.
9. Artificial insemination of pregnant cows. As mentioned

earlier, such animals may occasionally come in heat without regard for the customary rules of behavior. Poking an inseminating tube through a sealed cervix is inviting trouble, particularly when cows are in the early stages of pregnancy.

10. Damage to the lining of the uterus. This is usually due to infection that can be traced back to troubles at previous freshenings. In combination with "pulling" of calves, careless manual "cleaning" of afterbirth, and similar occurrences, it is often to blame for destroying some of the "buttons" or areas of the uterine wall. Such damage may make it physically impossible for calves to be supplied with proper amounts of food and oxygen after they have developed to a certain stage. Consequently they die and are aborted.

11. Various kinds of drugs. Some are medicines like the iodides used against lumpjaw and "wooden tongue." Others are recognized poisons like lead, arsenic, mercury, etc., used in paints, sprays, fertilizers, etc., commonly found on farms.

12. High body temperatures that commonly accompany diseases like shipping fever, red nose (IBR), anaplasmosis, and a number of others. Unborn calves are literally roasted to death as well as being poisoned by bacterial products in the blood.

13. Nutritional deficiencies, particularly in heifers that were bred when they were underdeveloped and not ready for the burden of reproduction. Cows live first and have calves afterward, so the babies are apt to be aborted when there isn't food enough for both dam and offspring.

14. Excessive bleeding. This is because blood is needed to carry food and oxygen to unborn calves as well as for the removal of waste products that they give off while developing. A lack of it can mean the death of calves through suffocation and poisoning, and their later abortion is to be expected. Severe loss of blood may follow careless dehorning, bad wire cuts, or sweet clover poisoning.

15. So-called "lethal factors" which are probably found oftener in cattle than in any of the other farm animals. They include such things as "doughnut skull," "bulldog head," "short spine," and others that probably haven't been recognized because they don't cause hideously deformed calves. These factors are inherited.

16. A specific type of germ referred to as a hemolytic streptococcus has recently been identified as the cause of numerous
abortions in Illinois and Wisconsin herds. It may or may
not represent a contagious disease of some kind.

Failure To "Settle"

There are generally three classes of cows that fail to conceive
when they are bred. There's the kind that comes in heat at abnormally short intervals and another kind that comes in heat at
abnormally long intervals, often after they were thought to be
pregnant. Both of these types have been discussed earlier under
the heading of "Irregular Heat Periods." The third kind is composed of cows that come in heat regularly at normal intervals, but
simply fail to "settle," even when bred repeatedly. There are ten
more common causes of such trouble:

1. Some kind of reproductive disease is most likely to be
   involved. Included are vibriosis, Bang's disease, trichomoniasis, and probably vaginitis. Infection of this kind must
   always be considered as a possibility since it can easily
   cause failure to settle without interfering with the regular
   appearance of heat periods.

2. Impotent bulls are probably the next most common cause of
   failure to conceive. A sterile sire can't be expected to settle
   cows, regardless of how healthy the females may be.

3. Inheritance is another cause of breeding troubles, and is
   probably more important than generally believed. Some
   cows are born with a natural tendency to "shy breeding"
   just as others are highly fertile and settle with little trouble.
   It seems logical to assume that breeding abilities are inherited just the same as type, test, and milk production.

4. Vitamin deficiencies may be present, even though the ration
   seems entirely adequate. At least, the addition of vitamins
   A and C have been reported at various times as useful in
   settling shy-breeding cows. This may well be true, for breeding efficiency often seems to be helped when cows are turned
   out to vitamin-rich green grass in the spring of the year.

5. A deficiency of trace elements like cobalt and manganese
   may also be related to breeding troubles. In spite of the
   arguments still raging over their importance in bovine reproduction, it is likely that the minerals may be of value in
   at least some areas.

6. Cows may be bred too early in their heat periods. Bovine females normally release eggs from the ovaries about eighteen hours after they go out of heat, so it is usually regarded as desirable to breed them as late as possible in their heat periods. If breeding is done too early, many of the spermatazoa may die before they have a chance to fertilize the egg.

7. Cows may be bred too late in their heat periods. Late breeding won't be satisfactory for all cows, since some of them ovulate much earlier than they're supposed to. In a case of this kind the egg may pass from the uterus before it has a chance to be fertilized.

8. A lack of hormonal balance may make it possible for heat periods to occur without ovulation or release of eggs from ovaries. Without an egg to fertilize, pregnancy is impossible, of course.

9. An acid condition in the vagina may be strong enough to kill spermatazoa before they can enter the uterus to fertilize an egg after service. Such acidity is frequently due to the presence of certain molds and yeasts as well as various types of bacteria.

10. Damage to the uterine lining through past injuries and infection due to retained afterbirth may cause breeding trouble even when heat periods are regular. An illustration can be furnished by fallopian tubes that have grown together so that eggs can no longer pass through them from the ovaries into the uterus.

Treatment is entirely dependent on the cause, of course, and in some cases there may not be any. After all, it isn't easy to do anything about pedigrees and ancestors that determine inherited characteristics. There just aren't any miraculous "shots" or "tonics" that will work on all problem cows, so you hadn't better waste your time and money trying to find such a product.

Sterility in Bulls

Questions are frequently asked about sterile bulls. Trouble is usually noted after a period of satisfactory service, but an occasional owner complains that not a single cow has been settled by a certain sire. Sometimes the bull in question will serve cows in a normal manner, while in other cases he doesn't show the slightest interest in the females. He may mount the cows without being able to breed them, or he may not even be able to get his front feet off the ground. Whatever the circumstances, the cows aren't being settled, and the owner wants to know why.

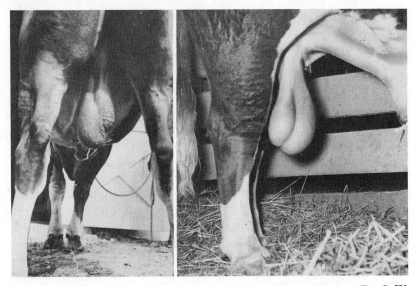

Left: Atrophy of right testicle following injury. (Picture, courtesy Dr. J. W. Gibbons, A.P.I., Auburn, Ala.)

Right: Orchitis or severe inflammation of testicles following an injury that resulted in permanent sterility.

When the cows are serviced satisfactorily, but fail to settle, there are eight possible causes to consider:

1. Over-use at some time may have made the bull sterile, especially when young animals are involved. In such cases the first few cows usually settle before a steady stream of "repeaters" appears.

2. Diseases like Bang's, trichomoniasis, etc., can cause similar symptoms, with troubles appearing only after infection occurs.

3. A similar history of sudden trouble may go along with an account of injury to the testicles. They may either shrink of swell afterward, but in either case they are prevented from producing spermatazoa to fertilize eggs.

4. Faulty rations may be to blame. A lack of certain trace elements and vitamins A or C is seemingly able to affect the breeding efficiency of bulls.

5. An infection of the prostate or Cowper's glands as well as

the seminal vesicles may cause sterility, even though the bull continues to serve cows in a normal manner.

6. As in the case of cows, heredity may be a factor affecting the breeding capabilities of bulls.

7. A serious illness like scours or pneumonia occurring in calf-hood may affect a bull's breeding efficiency in later life. This is usually because of irreparable damage done to the testicles at the time of sickness.

8. Old age may be to blame, even though bulls continue to breed cows in a normal manner. Older sires simply don't produce as many spermatazoa as young ones, so the chances of conception are decreased accordingly.

When bulls don't breed the cows, regardless of whether or not they try, there are again eight possible causes to consider:

1. Improper feeding and watering may permit bulls to become overly fat or "pot-bellied" so they are sluggish or physically unable to serve cows.

2. Sore or improperly trimmed feet may hurt a bull so much that he won't even try to complete the service act.

3. Broken bones or injured joints may make breeding a physical impossibility for the sire.

4. Fear of slipping may cause a bull to refuse serving a cow on concrete flooring or "across the gutter." A bull that has once injured his penis on a cow that didn't stand properly may refuse to mount another one that jumps around under him.

5. Wire cuts, infection, tumors, or injuries may make the penis so sore that a bull is unwilling to attempt service.

6. A lack of hormonal balance may cause lack of sexual interest, even in young bulls.

7. Lack of exercise is a common cause of sluggishness in bulls, generally because inactivity permits them to become overly fat.

8. Old age may be included in this list as well as the first one, since the time eventually comes when all bulls lose their interest in cows.

Treatment is dependent on cause, and a glance at the two lists will show that no single one can be expected to remedy all cases. Animals that have become sterile through over-use may improve after a long rest, but this doesn't help in most cases, either. Some causes, like old age and Bang's disease, just can't be remedied. Others may require only changes of management along certain lines related to care and feeding. Accordingly, it's a good idea to be sure of what's causing sterility in a bull before money is spent on tonics and drugs and hormones and vitamins that may not be needed at all.

Retained Afterbirth

CAUSE. Usually an infection of the uterus that leads to swelling and inflammation of the uterine "buttons" and keeps the fetal membranes from coming loose in a normal fashion after calving. The exact type of infection isn't always known, but genital diseases like Bang's, trichomoniasis, and vibriosis are frequently involved. It is not generally believed that a lack of minerals or vitamins will cause the retention of afterbirth, but the trouble is often associated with the breeding of under-developed heifers that are physically unprepared for the burden of reproduction.

TREATMENT. It is generally best to allow cows twenty-four hours in which to get rid of the "cleanings" without help. After that, the afterbirth may be removed manually whenever it can be easily separated from the uterine "buttons." No definite time can be set for this job, because there is great variation in cases, with some cows ready to clean in twenty-four hours while others require several days. Trying out a "button" or two will serve to show when the afterbirth can be easily detached. Scrupulous cleanliness should be observed in order to prevent the introduction of additional infection, and the vulva and surrounding area is best scrubbed with a mild disinfectant solution first. A rubber sleeve is advisedly worn for protection against Bang's germs that may cause undulant fever in human beings. If a sleeve isn't available, the hands and arms can be coated with mineral oil or lard for protection. Such agents will also act as lubricants when the hand is inserted in the uterus. When a sleeve is worn a mild soap is best used as a lubricant, since oils and greases destroy rubber. Once inside the uterus, the forefinger is worked between the afterbirth and each button to peel it off at that point. A little pulling with the other hand on the exposed part of the afterbirth will often help, but it must be done gently to avoid tearing off the caruncles along with the afterbirth. If this occurs, fatal bleeding may result, or the future breeding ability of the animal may be damaged. If the membranes don't "unbutton" easily, they should be left until they do.

In such cases a uterine capsule may be inserted in the uterus to keep down infection during the waiting period. One or two of the capsules are advisedly inserted immediately after the afterbirth is removed, too. Some owners prefer to use the capsules alone, inserting one every day until the membranes come away by themselves. However, membranes that are left in the uterus for long periods may cause severe sickness and even death due to generalized blood poisoning through an accumulation of pus in the uterus. Consequently, we feel that cows should be "cleaned" as soon as possible after calving. Several types of uterine capsules are available through veterinarians, or BFI powder may be put up in one ounce gelatin capsules for the purpose by druggists. Regardless of type, these capsules won't "clean" cows, but merely dissolve and spread through the uterus to act as germ-killers until the rotting afterbirth is removed or comes away by itself.

When given early, stilbestrol or posterior pituitary extract injected subcutaneously in 5 cc. doses may serve to contract the uterus. However, it is doubtful if such agents actually decrease swelling of the "buttons" so that the afterbirth comes away any earlier.

PREVENTION. No certain method, but a program of delayed breeding will prevent a great many cases of retained afterbirth. This is simple and practical for all cattlemen, since it merely calls for giving cows 60 to 90 days' rest before they are bred back after calving. This procedure gives the uterus a chance to clean up and get rid of any existing germs before they are sealed in to grow with another calf during the gestation period. Cows that have been sick with various ailments will usually require more than the recommended two or three months' rest period.

Clean bulls are not to be used on diseased cows, nor are clean cows to be bred to diseased bulls. In either case infection is thus given a chance to spread through a herd so it can cause trouble with retained afterbirth at calving time.

The breeding of under-developed heifers should be avoided, since this practice may contribute to the retention of fetal membranes, too.

"Free Martins"

This is a term that is given to female bovines that have been born with all or some of their reproductive organs missing. The usual animal has a vulva and vagina, but no uterus or ovaries. They are generally born twins to bulls, and an explanation of their cause is given under "About Twins" which appears in the Calf Troubles section of this book. The animals usually fail to come in heat and gradually assume a coarse appearance so they resemble steers as they grow older.

Eversion or Prolapse of the Vagina

CAUSE. Usually unknown, but the lining of the vagina loosens and stretches so that there no longer is room for it within the body. Reproductive diseases and lack of exercise are often factors in causing flabbiness of the vaginal lining, while the weight of calves in advanced pregnancies generally helps to force the tissues out of position. In beef cattle the condition is often due to large deposits of fat beneath the lining.

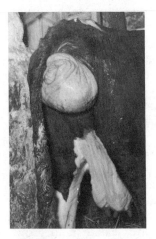

Prolapse of the vagina.

SYMPTOMS. Usually starts with the protrusion of a small part of the vaginal lining which is seen only when cows lie down. This has the appearance of a smooth, dark pink ball, which recedes out of sight when animals stand up again. The condition grows worse with time, and more and more of the lining is forced out, especially during the late stages of pregnancy. When the prolapse appears in one pregnancy, it is pretty sure to be worse in succeeding gestations. Eventually the condition becomes so bad that the tissues will no longer return by themselves when cows stand up, and the large mass must be replaced manually. In this stage the prolapsed lining usually becomes inflamed, swollen, covered with manure, and often is torn or infected. Affected cows may be unable to pass urine because of the vaginal lining being folded over the urethral opening. Once the condition has become established, it may appear in cows while they are open as well as when they are pregnant.

TREATMENT. Surgical removal of the surplus vaginal lining is the most practical, and corrects the condition permanently. It is best done in the early stages of pregnancy so that vaginal healing is complete before the calf is born.

An alternative consists of thoroughly cleaning the prolapsed lining, coating it with mineral oil, and replacing it. Once returned, it can be held in position by:

1. Keeping the hind end of the cow higher than the front at all times.
2. Placing some type of rope or strap harness over the vulva so a recurrence of the prolapse is prevented.
3. Placing stitches of heavy cord across the vulva for the same purpose. The stitches should go through the skin near the pin bones instead of through the vulva itself.
4. Setting two or three ordinary hog rings in the skin near the pin bones on each side and lacing heavy cord through them across the vulva to retain the prolapse.

All of these devices must be removed at calving time, of course, or severe tearing of the vagina may result. Decreasing the amount of roughage in the diet is also helpful in any treatment of prolapsed vagina. This is because such feeding means that less space is required by the digestive organs, and so causes less crowding of the vaginal lining.

Eversion or Prolapse of the Uterus

CAUSE. Usually some kind of infection in the reproductive tract that causes straining to result in the uterus being turned wrong side out and following the calf through the vulva. Such things as injuries or retained afterbirth may cause irritation that leads to excessive straining, and the condition often occurs in connection with milk fever or acetonemia. In the case of these two diseases the prolapse is probably due to the paralysis of muscles that normally hold the uterus in place. Aside from the above causes, it seems that injuries to various nerves may sometimes be responsible for trouble, for the cows aren't sick and prolapse occurs without any noticeable straining.

SYMPTOMS. A wrinkled red mass is found protruding through the vulva shortly after calving. It is covered with a large number of mushroom-like "buttons" which are enough to distinguish it from the smooth surface presented by a vaginal prolapse, and the afterbirth is frequently still attached to these elevations. The mass has a tendency to become larger, for the arteries pump blood into it while the veins are largely constricted to prevent its return. Consequently the uterus becomes greatly distended with blood, often approaching the size of a bushel basket.

TREATMENT. Replacement if the uterus hasn't been damaged by freezing, trampling, or other injuries. The organ is thoroughly cleaned first, the afterbirth removed, and a liberal coating of mineral oil or unsalted lard is applied. An old sheet or tablecloth is placed under the uterus for support, and the animal is made to stand on its feet if at all possible. The ends of the supporting cloth are grasped by a man on each side of the cow and the uterus is raised as high as possible so the blood will drain out and decrease the size of the organ. Reduction is further helped by gentle massage, and patient manipulation will usually effect replacement through the vulva. Once returned it can be smoothed out by inserting an arm full length in each horn. Great care must be used throughout the pro- cedure to avoid tearing off the exposed "buttons" and causing the cow to bleed to death. Fists are better for handling the uterus than open hands, since fingers may poke holes in the organ and cause serious injuries. Hands and arms should be kept clean throughout. Whenever there is a chance of Bang's disease being involved, they should be well oiled as well, for personal protec- tion against undulant fever.

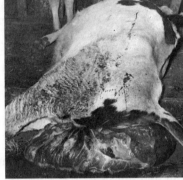

Prolapse of uterus following calving.

When animals are unable to stand up by themselves, the hind quarters may be raised with a block and tackle after applying a rope sling as described in the Practical Pointers section of this book. Time is well-spent in get- ting animals in such a position, for gravity will then help the uterus to practically fall back inside the cow. On the other hand, the job may approach impossible proportions when a cow is down and the uterus has to be pushed back uphill against her straining efforts to prevent replacement.

If the uterus has been badly damaged while out it is usually best to butcher the cow and salvage her for beef as soon as possible. Amputation of the uterus is an alternative, but the operation re- quires considerable surgical skill in tying off important blood ves- sels so the cow doesn't bleed to death afterward. The operation doesn't give animals a very good chance of survival under the best of conditions.

PREVENTION. About all that can be done is to see that the hind quarters of cows are kept slightly elevated or at least level with the rest of the body for a while after calving. Animals that are allowed to calve in stanchions with their hind ends dropped in gutters always have a good chance of turning themselves wrong side out at parturition time. This fact provides another reason why a box stall should be available for cows when they freshen.

Discharge from the Vagina

CAUSE. Usually infection that is present in the vagina or uterus, but sometimes a diseased condition of the urinary tract. Infection of the reproductive tract is generally associated with diseases like Bang's, vibriosis, and trichomoniasis, so discharges occurring at any stage of pregnancy may be due to abortion. In addition they may be due to infections of the vagina that are not related to abortions at all. Clear secretions resembling egg white are normal discharges at time of heat, and so are the bloody ones following heat periods and calving. White or grayish discharges usually contain pus which is indicative of dangerous infection either in the urinary or reproductive systems. They are commonly associated with injuries at calving time, metritis, or retained afterbirth. Discharges that smell badly warrant an immediate investigation to determine the source.

TREATMENT. Pretty much dependent on the cause, with management being more important than medicines in relation to causes like reproductive diseases. When infection is localized in the vagina it can be treated as described under Vaginitis in this book. If the uterus is involved, treatment can be followed as described for Metritis.

Metritis or Inflammation of the Uterus

CAUSE. Almost always some type of infection. Generally seen as a result of difficult calving or retained afterbirth, but often associated with abortions due to various causes.

SYMPTOMS. Animals go off feed, act generally droopy, and frequently run high temperatures. Weight is lost, milk production decreases, and movements are slow. There may or may not be straining or arching of the back, but there is generally a foul-smelling brownish or bloody discharge from the vagina. Sometimes there are considerable amounts of pus in the discharges. Generalized blood poisoning may get bad enough to even cause death, and affected animals are often left permanently sterile after an attack.

TREATMENT. Primarily aimed at destroying the infection that is causing trouble. Various of the sulfa or mixed sulfa solutions are generally given intravenously in 500 cc. doses for the sake of faster action. Sulfanilimide, sulfathiazole, or sulfamethazine tablets may be given orally at the rate of a grain per pound of body weight daily for not over three days. Million unit doses of penicillin in oil and wax may be given intramuscularly each day in combination with the sulfa treatments.

When there are considerable amounts of fluids in the uterus it is desirable to pass a small rubber tube and siphon it off. A pint of sulfanilimide in oil may be injected directly into the uterus every other day for a week if needed for that long. Penicillin or streptomycin in oil may also be introduced into the uterus, and various of the uterine capsules used in the treatment of retained afterbirth may prove effective in destroying infections involved in metritis. Douching of the uterus is not generally recommended since water is likely to have an irritating effect on the uterine lining. Intravenous injection of antihistamine solutions in 10-40 cc. doses may aid in restoring animals to a normal condition by blocking the effects of dangerous histamines produced by the infective processes.

Torsion of the Uterus

CAUSE. Not definitely known, but the lurching manner in which a cow raises her hind end first and then gets to her feet has suggested that this may be to blame. Being fastened at only one end, the uterus has a good chance of being twisted by such a motion. Since the pregnant uterus is more or less filled with fluid, twisting generally occurs behind the cervix in the front part of the vagina where there is nothing to hold the walls apart. The twisting may be either to the right or left, and can be compared to twisting the top of a sack. Torsion of the uterus sometimes occurs at parturition time, when it seems likely to be caused by the calf falling back into the abdomen after having once been raised into the pelvic cavity.

SYMPTOMS. Sometimes none at all until parturition time when the twisted condition of the uterus is revealed as preventing passage of the calf. At other times the cow goes off feed, acts dull, loses weight and fails to do well generally. In cases of long standing the twisting may cut off the circulation of blood so the uterus becomes gangrenous or ruptures to let the calf drop out on top of the digestive organs. Under such conditions peritonitis generally develops with the symptoms given earlier for that trouble.

DIAGNOSIS. Made through a rectal examination that reveals the twist in the front part of the vagina. The twist can be felt, and tracing of the uterine arteries will show how they have been carried over or under from their proper positions. The ovaries are similarly displaced, as they are carried along with the respective horns of the uterus when it revolves. The condition is most common in advanced pregnancy, but has been reported as early as the fifth month of the gestation period. Symptoms alone may cause the trouble to be confused with acetonemia, milk fever, hardware trouble, indigestion, or peritonitis due to other causes.

TREATMENT. Usually consists of rolling the cow to untwist the uterus. The animal is cast on the same side as the direction of the twist, so when the twist is to the right the cow is thrown on the right side. The animal is laid flat on her side with the feet extended. The front feet are then tied together and the hind feet likewise fastened together. The cow is then rolled over with a quick jerk in the direction of the twist, so a cow that is cast on her right side is turned completely over on her back and brought to rest again on her left side. A rectal examination is then made to see it the twist has been relieved. If not, the feet are bunched under the animal and she is slowly turned over on her belly until she is again resting on her right side. Then the legs are extended and the quick roll to the right repeated. This is continued until the twist has been corrected, with the rapidity of the roll being important to success.

Torsion of the uterus can also be corrected by surgery on the standing animal. If the twist is to the right, an incision is made in the right flank. An arm is then introduced, the fingers are placed beneath the calf, and uterus and calf together are turned back in the proper position. An incision is made in the left flank when the twist is to the left.

Mummified Calves

CAUSE. Unknown, but generally related to something that causes bleeding inside the uterus. The blood serves to separate the fetal membranes from their attachments to the "buttons," and the calf naturally dies from lack of food and oxygen. The blood eventually clots and is absorbed, although much of the coloring matter is left behind to account for the characteristic dark color of mummified calves. Infection of the uterus by germs like B. abortus and V. fetus has been blamed for causing some cases of uterine bleeding, but mummification of calves has occurred in the absence of any known germs.

SYMPTOMS. There are usually no symptoms save the failure of a cow to deliver a calf or show pregnancy at the expected time.

DIAGNOSIS. Made through a rectal examination that reveals the shriveled body of the calf in a uterus that is devoid of fluids usually associated with pregnancy. There is no evidence of rotting of the calf or metritis. Mummification seems more common in first calf heifers at 4-6 months of the gestation period.

TREATMENT. Ordinary animals are best sold for beef. Others may be aborted by removing the yellow body of pregnancy from the ovary by means of manipulation through the wall of the rectum. An alternate method consists of injecting stilbestrol intramuscularly in doses that are repeated at four day intervals as needed. After abortion has been produced, involved animals should be given a three or four months' rest before being bred again. Most of them will conceive without too much trouble and carry their next calves to term.

Overlong Pregnancies

The length of the normal gestation period in cows varies considerably, ranging between 260 and 296 days, with an average usually being figured at about 282 days. Although bull calves are likely to be carried longer than heifers, even then they are generally born fairly close to the 282-day average gestation period. However, abnormally long gestation periods are sometimes reported, with the calves that are being carried always being extremely large so that they cause serious trouble at freshening time. These calves show evidence of an extra-long period of development by such things as long hair and an advanced stage of tooth growth. Cows may be badly injured by attempts to "pull" such calves with a wire-stretcher or tractor, and they can often be successfully delivered only by a caesarean operation. Practically all the calves from these overlong pregnancies are either born dead or die shortly after birth.

The cause is not definitely known, but it is generally believed to be an inherited factor. Research indicates that a normal gestation period is dependent on hormonal balance between the cow and her unborn calf. Accordingly, over-long pregnancies are assumed to be caused by some kind of a hormonal upset. A so-called "mutant" gene appears to be the cause of such trouble. When this "mutant" gene is not involved, cows go through normal gestation periods.

Nine calves out of a certain bull were reported as being carried for abnormal periods ranging up to 320 days. A cow that was mated to another bull had a gestation period of 369 days and was slaughtered because she was found to be carrying a calf that weighed 217 pounds. A few years ago an investigation of a single herd revealed 30 over-long pregnancies when the 282-day period was used as a base.

These over-long pregnancies usually follow pretty much the same sort of pattern. The first seven or eight months are likely to be perfectly normal, but the changes naturally expected at about the 280th day are absent. There is no udder development, the pelvic ligaments fail to relax, and there is no indication of pregnancy other than increased body size. Cows eat and appear perfectly healthy until labor begins. This may start at almost any time, sometimes as much as three months after the expected calving date. When labor does begin, the cow still will not be relaxed in a natural manner.

A little caution must be used before deciding that a cow is going through one of these over-long pregnancies when she does not calve at the expected time, for there may be nothing wrong with her reproductive cycle at all. It frequently happens that a cow's breeding date is recorded, and a much later service is then forgotten. Such an omission naturally leads to expecting a calf at the wrong time. It is also possible that the breeding date is correct, but that the calf has become mummified. Another possibility concerns a twist in the neck of the uterus which makes it impossible for a calf to be born normally. The cow may not have settled to the recorded service at all, and for one reason or another has not come in heat since so the owner assumes she is pregnant. Finally, the cow may have actually conceived, but then aborted the calf without being noticed. If she does not come in heat again, she may be credited with carrying an over-time calf.

In case this trouble really does show up in a herd, an owner will do well to review his breeding program. Certain cow families may be revealed as more susceptible to over-long pregnancies than others, thus indicating they are carriers of the undesirable "mutant" gene. Bulls that sire these giant calves might well be removed from service.

Fetal Monsters, Freak Calves

These are names that are given to abnormal or badly deformed calves. They are usually born dead, but occasionally are alive at birth. Living or dead, it is often impossible to remove them in a natural manner. Some of the commoner defects are:

1. Hermaphrodites. Calves are neither male or female, but have some of the genital organs of both sexes.
2. Brain rupture. Brain escapes under the skin through an opening of the skull in the face region.
3. Bighead or Hydrocephalus. An accumulation of fluid in the brain causes enlargement of the head.

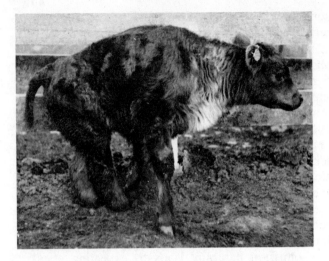

An example of a congenital defect caused by the amputated legs factor.

4. Bulldogs. In an extreme form calves may have extremely short legs, bulging forehead, dished nose, and undershot lower jaw. A calf that inherits the causative gene from only one parent may be shortlegged with a normal head.
5. Dwarfs. Heads usually a little large and legs a little short.
6. Andy Gumps. The lower jaw is shortened, incompletely formed, or entirely missing.
7. Missing upper jaw.
8. Parrot mouths. Back teeth are crowded in lower jaws, which are narrow, shortened, and often broken.
9. Muscle contracture monsters. Part or all of the body joints are stiff, with legs rigidly folded to interfere with birth.
10. Blindness. Eyeballs may be completely missing, or the eyes may be sightless and only slightly smaller than normal.
11. Glass, Watch, or Wall Eye. One or both eyes may have a gray or bluish iris.
12. Cleft Palate. Calves are unable to suck.
13. Waterlogged. Calves are swollen out of shape by accumulations of water under the skin.
14. Mummies. Calves are dead, shriveled, and dried up.
15. Amputated legs. May be missing at elbow or hock joints.
16. Raw feet. Skin is lacking so areas appear bloody. Lining of the mouth and nostrils may also be missing.
17. Extra legs. Usually grow out of the shoulder area.
18. Two heads.
19. Siamese twins. Calves joined either at the brisket or back.

20. Schistosomus reflexus. Internal organs lie outside the body.
21. Clubfoot. Tendons may be contracted so feet are drawn back at the pasterns, and hind legs may be straight with no crook at hock.
22. Rubber feet. Calves are unable to stand because bones in pastern region are missing.
23. Horny hide. Skin covered with horn-like scales.
24. Atresia ani. There is no outer opening of the intestine. Heifers may pass manure through the vulva.
25. Buffalo calves. Humps are caused by abnormally long spinal processes on backbone in shoulder area.
26. Cryptorchids. One or both testicles remain inside the body.
27. Posterior paralysis. Hind quarters are paralyzed.
28. Umbilical hernia. Intestines escape under skin at navel.
29. Scrotal hernia. Intestines escape into scrotum with testicles.
30. Flank hernia. Intestines escape under skin of lower flank.

All of these freak calves are due to either faulty development or inherited causes. The birth of a single freak calf will usually represent a developmental failure, while the birth of several similar freaks in a herd is strong evidence of an inherited condition. In doubtful cases an owner should contact his local veterinarian, county agent, state agricultural college specialists, or breed association fieldmen for help in identifying the defect.

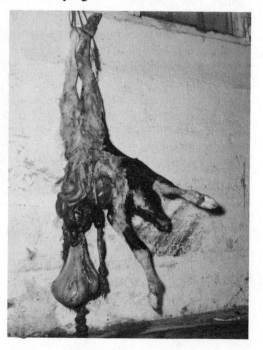

Schistosomus reflexus calf.

When an involved bull is a purebred, the secretary of the breed association should be notified and furnished with a complete description of the defect, including the names and registration numbers of the parents.

Uterine Dropsy or Hydrops Amnion

Calves normally are carried inside of one "water bag" that in turn is carried inside a larger "water bag" within the uterus. The smaller one usually holds about a gallon of fluid and the larger one about three times as much. For unknown reasons the amount of this fluid sometimes increases tremendously, with a total of forty or fifty gallons not being uncommon. This causes the cow to get bigger and bigger as the fluid gradually accumulates. The excessive pressure makes her uncomfortable, she fails to eat well, and shows her pain by constant shifting and groaning. Eventually the time comes when the great extra weight keeps her from getting back on her feet after she has laid down. The cause is essentially unknown, but a diseased condition of the uterus or loss of "buttons" at a previous calving has been suggested as contributing to the condition. In one of our own cases, a post-mortem examination showed that the calf had been strangled with its own navel cord in the uterus. However, it was not known whether or not the event was associated in any way with an excess of fluid that was estimated at about forty gallons.

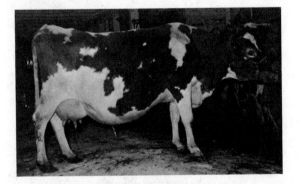

Guernsey cow in advanced stage of uterine dropsy.

When discovered in the early stages, the most practical treatment consists of delivery of the calf by means of a caesarean operation. Cows then have a 50-50 chance of recovering and continuing later as successful breeders. Draining of the fluids through "tapping" is not generally effective, since the large amounts of fluid have a tendency to reappear within a short time. Animals that are slaughtered in the late stages are apt to be condemned as unfit for human food and sent to the "tank" in packing houses because of dark-colored meat caused by absorption of the dropsical fluid.

"Breaking Down" Heifers

The use of heavy mature bulls on heifers sometimes causes severe injuries through broken bones. These can be avoided through artificial insemination or the use of young bulls. Another method consists of using a special chute for breeding the heifers. This has a stanchion at one end and is just wide enough for the heifer to stand in. A ramp about a foot wide is built on each side of the chute from the ground up to about shoulder level of the heifers. When mounting for service the bull will then stand on the ramps with his front feet so his weight is taken off the heifer entirely.

Infectious Pustular Vaginitis, Pustular Vaginitis

CAUSE. The same virus that causes the Mucosal Disease Complex, although there may be two or more diseases that show practically the same symptoms. For example, a contagious catarrhal vaginitis caused by a virus is known to exist in California, but it is different from other types because it is recognized only through breeding troubles or a vaginal discharge, with no evidence of pain. Although it has been reported from several different states within the past few years, no conclusions can be drawn at this time in regard to the importance of the disease in North America.

MEANS OF SPREAD. Not always known, but evidently sometimes spread through infected feed or water. There is also a possibility that the virus may be air-borne, with poorly ventilated barns favoring its rapid spread through a herd. The California type of disease is apparently spread to at least some degree through the mating act, with infected bulls serving to carry the virus from cow to cow.

SYMPTOMS. Limited in the California type to a vaginal discharge, evidence of breeding troubles, and a non-painful swelling of the vaginal lining. In other types of the disease urination may be frequent and painful as shown by backing up, kicking, switching the tail, and lying down and getting up again in a few minutes. Although animals continue to eat well, milk production goes down about a third when dairy cows are involved, and beef heifers lose weight, probably because of pain that keeps them moving and interferes with normal resting periods. An examination of the lining of the vulva and vagina will show it to be swollen, inflamed, and very sensitive. Practically all affected animals will show evidence of a white vaginal discharge, and in some cases the lining will be pocked with cheesy yellow ulcers. The disease may appear highly contagious in some outbreaks, and affect only a few animals in others.

TREATMENT. In case of an outbreak, it is recommended that a 3 per cent solution of potassium permanganate be applied twice daily to the lining of affected vaginas and vulvas. A soft brush can be used for making the applications. In the case of beef cattle, it may be easier to apply the solution as a douche by using a bulb syringe. The average case will improve within three or four days. In advanced cases it may be desirable to give intramuscular injections of penicillin and streptomycin for the control of secondary bacterial infection. Treatment is best continued for a week, since recurrences are likely if medication is stopped too soon. It will also be advisable to breed all cows in the herd artificially for six months or more in order to avoid the danger of infecting bulls that will then be able to continue spread of the disease.

PREVENTION. No measures can be recommended.

Lowland Abortions

CAUSE. On the basis of research work at the University of Wisconsin, believed to be nitrates in certain weeds growing on unimproved marsh lands. Red-berried elder, certain species of goldenrod, stinging nettle, white and purple boneset all store nitrates in dangerous amounts and seemed to be the weeds responsible for most of the trouble in the Wisconsin pastures that were investigated. Bull thistle, Canada thistle, murdock, lambsquarter, pigweed, and young plants of cinquefoil are also included in the list of weeds that store nitrates, but these plants were not always present in pastures that were studied. This trouble gets its name from the fact that abortions occur only when cows are pastured on marshland or swamp ground that has been cleared and then allowed to produce whatever plants come up naturally afterward. Once believed to be largely confined to Wisconsin, these lowland abortions have been reported from various other states in recent years.

SYMPTOMS. There are no symptoms of sickness or ill-health other than the abortions. These may occur at any stage of pregnancy, although they are commonest between the fourth and sixth months. Cows of all ages are susceptible, and abortions have been reported in beef and dairy herds alike. Calves may be lost at any time during the pasture season, and as late as October. However, losses are usually heaviest during May and June or September.

DIAGNOSIS. Properly begins only after the elimination of contagious diseases like vibriosis, brucellosis, and leptospirosis. Since abortions may go along with ailments producing high body temperatures, diseases like those of the mucosal disease complex should also be eliminated as possible causes. Then there are probably other plants that may cause abortions, and these plants need not necessarily be high in nitrates, either. For example, a species of broomweed has been reported as responsible for many abortions in range areas of Texas. Finally, the quality of pasture and availability of minerals should be considered, for deficiencies of various minerals and vitamins are capable of causing abortions, too. If not due to any of these other causes, and if the cows have been running on wild lowland pastures, it may well be that nitrate-bearing weeds are to blame for the abortions.

TREATMENT. None recognized at this time other than taking cows off suspected pastures.

PREVENTION. Wisconsin research workers have offered the following recommendations:

1. Spray weedy areas with 2, 4-D and if there is much brush, some 2, 4, 5-T in the mixture will help get a good kill.
2. Avoid pasturing after spraying until the grass has made a good growth and the weeds have dried down, because the killed plants may still contain large amounts of nitrate.
3. Feed good supplementary rations, for cattle are usually reluctant to eat trouble-making weeds unless starved to it.

When spraying is impossible, they recommend the following:

1. Breed cows to freshen shortly after the pasture season begins.
2. Then do not breed them again for at least three months after calving. By that time the pasture season will be pretty well over.
3. If possible, pasture pregnant cows on uplands all the time.
4. When it is impractical to pasture uplands, keep pregnant cows on "tame" lowland pastures.
5. Renovate "wild" lowland pastures as soon as possible.
6. Seed down these pastures with improved pasture grass mixtures.
7. Have soil samples analyzed, and fertilize the soil according to actual needs to minimize the danger of applying too much nitrogen.

8. Supplement cow rations with a simple, adequate major mineral mixture.

9. Feed trace-mineralized salt, and feed it only in loose form.

That "Cystic" Cow

The so-called "cystic" cow isn't always recognized, for she does not always show the same symptoms. She isn't hard to notice when displaying the commonest symptoms, for she then has a heat period that lasts for two or three days instead of the customary few hours. She finally goes out of heat, but in a week or two shows signs of being in heat again. This routine is repeated again and again, with the heat periods coming closer together and lasting a little longer each time. Finally she is in heat all the time so that she may become known as a "chronic buller" described on page 290 of this book.

At the other extreme, the "cystic" cow may not come in heat at all, thus becoming known as a "shy breeder" or being classed as a sterile animal. As another possibility, she may actually be pregnant, but with the cysts causing her to come in heat at irregular intervals.

These various possible symptoms are all due to a blister-like follicle on the ovary that goes wrong. Under normal conditions such a follicle matures about every three weeks and releases a hormone into the blood stream so that symptoms of heat are shown. When it ruptures, the cow quiets down and doesn't come in heat again until another follicle matures. When the follicle fails to rupture, it usually increases in size to become a cyst. Under such conditions the heat-producing hormone may not be produced at all, it may be produced continually, or only at irregular intervals to account for the various symptoms described.

These "cystic" cows can usually be cured if treatment is started early enough, but the chances of recovery decrease according to the length of time the animal has been affected. The most successful treatment consists of injecting a hormone preparation into the blood stream at the same time that the ovarian cysts are ruptured by means of rectal manipulation. Several different hormones are available for treatment, but the choice of products is best left up to a veterinarian who has had a chance to examine the cow. One treatment is usually enough, but extra ones are sometimes needed in exceptionally bad cases. The matter isn't as simple as it sounds, though, for some cows won't respond to treatment of any kind. In these cases it often happens that the adrenal glands are affected to account for the formation of cysts.

At the present time it will usually pay an owner to gamble a few dollars on treatment, especially on cases that haven't lasted very long. In the event of failure, he should be ready to make beef out of the animal just as he would a cow that is non-productive for any other reason.

Improving Results from Artificial Insemination

An owner will need to know more than how to tell when a cow is in heat, for some cows will require repeat breedings simply because they have been bred at the wrong time in their period. In order to have the best chance of calling the technician at the proper time, the owner will also need to know that:

1. The average cow shows signs of heat for about 18 hours.
2. A cow doesn't usually ovulate or release an egg from an ovary until about 12 hours after she has gone out of heat.
3. When a cow is bred too early, most of the spermatazoa from the bull may be dead before ovulation occurs to make conception possible.
4. When a cow is bred too late, the egg may have escaped from the fallopian tubes where fertilization usually occurs, or even passed out of the uterus entirely.
5. The chances of fertilization are usually best up to 6 hours after cows go out of heat.
6. However, occasional cows may ovulate abnormally early or late so different breeding times will need to be used on them.

With the above facts recognized, the average owner can increase the breeding efficiency of his herd by:

1. Calling the technician promptly and telling him when signs of heat were first noticed. Cows can then be bred shortly after they go out of heat to increase the chances of conception.
2. Being sure to call promptly, for cows that are in heat in the morning are best bred in the late afternoon of the same day. On the other hand, cows noted in heat during the afternoon are advisedly bred the next forenoon. Prompt calls give the technician a chance to lay out his stops to best advantage.
3. In the case of "repeat" breeders, being sure to tell the technician the time when the cows were bred in past heat periods. It may be desirable to breed such animals earlier or later than usual on the chance that they represent an exception that proves the rule in regard to the best time for inseminating cows.

Artificial Insemination, Pro and Con

For some time we've been aware that there is considerable difference of opinion in regard to the artificial insemination of cows. Most of these differences have been over the comparative conception rates following natural and artificial service, and opinion seems pretty well divided. Disregarding the efficiency angle completely, though, it is only fair to acknowledge that artificial insemination has both advantages and disadvantages. They just about balance, with five pros and five cons, and they look like this:

Advantages

1. It permits wider use of sires. The semen needed for a single natural service may be diluted and used on a hundred or more cows. This is particularly important in the case of valuable proven sires that would be unable to stand the strain of heavy natural service. In addition, valuable crippled sires may be used even after they are no longer able to mount a cow, with semen being secured by rectal massage.

2. It provides valuable sires at a reasonable cost. It not only permits the use of bulls that the average owner can't afford to buy, but it theoretically shortens the time required for herd improvement.

3. It saves the amount needed for keeping a bull. The room and feed needed for him can then be used to keep an extra cow. Even after the deduction of service fees, such a change will often show a profit. In addition, it avoids the danger of a bull breaking loose to kill someone or breed a neighbor's prize cow of a different breed.

4. It may help prevent the spread of genital diseases like trichomoniasis and vibriosis. When a bull breeds an infected cow naturally, he has a good chance of acquiring the disease, and after that he is likely to infect every cow he breeds. With treated semen and a sterile tube being used for each service, this danger is eliminated.

5. It improves stock in entire areas to attract distant buyers. It's a good thing when an entire community or county develops a reputation as a source of good cattle. Buyers like to purchase in truckload lots, and the ability to get them in small areas saves them time and expense. These savings are often passed on to the breeders in the form of better prices for their animals.

Disadvantages

1. It may disturb breeding programs. If semen from a certain bull is unavailable on the date a certain cow is in heat, she will have to be skipped or bred to a different bull. This sort of thing makes it difficult to follow specified blood lines in a herd.
2. It may permit a single diseased bull to infect a large number of cows in a large number of herds. Unless treated with antibiotics, the semen of bulls is perfectly capable of spreading diseases like vibriosis, trichomoniasis, and brucellosis.
3. It requires a well-trained manager and staff of technicians to do the actual inseminating. Lacking such personnel, poor conception rates and general dissatisfaction may wreck a project and cause loss to its stockholders.
4. The breeding of pregnant cows may cause abortions, especially those in the early stages of pregnancy. It is not uncommon for pregnant cows to come in heat, and while natural service does no harm, pushing an inseminating tube through the cervical seal is very likely to result in an abortion.
5. A heavy turnover of bulls may make an artificial breeding unit pretty expensive to operate. Animals are worked hard, and many of them won't stand the pace. Bulls that become sterile hurt breeding programs when they have to be retired from service. In addition, it costs money to replace them, and this expense can really add up.

Maybe you are now using a bull naturally and aren't exactly pleased with results. Or you may be using artificial services without being too well satisfied. In either event you are probably considering the advisability of making a change. Before you make up your mind, just remember that artificial insemination has both advantages and disadvantages like everything else. Studying our lists may help you decide what is best for you.

Epizootic Bovine Abortion (EBA, Foothill Abortion)

CAUSE. One of the psittacosis-lymphogranuloma-venereum (PLV) group. The agent was isolated in 1959. Since it is commonest in the U.S. in cattle which pasture in the foothills of mountains, it is often called "foothill abortion." The disease is particularly well known in California, but is widespread in the western states and the Rocky Mountain states. It has also been reported in a mild form from Spain and Germany.

MEANS OF SPREAD. Unknown at this time, for the infection has been reproduced only by inoculation so far. This leads to suspicion that the natural means of spread may be through ticks or biting flies. Although PLV organisms have been isolated from ticks in California areas where EBA has appeared, there is no definite proof that they are spreaders of the disease.

SYMPTOMS. Not likely to be any other than abortion, although experimental animals develop a high fever within two days after inoculation with the causative agent. This fever lasts for two or three days, but the animals appear normal during this period and until abortion two or three months later. The disease appears in both beef and diary animals, but seems to be more severe in beef herds. Abortions almost invariably occur during the last three months of the gestation period. Calves may occasionally be born alive, but are so weak that they live only a short time.

Although most abortions occur during the late summer or early fall, this fact is believed to be related to breeding so that calves are born during the late fall and winter months rather than indicating a seasonal factor. It has been noted that abortions occur only during the first pregnancy of animals native to areas where EBA has appeared. On the other hand, imported cattle of all ages may abort if they come from areas where EBA has been unknown. Cows seldom abort more than once, indicating that an attack gives immunity. However, it has been shown that cattle moved from an area subject to EBA to one where it is unknown apparently lose such immunity. This suggests that the first immunity is maintained only through constant reexposure to the disease. The abortion rate may run anywhere between 20 and 75%. Although retained afterbirth may occur, the breeding ability does not seem to be affected in aborting animals.

Opening an aborted calf may show any one or more of several things, but no certain one in all cases. There may be swelling and hemorrhage of the eye tissues, the under side of the tongue, and the lining of the windpipe. The skin may show reddened blotches, and the abdomen may be bloated with a blood-tinged liquid. The liver is usually enlarged, extremely friable, and granulated in appearance. Its color may range from pale red to reddish-orange.

DIAGNOSIS. Very difficult, even in the laboratory, because by the time abortion occurs the causative agent is gone or exists in very small concentrations in the calves. A tentative diagnosis might be made on the basis of lesions or a herd history of animals having been kept in an area where EBA was known to exist. From a practical standpoint, the elimination of other possible causes of abortion should be considered. This would include diseases like brucellosis, leptospirosis, vibriosis, IBR. and BVD.

TREATMENT. None recognized. Because of its self-limiting nature and the absence of generalized sickness in affected animals, none is likely to be needed, anyway.

PREVENTION. Even though there is evidence that immunity develops after an abortion, no successful vaccine has been developed so far for use against EBA. The use of chlortetracycline in pelleted ·feed has given excellent results in experiments. However, no practical method has been devised for providing cattle on isolated ranges with continuous access to the medicated feed at satisfactory dosage levels. Such a procedure would have no such drawback in the case of dairy herds, of course.

Tumor of the Penis

Tumors may occur on the glans or other parts of the bull's penis. They are usually noted only after they have started to bleed following service, and have been mistaken for gaping wounds due to wire cuts or injuries. They are most effectively treated by surgical removal. After treatment is usually unnecessary, but bulls should be brought close to cows daily for a week or so afterward. This is so that protrusion of the penis will serve to prevent adhesions of the cut surfaces to the lining of the sheath. Animals should not be returned to service until the area is completely healed.

Broken Penis

This is a fairly common bull trouble that usually occurs when a female makes a sudden sidewise movement when service is being attempted. The accident may also happen in other ways as when bulls attempt to jump gates or other obstructions. The injury is frequently caused by including the penis in a half hitch around the body when a bull is to be cast.

Although the condition is commonly referred to as a "broken penis," the organ really isn't broken at all. Instead, a major blood vessel is broken, and blood escapes to form a large swelling. Since this usually forms on one side of the penis, the organ then appears crooked as though actually broken and bent at the break. In some cases there is a swelling that appears just in front of the scrotum to make an owner afraid that the bull has been ruptured in that area. Regardless of the exact location, this swelling varies a great deal in size according to the extent of the injury and the amount of blood that has escaped. The swelling is extremely sore shortly after an injury has occurred, but the inflammation gradually subsides so the area is no longer sensitive.

A diagnosis is made on the basis of an examination that reveals the swelling as involving only the penis. Without such an examination it might be possible in some cases to confuse the condition with something entirely different like a hernia that has allowed some of the intestines to escape from the body and bunch up under the skin. A similar swelling might result from a bad bruise of tissues not involving the penis, or show up as the beginning of an abscess in the belly wall.

The correct treatment will depend pretty much on the size of the swelling. Many of the smaller ones require no treatment at all other than removal of the bull from service for a few weeks. In these cases the swelling gradually goes down as the blood is resorbed by the body. The penis may be left as appearing crooked, but the bull will usually be able to breed with no trouble anyway.

In severer cases it will be necessary to remove the clotted blood by surgery. This operation should be attempted only by a veterinarian so that every last bit of the clotted blood is removed to prevent infection. Otherwise, any blood that is left in the pocket furnishes an ideal place for bacteria to grow so that pus forms and an abscess develops. After the clotted blood is removed, the incision is closed with catgut stitches to hasten healing.

In some of these cases it may be desirable to remove the bull from service for a few weeks after the operation. However, some veterinarians advocate putting the bull back in service within a couple of days because inactivity may aid in the development of adhesions that will interfere with normal protrusion of the penis. At least one man recommends using a steel wire which is inserted through the penis a few inches back from its tip. This wire is then used to pull the penis out of the sheath a few times each day to prevent adhesions. A more practical method of accomplishing the same purpose consists of allowing the bull to come close to cows or heifers for a short time every day. This can easily be done by bringing the females close to the fence of his corral or pen. Most bulls will then be stimulated to protrude the penis a few times to break down any adhesions that may be forming.

11.

MISCELLANEOUS TROUBLES

Lumpjaw (Actinomycosis)

CAUSE. An organism known as *Actinomycosis bovis* that is normally found in soils and on vegetation almost everywhere. It probably gets into mouth tissues through ulcers, piercing by awns like barley beards, or during periods when temporary teeth are being shed. Regardless of how infection starts, the jaws and other bones of the head are eventually invaded to result in their destruction.

SYMPTOMS. Usually starts as a painful bony swelling on either the upper or lower jaw which is often thought due to a blow or injury. However, the swelling continues to grow, sometimes involving the whole side of the face within a month or two. Examination of the mouth will then generally show generalized swelling, inflammation of the gums, and sometimes openings that are draining pus. Various of the back teeth may also be loosened, while enlargement of the nasal bones frequently causes noisy or difficult breathing. Chewing is difficult because of the sore mouth and loose teeth, so constant slobbering is a common symptom. Swellings and abscesses may break at various points along the outside of the jaws to discharge pus and bloody material. Growth is likely to continue for a year or more, and often stops after a large size has been reached and bones are hopelessly honeycombed. Growths sometimes remain small, with little damage being done to animals. As a general rule, though, inability to eat properly soon leads to extreme loss of weight so animals become little more than walking skeletons. The disease has a tendency to appear in younger animals that are two or three years old, but is rarely seen in those less than a year of age.

DIAGNOSIS. Definite only when the organisms are demonstrated under the microscope. May be confused with bruises, bad teeth, abscesses, "wooden tongue," and occlusion of the parotid duct.

TREATMENT. None completely satisfactory, for results have been inconsistent. When caught in the early stages, infection can sometimes be controlled by intravenous injection of 150—250 cc. of 20% sodium iodide solution. This is repeated at ten-day intervals as needed. An alternate method consists of giving 5–10 grams of potassium iodide in water by mouth every day until symptoms of iodism appear. The treatment is then stopped for ten days and repeated again if considered desirable.

Symptoms of iodism are shown by watering of the eyes, excessive scaly dandruff. and loss of appetite. Iodide treatments can cause abortions, so these compounds should not be used on pregnant animals. Organic iodides are available, and are reported as being equally effective, more palatable, and not as dangerous as sodium and potassium iodides.

Other treatments consist of painting the swelling daily with iodine or injecting small amounts of Lugol's solution in several places around the base of the swelling every three or four days as indicated. Penicillin has been reported as of value, and a combination of streptomycin and penicillin can be injected directly into the body and around the edges of the swelling. Streptomycin in combination with surgery and potassium iodide may prove effective, with the antibiotic being injected around the edges of the lesion every day for five days.

In the case of valuable animals it may be desirable to try treatment with x-rays. Although this may help in controlling the growth of actinomycosis, it cannot be depended on to effect a permanent cure. Growth may be temporarily stopped, but the lesion will usually become active again.

Regardless of the treatment tried, infected animals which are discharging from affected areas should be isolated from others, and steps should be taken to avoid the exposure of human beings to affected animals.

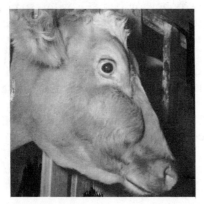 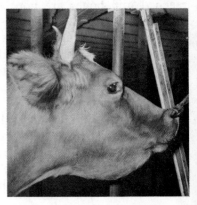

Lumpjaw of the upper jaw.   An early case of lumpjaw.

"Wooden Tongue" or Actinobacillosis

CAUSE. An organism known as *Actinobacillus lignieresi* which is widely distributed in soils and on forage. It probably gains a start in animals through the same avenues as used by A. bovis.

SYMPTOMS. Swellings in head and throat muscles instead of bone enlargements as in the case of lumpjaw. These may affect the tongue or appear between the lower jaws and in the region of the upper throat. They are usually painless and movable, although sometimes quite hard. Ability to move a swelling may help to distinguish it from an A. bovis infection. Actinobacillosis frequently occurs as a small hard swelling about the size of a hickory nut which appears under the skin part-way between the eye and the corner of the mouth. Although not seen until dead animals are opened, A. lignieresi may also attack various internal organs of cattle to cause actinobacillosis of the liver, rumen, etc. Symptoms are then those of a generally wasting away and loss of weight.

When the tongue is affected there is profuse slobbering and increasing difficulty in eating that makes the animals grow thin and weak. Examination will often show swelling along the sides and under part of the tongue. Enlargements feel solid and appear painful when movements of the tongue are attempted. In advanced cases the tongue is often so badly swollen that it protrudes from the mouth in a helpless fashion. The typical appearance and partial paralysis of the tongue are responsible for the descriptive name of "wooden tongue" that has been given to this disease. Depending on the area and extent of enlargement, there may or may not be interference with breathing.

DIAGNOSIS. Definite only when *A. lignieresi* can be demonstrated under the microscope, but the location and appearance of swellings will often provide a hint as to their nature. The condition may be confused with the same troubles listed earlier under lumpjaw.

TREATMENT. Pretty much the same as already given for lumpjaw, although the tongue shouldn't be painted with iodine, of course. Nodules under the skin may be removed surgically, while abscesses close to the surface can be opened and drained. When necessary the abscess cavities can then be packed for twenty-four hours with gauze that has been soaked in iodine. The gauze is then removed to allow healing. Treatment of any kind may have to be repeated, since infection may recur. This condition is usually curable, and in general is much less serious than lumpjaw.

Mucormycosis

CAUSE. Molds of the *Mucor, Rhizopus,* and *Absidia* genera. Although not an important disease of cattle, it has been increasing in occurrence. It has been suggested that the increased incidence of this disease may be due to the use of antibiotics which have decreased bacterial growth to permit increased development of fungi which are not affected by the antibiotics. The method of infection is unknown.

SYMPTOMS. Usually either abortion or various signs of pneumonia, but it is believed that various kinds of nervous symptoms like staggering and walking in circles may be the result of brain infection. Abortion is most likely to occur during the last two months of pregnancy, but they have been reported as occurring as early as the third month. Opening a dead animal may show no specific lesions, but in one case calcified necrotic nodules were found throughout the carcass of a yearling heifer.

DIAGNOSIS. Definite only through demonstration of the causative fungus under the microscope.

TREATMENT. No measures can be recommended at this time for either treatment or prevention.

Cryptococcosis

CAUSE. A fungus called Cryptococcus neoformans (*Torula histolytica*). In the United States it has been identified in man, cattle, horses, cats, dogs, and several kinds of wild animals. In cattle it has been reported as related to lung infections, pus in lymph nodes, and mastitis. The means of infection is unknown.

SYMPTOMS. In cattle the most important ones are those of mastitis. One or all four quarters may be involved, with swelling and inflammation often being noticed first in the upper part of the udder and then working down. The appearance of the milk may not be abnormal in the beginning of an attack, but small flakes are not long in showing up. In severe cases the amount of milk produced drops off drastically in a short time and the milk itself takes on a grayish white color while becoming quite thick.

DIAGNOSIS. Definite only when C. neoformans can be demonstrated in milk samples following special culturing processes in the laboratory.

TREATMENT. None can be recommended at this time, for treatment with various antibiotics and antifungal agents has not been very successful.

Histoplasmosis

CAUSE. A fungus by the name of *Histoplasma capsulatum*. It is common in the soil over much of the world, and most of the river valleys in the temperate and tropical zones are believed to be infected. Many kinds of domestic and wild animals have been found to be diseased, including dogs, cats, cattle, horses, sheep, rats, mice, skunks, foxes, raccoons, and opossums. Human beings are also susceptible, and it has been estimated that 500,000 people acquire the infection every year in the U.S. alone.

MEANS OF SPREAD. Entirely by inhalation of the fungus, either alone or in dust that has been stirred up by various causes.

SYMPTOMS. Dependent on whether infection is confined to the lungs or spread throughout the body. When only the lungs are involved there will usually be no serious trouble because healing is followed by sealing off and often complete calcification of the affected area.

When the infection involves other body areas, symptoms may include loss of weight, persistent diarrhea, coughing, weakness, and intermittent fever. One cow lost weight for several months before she showed signs of difficult breathing, diarrhea, grinding of the teeth, swelling of the brisket, and a rough haircoat. One calf was found dead of the disease without having shown any previous signs of sickness at all.

Opening a dead animal may reveal lesions of various kinds, including swollen lymph nodes, thickened walls of the small intestine, enlargement of the liver and spleen, yellowish fluid in the body cavities, tumor-like growths, fibrinous deposits on the lung surfaces, and ulceration of the mouth tissues. Organs like the spleen, liver, pancreas, kidneys, and adrenal glands may be splotched and contain nodules. Only a small number of infected cattle can be expected to die.

DIAGNOSIS. May be difficult because symptoms are not always shown. However, histoplasmosis may be suspected when animals develop a persistent diarrhea and steadily lose weight. These animals may be skin tested with histoplasmin much as cattle are tested for tuberculosis with tuberculin, except that the side of the neck is used as an injection site instead of the under side of the tail. It should be noted, though, that in areas where there is a great deal of histoplasmosis, apparently healthy animals will often react to the test. In addition to the blood test, blood samples may be drawn and subjected to laboratory testing for histoplasmosis.

A definite diagnosis can be made only by culturing the organism from tissue specimens or demonstrating it in tissues under the microscope. The disease is not transmitted to man from animals, and infected cattle only indicate that the fungus exists in soil of the area. Skin-test surveys have shown that histoplasmosis exists on a large scale in cattle, and that infection without evidence of ill health is common.

TREATMENT. Experimental work indicates that amphotericin B is the best antibiotic available at this time for the treatment of histoplasmosis. This product has no effect on bacteria and it must be given intravenously. The daily dosage and schedule for treatment has not been established for cattle.

PREVENTION. Entirely a matter of lessening exposure to infected dust. The oiling or paving of feed lots would help in this respect, but the sterilization of soil or other material containing the fungus is impractical at this time. No vaccines are currently available for the prevention of histoplasmosis.

Foot Rot

CAUSE. Generally believed to be a germ called *Actinomyces necrophorus,* or the same one that is to blame for calf diphtheria. It is commonly found in mud or filth, and causes trouble after the skin has been broken by some kind of an injury to provide a way for it to enter underlying tissues.

SYMPTOMS. Usually starts with lameness. The foot may be raised and shaken by the animal as if something was lodged between the claws. Examination may show nothing at all, or a reddening and swelling of the skin between the toes. The heels or soles may be sensitive, or painful areas may be found around the top of the hoofs. In advanced cases pus may be discharged through an opening at some point, or the entire foot may become a swollen, stinking mass of rotting flesh. Sometimes the feet may simply be sore and swollen so that cows spend most of their time lying down. Failure to eat naturally causes rapid loss of weight, and cows may become extremely thin within a short period of time.

DIAGNOSIS. Pretty much through the elimination of other troubles that are capable of causing lameness. These include foreign bodies in the foot, cuts, broken bones, untrimmed hoofs, sprains, bruises, prolonged standing on concrete floors, and inflamed tendons or tendon sheaths.

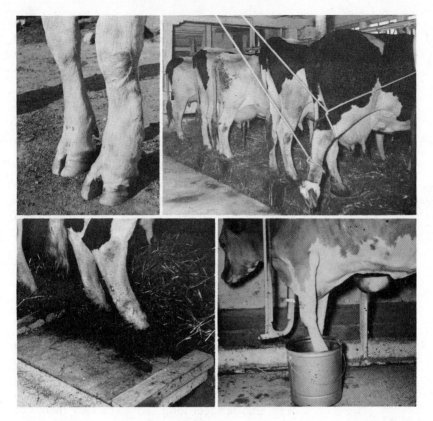

Top left: Bad case of foot rot in front foot.

Top right: Raising hind foot of cow in stanchion to permit treatment and bandaging of sore foot.

Bottom right: Treating foot rot with a pail to hold solution.

Bottom left: Platform prevents the animal from standing in the gutter and aids in the prevention of foot rot.

TREATMENT. At one time or another, all of the following have been demonstrated as effective against this disease:

1. Soaking affected feet daily for 20 minutes or more in some kind of antiseptic solution. Common ones are 2% copper sulfate, 5% chlorine, 5% potassium permanganate, 2% creolin, 2% lysol, and 5% formalin. A half-barrel with a loop of wire attached for moving it makes a practical foot bath for such treatment. When foot rot is a herd problem, it may be desirable to build a cement-floored pen. A four-inch curb completely around the bottom of the pen will make it water-tight, so that a couple of inches of solution

can be held there. Animals can then be placed in the pen for a half hour or so at a time. A piece of half-inch pipe can be inserted through the curb at floor level, with a cap on the outside end to make draining and cleaning of the pen an easy job.

2. Treating with powdered copper sulfate. The affected hoof is first trimmed and cleaned, with all the dead flesh being removed. The lesion is then dusted with copper sulfate, covered with cotton, and bandaged. A gunny sack can be used for bandaging as described on page 11 of this book. The bandage is removed after three days to prevent irritation. A few cases will require a second treatment.

3. Bandaging in a similar manner after the infected area has been treated with formalin, butter of antimony, iodine, other antiseptics, or various kinds of ointments.

4. Injecting animals intramuscularly with antibiotics like penicillin and streptomycin.

5. Injecting animals intravenously with solutions of sulfapyradine, sulfamerazine, sulfathiazole, and other sulfa salts.

6. Giving animals tablets or drenches of various sulfas.

7. Mixing solutions of sulfa salts with drinking water when outbreaks are a herd problem, especially in feed lots.

8. Driving animals once daily through a shallow box containing hydrated lime. This box should be about two feet wide, six inches deep, and ten feet long. Three or four inches of lime are placed in it, and the box set up in a narrow gate or doorway used by cattle to reach feed or water. The treatment is made better by mixing five pounds of powdered copper sulfate with every 100 pounds of the lime. The box will require regular cleaning and the frequent addition of more lime.

9. Driving animals through a similar, but water-tight, box containing four inches of a 10% copper sulfate solution. The addition of two or three gallons of white vinegar will help dissolve the copper sulfate in cold water. The solution should be discarded when it becomes dirty.

10. Seeing that animals in feed lots get vitamin A in some form. Since all growing plants are rich in carotene and have a high vitamin A value, cattle having green feed usually have plenty of this vitamin. In the feed lot vitamin A can be supplied by alfalfa pellets, commercial vitamin A concentrates, or leafy green roughage.

11. Supplying antibiotics. Aureomycin can be added to the feed at the rate of 0.2 mg. per pound of body weight. Water-soluble antibiotics may be added to drinking water at the rate of 1 pound per 50 gallons. (Water-soluble vitamins may also be supplied in the drinking water.)

12. Adding sulfa salts to the regular drinking water. These are best purchased in solution and added to the drinking water according to the manufacturer's recommendations.

13. Along with any other treatment that is used, it is a good idea to mix an iodine compound with the salt at the rate of one pound to every 50 pounds of salt and furnish it free-choice. In addition to being a valuable part of treatment, many owners believe that this type of salt mix helps to prevent many cases of foot rot.

14. In advanced cases, the joint capsules of the foot are likely to be hopelessly damaged, and it may be desirable to have a veterinarian amputate one of the toes to provide drainage of the infected area. The operation requires several weeks for healing, but does little actual damage, since cattle can get along with one toe on a foot about as well as they ever did on the two given them at birth.

PREVENTION. Properly begins with the elimination of mudholes and correction of filthy barnyards and feed lots in which necrophorus germs are usually found. Mudholes can be drained, fenced off, or filled with sand. Rough gravel or cinders can't be recommended as a filler, since fragments are then likely to cut feet and provide an entrance for germs. Filthy lots and barnyards are probably best remedied by covering them with concrete. The first cost may seem high, but the savings over a period of years will often pay for such an improvement several times over.

Some dairy cows form the bad habit of continually standing back in the gutter, and this practice sometimes encourages attacks of foot rot. It can be prevented by building some kind of a platform across the gutter to keep the animal out of it. The one shown on page 320 was made out of an old plank and some short pieces of a 2" x 4" beam. This type is easily removed and replaced with a manure fork when the gutter is being cleaned out.

Many cases of foot rot are started by neglected feet. In such cases the edges of the hoofs fold over into the bottom of the foot to cause lesions much like those following an ingrown toenail. In addition to making a susceptible sore, the cupped edge of the hoof collects and holds filth that is likely to contain millions of necrophorus germs. In view of this fact, any foot rot prevention program should include regular examination and trimming of feet.

During wet seasons cattle can be made to walk through a box of hydrated lime twice daily to dry their feet and make living conditions unfavorable for *A. necrophorus*. Hydrated lime can also be sprinkled around feed bunks and water tanks and hay racks.

Mixing iodine compounds with salt and grain is often considered as a good preventive measure. In one case the iodine was added at the rate of two pounds per ton of grain, and was fed to half a herd of feeder cattle in a lot where bad cases of foot rot were occurring. No new cases of foot rot occurred in the treated group during a 16-day test, and the four cases present at the beginning of the test cleared up without any other treatment. In contrast, 16 new cases of foot rot developed in the control group during the same test period. However, recent work at Colorado State University showed the use of iodine compounds for the control of foot rot in feeder cattle to be of questionable value.

Foreign Bodies In The Foot

CAUSE. Stepping on nails, splinters, stubbles, glass, stones, tin, etc., so the objects become imbedded in the deeper parts of the foot.

SYMPTOMS. Much like those just described for foot rot, with sudden lameness and swelling of the foot. An opening which discharges pus often appears at some point around the top of the hoof. Such openings are likely to heal up, break, heal again and rebreak for long periods until the foreign body is finally removed.

DIAGNOSIS. Usually through a careful examination of the foot that reveals the foreign body. All holes, cracks, and crevices of the hoof should be thoroughly explored, for a small object can sometimes cause a lot of trouble. Time is often saved by casting animals with a rope to make the examination easier for both man and beast. Methods of casting are described in the Practical Pointers section of this book.

TREATMENT. Begins with removal of the foreign body. The wound should then be thoroughly cleaned out with a mild disinfectant. Peroxide is especially good, since its boiling action helps to bring out small particles of dirt that aren't readily seen. Bandaging of the foot is desirable after cleaning has been accomplished in order to prevent recontamination, and animals are best kept out of mud and filth until healing is complete. Various kinds of healing agents can be used under the bandages to shorten healing time, with penicillin ointment like that used for mastitis treatment being especially recommended, and applications being made daily as needed. In the case of deep wounds it is always well to inject 1500 or more units of tetanus antitoxin as protection against possible attacks of lockjaw. Even though cattle are relatively resistant to lockjaw, there still is no excuse for an owner taking chances with the disease.

Tumors of the Feet

Wart-like growths representing a form of tumor are sometimes found around the top of the hoof and between the toes of cattle. The accompanying photograph shows them as they appeared on the hind feet of a young dairy cow, but the growths are much more often seen on the hoofs of beef cattle that are running in feed lots. They are generally considered as being harmless, although they may encourage foot rot or grow so large that they cause pain and difficulty in walking. The most practical treatment consists of surgical removal of the growths. There is little danger of recurrence afterward.

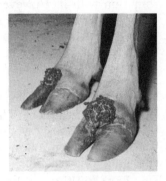

Wart-like growths, a form of tumor, around the top of the hoof.

Malignant Edema

CAUSE. A germ called *Clostridium septicum* which is commonly found in soil and often in the digestive tracts of perfectly healthy animals. Infection usually occurs through penetrating wounds, and has followed the use of dirty hypodermic needles as well as nail punctures and other accidental injuries. Like lockjaw, actual damage is done through a poison produced by the germs when they grow in tissues.

SYMPTOMS. Animals suddenly go off feed, stop producing milk, act dull, and move stiffly. High fevers that may approach 108 degrees are common. Various parts of the body may show extensive swellings which are soft and pit when pressed with the fingers. Cutting them open will show the swellings to be filled with a gelatin-like substance which is contained in the muscles as well as directly under the skin. The swellings sometimes resemble those of blackleg, but they contain little or no gas, and thus do not crackle under the touch. Bloating is frequently seen, and most affected animals die within a day or two after symptoms are noticed.

DIAGNOSIS. Definitely made only in the laboratory through the fluorescent antibody test or isolation of *C. septicum* under the microscope, but the typical symptoms are usually enough to indicate the true nature of trouble. Malignant edema may easily be confused with blackleg, and sometimes actually appears in combination with it. However, blackleg usually appears in cattle less than one year old, while malignant edema tends to affect animals over a year old, and this fact may help in the tentative diagnosis of outbreaks. Malignant edema has also been confused with anthrax.

TREATMENT. When caught early, massive doses of antiserum and penicillin may help, but most cases are not noticed until it is too late for treatment. The antiserum and penicillin are advisedly given intravenously at first to establish a high blood level immediately, and then followed by intramuscular injections to prolong the antibiotic reaction.

PREVENTION. Most practical through vaccination with a mixed bacterin which also gives protection against blackleg, and possibly other diseases. Calves are best vaccinated at weaning time, or when castration and dehorning are done. Earlier vaccination is not recommended because the immunity given by colostrum may interfere with proper action by the bacterin. Animals that are introduced into areas where the disease is known to exist should also be vaccinated. In case of an outbreak, all exposed susceptible animals should be vaccinated, although deaths may continue for another week or so. Carcasses of animals which have died of malignant edema should be burned or buried in quicklime to prevent the spread of infection as noted for the prevention of blackleg.

Aspergillosis

CAUSE. Fungi of several different Aspergillus species, including *A. flavus, A. clavatus, A. fumigatus,* and *A. glaucus* in feeds. At various times they have been identified in moldy sweet potatoes, moldy corn, and moldy peanut meal. Although recognized as a cause of abortion in cattle since 1929, and as a cause of pulmonary emphysema in cattle fed moldy sweet potatoes since 1945, aspergillosis attracted little attention as a cattle disease until the late 1950's. Since that time it has been reported with increasing frequency. Calves three to six months old seem much more susceptible than older animals, but the means of infection is unknown.

SYMPTOMS. Abortion that occurs chiefly in late pregnancy may be the only one. When aspergillosis affects the lungs, two different sets of symptoms may be shown. When the one caused by eating moldy sweet potatoes is involved, gasping for breath with open-mouth breathing, and swellings caused by air pockets under the skin over the neck, shoulders, and back are apt to be seen. This type of the disease always ends in death, sometimes within a day or two.

The other type is characterized by the development of nodules in the lungs, and is accompanied by evidence of chronic pneumonia. This includes such signs as loss of weight, coughing, nasal discharge, roughened hair coat, and muffled lung sounds during breathing. Like the first, this type also causes death, but it takes a little longer to occur.

In some cases aspergillosis is confined to the skin, and the only indication of infection is nodules that sometimes discharge pus and greatly resemble the lesions of skin tuberculosis.

Symptoms of aspergillosis following poisoning by damaged feed are largely dependent on the amount of toxic material eaten. Sometimes none will be shown other than a small loss of weight, and temporary drop in milk production. At other times, poisoning following the eating of moldy corn or peanut meal may cause more serious symptoms like going off feed, bleeding from the nose, bloody diarrhea, and general dullness. In addition, nervous symptoms like circling, grinding of the teeth, apparent blindness, ear twitching, trembling, and severe straining may be seen. Animals showing these nervous symptoms generally die within a couple of days.

Opening a dead animal may show little more than enlargement and emphysema of the lungs, but when poisoning has occurred, a yellow color and generalized jaundice is apt to be evident throughout the body cavities. There is also apt to be indication of bleeding throughout the digestive tract, and in the lungs, kidneys, and liver. The liver will usually have a yellow color, show a prominent lobular structure, and be sprinkled with necrotic areas.

DIAGNOSIS. Definite only through demonstrating the causative fungus under a microscope. When abortion is the chief symptom, it can often be found on the afterbirth or be cultured from the stomach contents of aborted calves. Poisoning will probably require microscopic examination of the liver, or chromatographic examination of the suspected poisonous feed. Lungs and skin lesions can be examined directly under the microscope for the fungus.

TREATMENT. None recognized. In case of trouble, the only effective control measure consists of identifying the causative feed and removing it from the ration. However, symptoms may continue to occur for two or three weeks after the feed has been eliminated.

Salt Sickness or Trace Element Deficiency

CAUSE. A deficiency of various trace elements; usually iron, copper, and iodine. These deficiencies may occur singly or in various combinations, and are due to feeding on plants from soils lacking the involved minerals. They cause trouble through anemia and a lack of hemoglobin in the blood.

SYMPTOMS. Affected animals are at first "picky" about feeds, often refusing good hay and grain in favor of filthy bedding, dirt, rags, wood, and bones. They grow sunken-eyed and rough-coated, steadily becoming thinner and weaker while the mucous membranes grow paler. Stunting is common, with two-year-olds sometimes being little bigger than normal yearlings. Heat cycles may be affected so that animals come around irregularly, and abortions may occur during the latter stages of pregnancy. A lack of trace elements may also be the cause of weak calves that die a few weeks after birth. There may be either constipation or diarrhea, but milk production is uniformly reduced. The pulse, respiration, and temperature usually remain normal throughout, with affected animals dying after a period of several weeks. Symptoms are commonest during the winter, with improvement often following turning out to pasture in the spring. In such cases the trouble has a tendency to reappear in the late summer as grazing becomes poorer. Cattle of any age may be affected, but trouble seems commonest in heifers shortly after the birth of their first calves. Trace element deficiencies are most likely to appear in Florida, Michigan, Wisconsin, and various of the Coastal Plains States, but may show up almost anywhere, particularly in areas where the soil has been badly depleted.

DIAGNOSIS. Eliminating other possible causes and then feeding the trace minerals to see if improvement follows. Results are some-times dramatic and almost miraculous after small amounts of the minerals have been supplied. It may be confused with infestation by worms, Johne's disease, coccidiosis, metritis, and other forms of generalized blood poisoning.

TREATMENT. Supplying the minerals through a trace-mineral-ized salt that is provided free-choice. A home-made mix can be made by combining 100 pounds of iodized common salt, 25 pounds of red iron oxide, one pound of powdered copper sulfate, and eight ounces of cobaltous chloride. Animals in extremely bad condition may be given a liquid made by dissolving one pound of ferrous sul-fate, two ounces of copper sulfate, and one ounce of cobaltous chloride in a gallon of water. The dose is ½ ounce daily as needed.

PREVENTION. Providing trace-mineralized salt free-choice is probably the most practical method. It may be placed loose in weather-proof boxes or supplied in block form.

Cobalt Deficiency

CAUSE. A deficiency of cobalt in the ration. It may occur either singly or in combination with other deficiencies.

SYMPTOMS.   Often the same as given for SALT SICKNESS. In borderline cases a cobalt deficiency can sometimes be suspected when animals fail to do well, even when on apparently adequate rations.

DIAGNOSIS.   Best made by supplying suspicious animals with a cobalt supplement. In serious cases improvement will be noted within a week, although mild cases will show no change. The cobalt can be supplied in salt, but this method has little diagnostic value. Animals may not eat the salt in large enough amounts, or regularly enough for a good test. In addition, when salt is used for diagnosis, one pasture is needed for test animals and another one for those not getting the salt. The pastures may easily differ enough to make the results unreliable. Forage can be analyzed for a cobalt deficiency, but the method is not very dependable because many different factors affect the ability of plants to take up cobalt from the soil. Accord-ingly, one plant might show a deficiency of cobalt while a different one growing beside it might show an excess. In recent years so-called cobalt "bullets" have come to be recognized as an excellent aid in diagnosing cobalt deficiency. They can be given to half a herd while the other half does not get any, and the animals then run together on the same pasture to eliminate possible forage differences. If a cobalt deficiency is involved, the animals getting the bullets will do better, of course.

TREATMENT. Supplying the cobalt through a trace-mineralized salt furnished on a free-choice basis. The cobalt bullets may also be used as a treatment, but there is some question about the comparative effectiveness of them and the salt. Since the bullets cost more, they would have to produce slightly better results in order to justify their use instead of the salt, and there has been no accurate comparison of the two under field conditions. Experimental work in South Dakota has been quoted as showing that steers getting cobalt bullets did much better than controls, but the results were misinterpreted because the control animals had no source of cobalt other than their feed. Under ranch conditions they would have had access to trace-mineralized salt, and the results might then have been much different. This experiment showed a need for cobalt rather than a need for cobalt bullets.

PREVENTION. Either through giving animals cobalt bullets or supplying them with trace-mineralized salt on a free-choice basis.

Freezing

Freezing is not usually a serious problem in cattle, but there are times when it causes trouble. The most common occurrences are frozen teats of cows or ears and tails of new-born calves. Occasionally the scrotum and testicles of bulls are frozen. Thawing out of the affected parts is the most important part of treatment, for it must not be done too fast. Accordingly, the application of snow or shaved ice is recommended for this purpose. The severity of freezing will determine the after effects and treatment, for damage may range all the way from slight peeling of skin to gangrene and sloughing of entire areas.

Regardless of where freezing has occurred, treatment is usually limited to thawing and the subsequent application of oily dressings to prevent chapping and to keep scabs soft while healing takes place. Glycerin is good for this purpose, and so is either zinc oxide or penicillin ointment. Even plain vaseline or wool fat can be used with good results. Whenever possible it is advisable to cover frozen areas with gauze after treatment in order to prevent infection.

Since most cases of freezing are associated with moisture of some kind, many of them can be prevented. Cows shouldn't be turned out with wet teats in cold weather, but this may happen shortly after calves have sucked or udders have been washed after milking. New-born calves should be carefully dried and protected in zero weather, even if it means moving them into the kitchen for an hour or so.

Broken Bones

CAUSE. Usually an injury of some kind like blows, stepping in holes, breaking down of heifers by bulls, animals doing a "split" when falling or trying to get up while in a weakened condition, etc. Some cases are due to hereditary weakness of bones or a lack of minerals that causes abnormal softening or brittleness.

SYMPTOMS. Dependent on location of breaks. In legs there is pain and inability to support weight on the limb. Sometimes it can be moved into normally impossible positions, but this isn't true when fractures don't extend completely through the bone. A grinding sensation can sometimes be detected when broken bones are moved. A broken back is likely to result in paralysis and lack of feeling beyond the point of injury. Breaking of the pelvic bones is apt to cause paralysis of the hind legs, while bleeding from the ears usually goes along with a fracture of the skull. Regardless of location, there is generally swelling at the point of a break because of bleeding and injury to adjacent tissues.

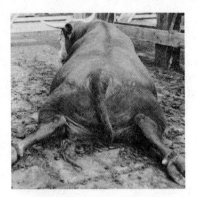

"Spreader" steer with fractured pelvis following slip and fall in icy yard.

DIAGNOSIS. Through careful examination and elimination of other possibilities. May be confused with foot rot, objects in the foot, nerve injuries, bruises, sprains, and dislocated joints.

TREATMENT. Fractures of joints, the pelvis, backbone, and leg bones above the knee or hock are usually considered as incurable in mature animals. Successful healing has been reported following surgery and the use of metal pins in such locations, and a trial may be justified in the case of extremely valuable animals. However, such measures are not likely to be practical for the average owner. Bones broken below the hock or knee sometimes heal, but the process is a long one and the chances of success are strictly in the nature of a gamble. Broken ribs, the tail, or lower parts of the feet have a fair chance of mending satisfactorily. Younger animals always respond better because of faster growing of all tissues.

When bones are broken cleanly in a straight line, treatment begins with bandaging over cotton and waiting for a day or two until the swelling goes down. After that the edges of the break can be brought together and fastened in place with splints that extend from the joint above to the joint below the break. Depending on the requirements, splints may be made from wood, leather, stovepipe, or hardware cloth. Strips of cloth dipped in thin cement or plaster of paris may be used either with or without splints to prevent movement of broken bones. In all cases, cotton must be applied under the splints and bandages in order to prevent cutting off the circulation of blood in the area. Splinting and bandaging are impossible in certain areas, of course, and in such places the bones must be allowed to mend without treatment.

If bones have shattered or broken the skin over them, cleaning of the area and removal of all bone fragments is the first step. Thorough drying should be practiced following cleaning, since water has a tendency to retard healing. In fact, glycerin is a better cleaning agent than many others. Peroxide is especially useful in bad wounds. Once the area is cleaned out, the injury can be treated daily with something like penicillin ointment. If splints are used, an opening must be left so the wound can be easily exposed by unwrapping bandages for treatment.

"Knocked-Down" Hip

This is a condition caused by injuries, usually occurring because of crowding in narrow gates or doorways. It must really be considered as a broken bone, for the end of the ilium or point of the hip bone is broken off. The condition usually causes no harm other than an impairment of appearance, for there are no joints in the end of the bone, and it supports no important structures. The displaced bone fragment settles out of the way under the skin and after a few days of evident soreness in the area there is usually no further indication of trouble. The injury is best left alone unless symptoms of lameness persist. Surgery may then be necessary to remove the bone fragment from beneath the skin.

Broken Tail

This condition is usually due to a fall backward while affected animals have been "riding" others, but it may also be caused by twisting, bending, or pulling the tail while owners are trying to move animals or make them stand up. There may be complete paralysis of the tail when it is broken close to the root, with inability to get it out of the way when manure or urine is being passed. In such cases the base of the tail usually appears as flattened and broken down. When broken closer to the end the tail may be seen as crooked and swollen. Pain is generally evident, and grating may be heard when the tail is moved. Straight breaks usually heal without any treatment whatever. Injuries to the root of the tail are likely to cause permanent paralysis of the appendage because the spinal cord is generally involved. When the tail bones are splintered and have broken the skin, it is advisable to treat them as advised earlier under broken bones. If bad infection occurs that can't be healed, it may be best to amputate the tail at the point of breaking.

Deformities of the Backbone

Deformities of the backbone frequently cause animals to become either "swaybacked" or "humpbacked." In some cases the backbone is curved to one side or the other to impair the appearance. Trouble in young animals is generally due to poor feeding that permits the development of rickets, but deformities may also be due to injuries that have affected muscles, nerves, or the backbone itself. In older animals the usual cause is injuries, although the condition may also be due to increasing flabbiness of muscles that are no longer strong enough to hold the backbone in a normal position. In addition there is a belief that a tendency to spinal deformities may be an inherited characteristic just the same as sloping rumps, weak legs, and other objectionable features. Aside from preventing rickets through better feeding there is usually nothing to be done about such deformities.

"Pot-Belly"

This condition is frequently seen in connection with a "swayback" that allows abnormal sagging of the belly. In all other cases it is generally due to improper management. Young animals may be affected because of infestation with stomach worms or through faulty feeding. Too much roughage and a lack of exercise is generally to blame in the case of bulls that sometimes develop a paunch which prevents them from breeding cows. Treatment of such cases is merely a matter of removing the cause. Some animals are like people in having a tendency to become pot-bellied as they grow older, and aside from watching their diet there is little to be done for them.

Dislocated Joints

Several of the important body joints are capable of being dislocated under proper conditions, with symptoms being largely dependent on the one that's involved. The usual cause is an injury that tears the capsule and ruptures ligaments, although infection is sometimes involved through the weakening of ligaments that are ordinarily strong enough to hold the joints together. Certain families seem to have an inherited tendency toward the dislocation of particular joints. The condition is almost always painful, and unusual movements may result, or none at all be permitted. Considerable swelling and inflammation of the area is to be expected. Diagnosis is usually made on the basis of characteristic movements or the feeling of displaced joints, but X-ray pictures may be needed for those that are heavily covered with muscles. Such injuries are easily confused with bruises and broken bones. Treatment consists of replacing the joint as quickly as possible and keeping it from becoming dislocated again. This latter job is apt to be pretty hard in large animals, for the restraining ligaments are already broken or badly weakened to encourage recurrence of the condition. Sometimes it is necessary to use a general anesthetic for putting animals completely to sleep before a joint can be replaced. The anesthesia has the effect of relaxing muscles that otherwise would resist helpful efforts. Dislocation of the hip and elbow joint is not considered as having any practical treatment. Dislocation of the stifle joint may sometimes be corrected by pulling the leg forward as far as possible at the same time the stifle is pushed back into position. However, the dislocation is likely to recur again when movement is attempted.

Arthritis

CAUSE. Not always known, but often due to injuries, infections, and poor rations that cause inflammation of various joints. Navel ill and metritis are commonly involved, while infection of joints through penetrating wounds occurs quite easily. Body infection is sometimes so bad that pus is present in almost all of the joints.

SYMPTOMS. Usually severe lameness and pain shown by difficult movements. Joints are likely to be hot and swollen, with pus sometimes being discharged from them. In a chronic form the swellings may take the form of painless "windpuffs" that cause no trouble at all. Death may result when infection is widespread throughout the body.

DIAGNOSIS. Based on typical symptoms and the elimination of other troubles like broken bones, dislocated joints, sprains, and bruises.

TREATMENT. None practical when important joints like the hip and shoulder are involved and draining pus. Others may be washed out daily with mild antiseptics like peroxide or glycerin and penicillin ointment injected into the wound afterward. When no wound is present, affected joints may be helped by the frequent application of hot packs followed by painting with iodine.

PREVENTION. Since many cases of arthritis can be traced back to navel ill, it is well to make a practice of disinfecting the navels of all new-born calves.

Broken Horns

CAUSE. Usually a blow or injury received while fighting. The skull surrounding the horn may be broken or the outer covering of horn may be torn loose from the bloody horn core.

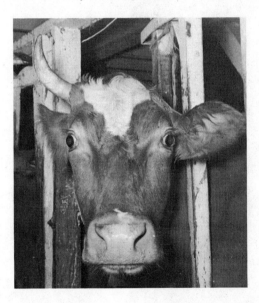

Broken horn gives head unbalanced appearance.

SYMPTOMS. When the skull is broken there is apt to be bleeding at the nostril, with tipping of the horn at an unusual angle and swelling around its base. When the outer shell has torn loose there is likely to be considerable bleeding around the base of the horn. Sometimes it comes off completely, leaving only the bloody horn core.

TREATMENT. The most practical consists of removing both horns to give the head a well-balanced appearance. Broken horns are almost impossible to arrange so they heal in a normal position. Different forms of splinting and tying have been suggested, but animals usually break them loose before healing can occur.

Bent Horn

For one reason and another it sometimes happens that a horn is bent so it persists in growing into the eye or side of the face. An inch or so may be sawed off the solid tip of the horn with no pain to the animal, but the job has to be repeated about once a year, since the horn keeps right on growing afterward. The condition can be permanently remedied by complete dehorning. It will generally be advisable to remove both horns at the same time in order to give the head a balanced appearance.

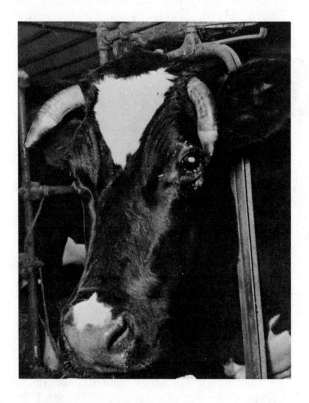

Bent horn growing into side of face requires dehorning.

Sinusitis After Dehorning

CAUSE. Infection that causes the formation of pus in the head sinuses opened by dehorning. This is often started by chaff, dust, and other foreign materials that manage to enter the dehorning wounds.

SYMPTOMS. Animals have a tendency to hold their heads low and to one side. They often go off feed and act dull, showing slight increases in pulse and temperature. In cases of long standing the pressure of pus may cause bulging of the facial bones, while interference with the brain and nerves may cause walking in circles and other signs of delirium. If pus happens to accumulate behind them, eyes may be forced partly out of their sockets. In milder cases the outstanding symptom is a discharge of white or grayish pus from the dehorning wounds.

TREATMENT. When caught early, reopening of the horn cavity to permit draining may be all that is needed. In other cases the sinuses may be thoroughly washed out with a mild disinfectant like a boric acid or 2% potassium permanganate solution. Tipping of the head will help to drain out loosened materials. One or two of the streptomycin bougies commonly used for mastitis treatment can be dropped into affected sinuses in order to destroy existing infection. In neglected cases of long standing surgery may be needed for boring holes through the skull to permit drainage at various places.

Monoliasis

CAUSE. Fungi of the genus Candida. The most important is *Candida albicans* (*Monila albicans*), but *Candida tropicalis* has been identified in mastitis outbreaks, and *Candida parapsilosis* has been reported as causing abortions in cattle. The method of infection is unknown.

SYMPTOMS. Dependent on the type of infection which occurs. When outbreaks occur in feedlots symptoms are always those of pneumonia. The earliest indication of trouble is difficulty in breathing and a moderate fever. The head and neck are extended, and open-mouth breathing is common, with slobbering also occurring. As the disease progresses, the saliva becomes thick and stringy, a brownish nasal discharge occurs, and the muzzle acquires a brownish crust. In the late stages a diarrhea may occur which results in a rapid loss of weight. Opening an animal dead of pneumonia is apt to show solidification of the lungs with cheesy yellow nodules scattered through the solid areas.

Outbreaks of mastitis in cattle have been identified as caused by *C. tropicalis*. In such cases the symptoms are those of mastitis which does not respond to antibiotic treatment.

Abortions have been shown as caused by both *C. parapsilosis* and *C. albicans*. In such cases the calves may either be aborted at various stages of development or born alive but so weak that they die within a short time.

DIAGNOSIS. Definite only in the laboratory through identification of the causative agent. Under farm conditions the infection might easily be confused with commoner troubles which cause symptoms of pneumonia, mastitis, and abortions. This may make tests for other diseases necessary so that a possibility of monoliasis is suggested through a process of elimination.

TREATMENT. None can be recommended, and until the means of infection is definitely known, preventive measures cannot be suggested, either.

Eversion or Prolapse of the Rectum

This condition is usually due to an irritation of the vagina that causes straining before, during, or after calving. Irritation of the rectum by diarrhea due to worms and other causes may also cause excessive straining, while the condition in beef animals is frequently due to deposits of fat in the perineal region. Treatment usually begins with thorough cleaning and oiling of the prolapsed part, followed by replacement. Stitches are best used to hold the rectum in place, since the prolapse has a tendency to recur. A single heavy cord or narrow ribbon can be inserted through the skin in several places while being passed completely around the anus in a fashion that leaves the two suture ends close together when stitching is completed. Pulling on them will then tighten the anus much as the top of a purse is closed by a drawstring. When drawn sufficiently tight the ends are tied together and the rectum is thus prevented from being everted again. Care must be used so the anus isn't closed so completely that the passage of manure is prevented. If the cause of straining is removed the stitches can usually be removed the next day. In neglected cases where the prolapsed rectum has been frozen or badly torn, the everted portion may need to be amputated. Blood vessels will require tying off in order to prevent excessive bleeding when such a step is taken.

Those "Downer" Cattle

Regardless of whether he raises beef or dairy cattle, the average owner has had experience with "downer" animals at some time or other. This term probably originated in stock yards and applies to animals that are down and can't get back on their feet. No single treatment will help all cases, for five major causes are generally recognized, with several possibilities included under each.

When placed in the form of a summary, they look like this:

DEFICIENCIES

1. Calcium. Involved in milk fever, rickets, and osteoporosis.
2. Magnesium. Involved in grass tetany, milk fever.
3. Phosphorus. Involved in milk fever, grass tetany, rickets, and osteomalacia.
4. Sugar. Involved in acetonemia.
5. Trace Elements. Involved in salt sickness.
6. Vitamin D. Involved in rickets, osteomalacia.

POISONING

1. Chemicals. Includes paint, sprays, fertilizers, etc.
2. Plants. Includes selenium, prussic acid, sweet clover, etc.
3. Medicines. Includes arsenic, strychnine, mercury, etc.
4. Bacteria. Usually in spoiled feeds to result in botulism.
5. Intestinal. Includes bloat, founder, and enterotoxemia.

CONTAGIOUS DISEASES

1. Anthrax.
2. Blackleg.
3. Shipping Fever.
4. Mastitis.
5. Mucosal Disease.

NON-CONTAGIOUS DISEASES

1. Lockjaw.
2. Leukemia.
3. Pyelonephritis or Kidney Infection.
4. Metritis or Inflammation of the Uterus.
5. Malignant Edema.

MISCELLANEOUS

1. Lightning Stroke.
2. Electric Shock.
3. Over-Heating.
4. Hardware Trouble.
5. Broken Bones.
6. Dislocated Joints.
7. Injured Nerves.
8. Pressure on Spinal Cord.
9. Starvation.
10. Liver Abscesses.

The next time one of your animals goes down, it may help to go over this list before you decide what is causing trouble. There may or may not be a remedy for your particular trouble, but it's certain that the wrong treatment won't help. On the other hand, the right kind may revive animals that are perilously close to death.

When Cattle have Sore Eyes

Cattle are often afflicted with sore eyes. Sometimes other symptoms are also shown, with eye trouble being indicated only by watering and mild swelling of the eyelids. At other times the eyes represent the only area of trouble, with many of the eyeballs being completely covered with a white or grayish film, and some of them showing a raised yellow spot or raw red ulcer. In such cases constant watering of the eyes may leave dirty streaks down over the jaws, and sometimes the hair falls out to give the faces a "scalded" appearance. Either one or both eyes may be affected, and animals may become practically blind and stand around humped up with the lids closed to keep out the light. There are several possible causes of sore eyes.

1. When the trouble is both severe and contagious, it is likely to be pinkeye.
2. When accompanied by other symptoms, contagious eye trouble may turn out to be an indication of malignant catarrhal fever.
3. When limited to a mild form, evidently contagious eye trouble may be discovered as being a symptom of diseases belonging to the mucosal disease complex.
4. When accompanied by evidence of skin lesions, eye trouble may be due to light sensitization or X disease.
5. Profuse watering of eyes is often due to irritation by dust or smoke or insect sprays.
6. Eyeworms sometimes cause symptoms of irritation.
7. It frequently happens that something is thrust into an eye to cut a lid or even puncture the eyeball.
8. At other times a foreign object in the eye may do no actual damage, but still cause a great deal of irritation and local reaction.
9. Either one of these last two conditions may be followed by secondary bacterial infection that greatly aggravates symptoms.

10. A deficiency of vitamin A can cause symptoms of eye trouble, particularly in cattle kept in dry lots for long periods.
11. Then there's always the possibility of a tumor or cancerous growth starting on the third eyelid or the eyeball itself. Secondary bacterial infection in such cases can then cause the true trouble to be overlooked.
12. Finally, it often happens that tiny tear glands located in the corner of the eye may become infected and enlarged so they look like tumors or imbedded foreign bodies.

Osteomalacia

CAUSE. A deficiency of phosphorus in the diet of mature cattle. Such a deficiency is most likely to occur when animals are on a ration composed almost entirely of roughage like hay, straw, or pasture. Hay alone contains sufficient phosphorus when it is grown on good soil, but may be very low in this mineral when it comes from poor soil. The grains are usually high in phosphorus, and their concentrates are even higher.

SYMPTOMS. Chiefly a shrinking and softening of the long bones. Animals often appear stiff, and have visibly deformed legs and enlarged joints. They grow thin, drop off in milk production, and appear particularly susceptible to broken bones that may cause them to go down in a more or less paralyzed condition. A depraved appetite often causes bone-chewing and the eating of material that will cause hardware trouble and liver abscesses. Affected cows may have a poor conception rate because of various breeding troubles induced by a phosphorus deficiency.

DIAGNOSIS. Usually through suspicious symptoms appearing in cattle that are on a low-grain or poor-quality roughage diet. However, a definite diagnosis may depend on chemical analysis of blood to show whether the deficiency involves calcium or phosphorus.

TREATMENT. Usually a matter of supplying phosphorus through correcting the ration and making a mineral mixture available on a free-choice basis. Feeds like cereal grains, cottonseed meal, and peanut meal are all high in phosphorus. The feeding of steamed bone meal is a practical procedure under ranch conditions, and either bran or the bone meal is satisfactory for supplemental feeding of dairy cows. A satisfactory home-made mineral mixture is described under RICKETS.

PREVENTION. Concerned with supplying animals with something like grain or bone meal to go along with their roughage.

Osteoporosis

CAUSE. A deficiency of calcium in the diet of mature cattle. Such a deficiency may occur when the roughage is poor in quality; when it is grown on calcium-deficient soil; or when too little roughage is fed to meet maintenance, production, and reproduction requirements. Legume forages are very rich in calcium, and there is usually no trouble if plenty of legumes are being fed.

SYMPTOMS. Practically the same as described for osteomalacia, especially in regard to softening of bones and enlargement of joints.

DIAGNOSIS. Largely through a history of affected animals having been on a calcium-deficient ration. However, a chemical examination of the blood may be needed to show whether it is a deficiency of calcium or phosphorus that is causing trouble.

TREATMENT. Pretty much a matter of supplying the calcium through good quality legume hay and a mineral mixture that is available on a free-choice basis. The home-made mixture referred to under Osteomalacia is also satisfactory for the treatment of this deficiency. In addition, from 10 to 20 pounds of some calcium product like finely-ground limestone can be added to each ton of the grain mixture.

PREVENTION. Usually nothing more than feeding a ration that includes plenty of good legume roughage. However, supplementary feeding of calcium products may be needed in certain areas where the soil is seriously deficient in this mineral.

When Cattle are Stiff-Moving

We once visited a farm where a two-year-old heifer was exceptionally stiff and slow in her movements. She had been brought off pasture and stanchioned a few days earlier, and appeared normal at that time. Since she showed no signs of actual sickness, we decided that the stiffness was due to the sudden change from pasture to a cement floor. This turned out to be true, for the heifer made a complete recovery shortly after she was again turned out. Similar cases often occur in older animals when they are brought inside for the winter. However, there are also other causes of stiffness in cattle.

The condition frequently resembles rheumatism in people, and seems to be brought on by lying in drafts or on cold, poorly-bedded floors. Joints may become infected by germs carried to them from other parts of the body when animals are affected with troubles like metritis, liver abscesses, mastitis, foot rot, and navel-ill to result in a painful condition known as polyarthritis. The joints may also be affected by the degenerative changes accompanying old age, and the same is true of joints when animals are affected with rickets, osteomalacia, and osteoporosis. Poor conformation may cause stiffness through poor weight distribution due to things like abnormally straight legs, excessively sloped pasterns, elongated toes, and wing shoulders. Joints or bones or nerves may be bruised, or a siege of sickness like shipping fever may be followed by infection of various muscles. Hardware trouble often causes cattle to move cautiously, and neglected hoofs may make animals footsore or throw them back on their heels to cause soreness in the tendons running down the back of the legs. It often happens that the exact cause of stiffness cannot be determined.

Symptoms vary considerably, of course, and range all the way from stiff movements to some degree of actual paralysis. Many animals walk with a peculiar, "string-halted" gait. Instead of taking a normal forward step with a hind foot, the foot is raised and half-drawn backward for a second or two. After a bit of trembling, the hind leg is finally jerked forward into proper position under the body. Either one or both of the hind legs may be affected, but this condition usually persists for only a few minutes at any one time. After that, the animal walks more or less normally until another attack occurs, usually when it gets up after having laid down for a while. Many of these stiff animals develop the habit of standing back in the gutter, probably because this position takes normal strain off certain joints and muscles. Mildly affected animals may simply show difficulty in backing up or moving the hind quarters sidewise in a stall. Bulls may be unable to breed cows, with the hind legs appearing too weak for supporting the body during service.

Treatment is naturally dependent on the primary cause, and a good foot-trimming job is often all that is needed. At other times, turning to pasture or into a soft-floored box stall will prove helpful. Hardware trouble may require surgery, and stiffness due to nutritional deficiencies may be remedied by better feeding. Following its successful use in cases of human arthritis, cortisone has been tried experimentally in a few cases, but it is hard to determine whether or not any permanent improvement can be expected. At any rate, the expense of such treatment is likely to make it impractical for the average owner. When the condition can be definitely traced back to certain blood lines, it will be best to try and eliminate them from future breeding programs.

Cases originating as injuries or joint infections often prove discouraging as far as treatment is concerned, although various sulfas and antibiotics are sometimes used with good results. However, many of these cases are completely hopeless because the stiffness is only an indication of wide-spread internal infection that has seriously damaged important organs like the heart, lungs, and liver.

Snake Bite Poisoning

CAUSE. Venom injected by various kinds of poisonous snakes. The rattlesnake, the cottonmouth moccasin, the copperhead, and the coral snake are the kinds found in the United States. The first three are classed as pit vipers and inject their venom through hollow fangs. The coral snake does not have a comparable fang system, and injects its venom while chewing. The coral snake belongs to the cobra family, and is the most poisonous of North American snakes, but its danger is decreased because it has a small mouth that does not allow it a very good hold on most parts of an animal's body. The venom of the Eastern or Florida diamondback rattlesnake is much more poisonous than that of the moccasin or the copperhead.

Although the chemical structure of snake venoms has not been established, their effects have been attributed to protein-destroying enzymes and paralyzing factors effecting the nervous system. The seriousness of any snake bite depends on the kind and size of the snake, the amount of venom injected, the toxicity of the venom, the size of the victim, and the location of the bite. Bites around the head, neck, and throat are the most serious for cattle. Since calves are notoriously curious, they are likely to become interested in a moving or rattling snake when they find one. Unfortunately, many of them are bitten while investigating, and almost always in the nose or upper part of the throat.

SYMPTOMS. Usually first shown by a swelling at the site of the bite. When cattle are bitten around the head, face, or throat, this swelling may cause difficulty in breathing. Suckling calves that have been bitten in the nose or throat may be unable to nurse because of a tongue that is swollen so badly that it protrudes from the mouth. Animals that have been bitten in a leg may be lame. Weakness, evidence of blindness, and partial paralysis may be noted, especially when a small animal is bitten by a large snake. Regardless of the location of the bite, sloughing of the tissues around it is likely to result in a few days.

DIAGNOSIS. Usually on the basis of swelling and the demonstration of fang marks. This last may be difficult unless the hair is shaved away, although oozing of blood from the skin punctures sometimes occurs to indicate the nature of trouble. This condition may be confused with swelling of the throat area due to wooden tongue, infection of the salivary glands, or occlusion of the parotid duct.

TREATMENT. Begins with locating the fang marks and clipping away hair in the area. If the bite is on a leg, a tourniquet should be placed on the leg above the bite and drawn tight to stop the circulation of blood. If antivenin is to be used within an hour, the tourniquet may be left on continuously, and discarded only after the antivenin has been injected. Otherwise, the tourniquet should be released for a minute or two every twenty minutes.

The fang wounds should be opened by deep cross incisions, and poisoned blood expelled by either sucking or squeezing the area. When available, the vacuum hose of a milking machine can be used as a suction cup for drawing out the blood. The wound may then be treated by washing it out with a potassium permanganate solution or hydrogen peroxide. As an alternative, silver nitrate can be applied. Ice packs are recommended for application to a large area around the wound, and these should be continued until definite improvement is noted. The ice packs deaden pain, and practically stop the enzyme action that causes sloughing of tissue around the bite. The early injection of antivenin is probably the most effective treatment known, but this product may not always be available. Antibiotics should be injected to control secondary infections, and the use of antihistamines is indicated when extensive protein-breakdown has occurred. Blood transfusions and intravenous injection of glucose or saline solutions may also prove helpful. The trachea may need to be opened from the outside to provide an inlet for air in case severe swelling of the throat threatens to cause suffocation of an animal. Suckling calves with badly swollen tongues may have to be fed through a stomach tube or with a spoon until the time when they are again able to nurse. Incision wounds should be kept open and draining until improvement occurs.

Stifle Injuries

CAUSE.

1. Bruising is probably the commonest one, with many of these injuries occurring when animals are fighting. Bruising can also occur when animals jump. over such things as wooden

gates or feed bunks and bump the front part of the hind legs during the last part of the leap.

2. Straining of joint ligaments can be followed by inflammation, with a great many of these injuries occurring when animals slip on ice or step unexpectedly into holes in the ground.

3. Wounds of various kinds that pierce the joint capsule may be followed by infection so the joint becomes inflamed. These wounds are usually combined with bruising of the joint and some degree of ligament straining.

4. Rickets in young animals or osteomalacia and osteoporosis in older cattle may cause the joint to be permanently injured.

5. Infection from some other part of the body may have been carried to the stifle by the circulating blood. In such cases trouble may have originally started as a liver abscess, hardware trouble, mastitis, or metritis. An occasional case is traced back to Bang's germs that have settled in the joint.

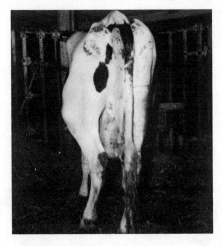

Stifle injury, a common cause of lameness.

SYMPTOMS. The area of the stifle joint is swollen, and there is evidence of severe lameness in the affected leg. When infection is involved, the animal may go off feed and run a fairly high fever. Little weight is placed on the foot, and the animal will often stand in a characteristic position with the fetlock half-doubled and the toes barely touching the ground to serve as a balance.

DIAGNOSIS. Usually on the basis of lameness and swelling of the stifle joint. Lameness alone might cause it to be confused with troubles like foot rot, calving paralysis, broken bones, and foreign bodies in the foot.

TREATMENT. Usually not very satisfactory when infection is involved, largely because the ordinarily smooth joint surfaces have been roughened and permanently damaged. Accordingly, animals are usually best sold for beef as soon as possible when this cause is to blame for trouble. In some cases it may be advisable to have a veterinarian drain the joint capsule, or to inject it with antibiotics. When injuries are due to bruising or straining of ligaments, the chances of recovery are fairly good. Hot packs or heat lamp treatments for several hours daily may help, and the same thing is true of frequent vigorous massaging with something like white liniment.

PREVENTION. Little that can be recommended, although proper feeding and the availability of minerals will reduce troubles due to rickets and osteomalacia. Management measures designed to prevent troubles like Bang's disease, mastitis, and metritis will help. help.

Sprains

CAUSE. Anything that will cause momentary separation of adjoining surfaces in a joint, with resultant injury to the joint capsule and ligaments of the joint. Accidents like slipping on ice, stepping in holes in the ground, sliding off rocks or gutter edges, and twisting when feet become caught are all likely to be causes at various times.

SYMPTOMS. The most outstanding is severe lameness and evidence of pain when the joint is moved or pressed. Although eventually present, swelling may not appear for some time after the injury.

DIAGNOSIS. Through an examination that eliminates the possibility of broken bones, bruises, foot rot, and other causes of lameness.

TREATMENT. Dependent on the amount of injury to the joint and related structures. In mild cases, rest, hot packs, heat lamp treatments, and massage with white liniment will prove helpful through promoting circulation of blood in the area. A supportive bandage is sometimes recommended for joints of the pastern region. There is little to be done in cases where joints are badly damaged, for a chronic arthritis is likely to develop, or the joints may grow together to make them permanently stiff. Antibiotics may be used in cases where the development of secondary infection is feared.

Laminitis, "Founder," "Stiff-Cow Disease"

CAUSE. Usually over-eating, but may also be caused by continued standing on a concrete floor, insufficient bedding, eating of spoiled feeds, excessive drinking of cold water, or by walking for long distances over rough or stony ground. In some sections of the country another type of laminitis is found which is not due to any of these listed causes. Although not definitely known, the cause of this type is believed to be some kind of a rust or mold on forage. Regardless of cause, trouble is directly due to substances formed in the animal's body which cause damage to the sensitive laminae of the hoofs. This structure is comparable to the so-called "quick" which underlies human toenails and fingernails.

SYMPTOMS.   The principal one is lameness, and the feet of animals may become so sore that they will crawl on their knees or spend most of their time lying down. Other symptoms are extreme stiffness, swelling of the fetlock region, and deformed, elongated, wrinkled, or misshapen hoofs after animals recover.

DIAGNOSIS.   Made through a careful examination of affected animals, consideration of feeding history, recent management, and the elimination of other possible causes of symptoms. Under farm conditions the sudden appearance of several cases might cause founder to be confused with other troubles like foot rot, fescue foot, foot and mouth disease, selenium poisoning, ergot poisoning, vesicular stomatitis, and mycotic stomatitis.

TREATMENT. Cases due to over-eating or the eating of spoiled feeds should first be treated with laxatives to empty out the digestive tract. Injections of antihistamines will generally help, especially in the early stages, and so will soaking the feet in cold water to relieve the congestion of blood. Animals can be stood in mud or water, or the feet can be bandaged and soaked with water every few minutes. Animals that have been standing on concrete floors or are suffering from bruised feet following travel are best moved out doors on sod. As an alternative they can be placed in a box stall that is floored with dirt or carpeted with several inches of silage or rotted straw. When the soreness and swelling have subsided, repeated trimming of the hoofs will help restore something like their normal shape as new growth is made.

When Cattle Die Suddenly

We recently visited a farm where a cow had died unexpectedly in the pasture. She had been all right the night before and the owner was sure she had been poisoned by something. However, an investigation revealed that death was due to a wire which had pierced the stomach much earlier. An abscess had developed around the wire, and the sudden death of the cow resulted when it ruptured and released a gallon or so of pus into the lungs.

A similar incident involved a dairy cow that was found dead in a pasture during the summer. Although she was at least 40 yards away from the nearest fence and the only tree was located at the far end of the pasture, it was finally decided that she had been struck by lightning.

Another case concerned three dairy cows that died quietly in their stanchions during a winter night. The animals stood side by side and the cause of their death appeared to be quite a mystery at first. It was solved when a checkup by an electrician showed a short circuit in the milking machine wiring. A leaking drinking cup had soaked the floor around them so the cows were electrocuted.

On another occasion a six-months-old calf was found dead in its pen one morning. A post mortem examination showed the abdominal cavity to be full of blood from a ruptured liver. The owner believed the injury had occurred when the hired man kicked the calf in the right flank the night before. Jamming in doorways, kicks by horses, collisions with cars, and other accidents can result in similar deaths from internal injuries.

Various kinds of contagious diseases can be responsible for the sudden death of cattle, too. One case involved two steers that were found dead in a feed lot as the first hint that anthrax was breaking loose on the farm. Another concerned a yearling heifer that died before we reached her and was being butchered out by the owner when we arrived. He reasoned that she would be all right to eat because of her sudden death, but changed his mind when we told him that the animal had blackleg. On another occasion a valuable pure-bred cow was bought at a sale and then trucked without a stop for several hundred miles. She was found dead the third morning after reaching her new home, and represented the beginning of a costly shipping fever outbreak. In recent years salmonellosis has been recognized as a possible cause of sudden death in young calves.

Although they aren't involved nearly so often as suspected, poisons are also a cause of sudden death. They can be divided into three classes: plant, chemical, or bacterial. The plants are represented by those containing prussic acid and various others that contain specific poisons, but spoiled sweet clover hay is also capable of causing sudden death. A typical case concerns a cow that calved normally one night and was found dead the next morning because of bleeding that didn't stop. Similar fatal bleeding may follow insignificant cuts and bruises when spoiled sweet clover is involved.

The chemical poisons include rat poisons, spray materials, and paint containing lead. Plain carelessness is usually to blame when they kill cattle. An illustration is furnished by the case of the owner who cleaned out his granary at threshing time and swept up a broken bag of nitrate fertilizer with spilled grain. The sweepings were then put out in a feed trough, and killed the two "boss" cows that drove off the others so they got all of the poisoned feed.

The bacterial poisons are represented by cases of botulism and enterotoxemia. Internal bleeding may be the unsuspected cause of sudden death, especially when there are no visible signs of blood. Such cases often occur at uneventful calvings when one of the uterine arteries is ruptured, but they may occur at any time when a major blood vessel has been weakened by something like an abscess or penetration by an internal parasite. After such weakening of the wall structure something like a bubble may form at the point of penetration. This continues to grow in size, with the wall growing thinner and thinner. Eventually the bubble bursts like a balloon, and the animal bleeds to death.

There are various other possible causes of sudden death that we haven't mentioned, but we hope that we've said enough so that owners won't be too sure of the exact cause when cattle die suddenly. A post mortem examination is usually needed to show the exact cause, and it may be something altogether different from what it was thought to be.

Brisket Disease (High Mountain Disease)

CAUSE. Basically a lack of oxygen in rarefied air which is made even more serious by excessive exercise which animals may be forced into while trying to get enough to eat at high altitudes. Regardless of the exact mechanics involved, emphysema of the lungs results in more resistance to the circulation of blood through them, and this in turn leads to overwork of the right side of the heart. Dilation of the right ventricle causes improper fitting of the valve between it and the right atrium so that something like leakage of the heart occurs.

The time required for development of the disease seems to depend on the altitude. One survey showed that about six months were required for this trouble to develop at 10,000 feet, while only about nine weeks were required at 12,500 feet. If factors like nutritional deficiencies, disturbances of metabolism, and various kinds of infections seem to be involved, it is likely that they are secondary causes. It is estimated that this trouble affects up to 3%

of all cattle in pastures 7,000 feet or more above sea level.

SYMPTOMS. Listlessness and a gradual loss of condition are usually noticed first. As time goes on the brisket region becomes enlarged, and a painless doughy mass finally extends up along the lower side of the neck to the jaws. The jugular veins become distended, often showing a pulse beat, and the abdomen may be enlarged with accumulated fluid. Edema of the stomach and intestines may interfere with fluid absorption so that animals develop a dark-colored diarrhea. Affected cattle tire easily, often cough, and pant for breath after the slightest exertion. Temperature and appetite usually remain normal, but the lining of the mouth and nostrils may appear somewhat blue in color. Opening a dead animal is apt to show a heart which is greatly dilated on the right side, and general edema of practically all tissues. The lungs are pale, emphysematous, and extremely light in weight. Large amounts of fluid may be present in the abdominal and thoracic body cavities, and will drip from cuts made in the tissues of the neck and brisket. The liver is enlarged and its veins are dilated. The course varies from one to twelve weeks, but animals usually die within a short time after advanced symptoms are shown. The condition affects both sexes and all age groups, but is seen oftenest in calves under a year old. From 5-10% of a herd may be affected, and most of the affected animals can be expected to die.

DIAGNOSIS. On the basis of typical symptoms appearing in animals that have been pastured at altitudes of over 6,000 feet. The ailment might be confused with hardware trouble, heart anomalies, tumors in the thoracic cavity, and infestation with internal parasites.

TREATMENT. The most practical procedure calls for moving affected animals to lower pastures, and this alone will effect recovery in about half the cases. They should be left alone as much as possible, and furnished with plenty of feed which is available with a minimum of effort. Animals that do not respond satisfactorily should be given antibiotics to counteract infections, particularly those that may attack the lungs. Colorado workers were able to help animals with oxygen, and some cases have been reported as helped by the use of digitalis. The drugs described for the treatment of udder edema in this book may help brisket disease by accelerating the removal of body fluids by increased kidney activity. Advanced cases may require surgery to drain accumulations of fluid from body cavities.

PREVENTION. Supplying food and water at convenient locations and in a restricted area to reduce the effort required to get them in high altitudes. Respiratory troubles should be treated promptly to eliminate danger of overworking the heart while it is trying to compensate for faulty lung action. Animals that recover from an attack should not be returned to high pastures because of the danger of recurrence of the disease.

Leukosis (Leukemia, Lymphomatosis)

CAUSE. Unknown. The disease has been transmitted with both cellular and cell-free material, and also bacteria-free material from affected cattle, so a virus is suspected. Virus-like particles have been found in cellular material from leukotic cattle. However, it is not definitely known if these were viral particles, or if they had anything at all to do with leukosis. Present information indicates that leukosis in cattle is similar to leukosis in poultry. Hereditary and environmental factors have been proposed as predisposing influences, but they have not been proven.

The most plausible theory has it that a causative agent is introduced into a susceptible animal, probably shortly before or after birth. This agent stimulates certain specialized body cells to produce a change in the blood cell composition and structure which may continue for years without producing any apparent symptoms of ill health. At the other extreme, the condition may gradually get worse until death finally results.

The disease is currently recognized as existing in three forms.

1. Chronic enzootic leukosis. The form was first reported in 1878, and it is the commonest form of the disease.

2. Juvenile leukosis. This form affects only calves and animals under two years of age. This is an uncommon type, with the incidence being estimated at about one case per 100,000 head of cattle every year. Since it has shown no tendency for transmission, it is not necessary to include it in an eradication and control plan.

3. Skin leukosis. The changes characteristic of this form occur in the skin. It has not been reported in calves, and most animals which become affected are two or three years old. However, older animals may also be affected. It is even rarer than the juvenile form, and has been estimated to occur at the rate of about 0.2 cases per 100,000 head of cattle per year.

MEANS OF SPREAD. Chiefly through the sale and movement of breeding animals. Enzootic leukosis has a tendency to become established in large herds and persist for years, sometimes causing the death of 2 to 5% of the older animals every year. These act as foci of the disease, and are known as "leukosis herds." Four to six years may pass after introduction of the disease into a herd before evidence of tumorous cases appears.

In addition, transmission of the disease seems linked in some way to the use of piroplasmosis vaccine. This is particularly true in Sweden, where a distinct relationship is shown between leukosis areas and those where piroplasmosis vaccine has been used.

SYMPTOMS. Since the other two forms are so rare, only the symptoms of enzootic leukosis will be considered here.

Enlargement of various lymph glands occurs under the jaws, in the flanks, and in front of the shoulders, with the animal otherwise appearing normal in the early stages. As time goes on the appetite is affected, weight is lost, dullness increases, and breathing becomes difficult. Lymph glands that are ordinarily too small to be noticed become visible in various parts of the body, with the eyes sometimes being caused to bulge from their sockets by growths behind them. Pressure by similar growths in other parts of the body cause such seemingly unrelated symptoms as bloat, constipation, delirium and paralysis. Anemia is always present and causes paleness of all the mucous membranes. Eventually the animal is covered with all kinds of various-sized enlargements that show the location of superficial lymph glands, and death results. Opening a dead animal may show tumors throughout the body or a few that are confined to a pretty small area.

Chronically affected animals may not show enlargement of the visible and palpable lymph nodes. In such cases tumor formation occurs very late, and only signs like weakness, lack of appetite, and loss of weight may be noticed. The general condition of many animals will remain unchanged even when they are carrying numerous tumors. Most cases showing tumor formation involve cows between four and eight years old.

DIAGNOSIS. Usually on the basis of typical symptoms involving most of the lymph glands. An examination of the blood may help through disclosing anemia and large numbers of immature white cells.

Rectal examination may prove helpful in making a diagnosis. This is because various of the internal lymph nodes and adjoining body organs can sometimes be detected as being abnormal before the superficial lymph nodes become noticeably enlarged. Tumors can be sectioned and examined microscopically in the laboratory for confirming a diagnosis of leukosis.

TREATMENT. None recognized at this time. Therefore, the control of leukosis is entirely dependent on preventive measures.

PREVENTION. Best illustrated by a program operating in Denmark. The first and most important part consists of locating the sources of infection or so-called "leukosis herds." When found, these are placed under public supervision.

The second part consists of requiring veterinarians to report all suspected cases of leukosis, regardless of whether they are found in private practice, in packing houses, or rendering plants. If an investigation verifies the diagnosis of leukosis, blood examinations are made on animals in the herd of origin. If other animals shown to be infected, the herd is placed under public supervision. If the blood examination does not reveal other infected animals, it is regarded as an observation herd, and blood examinations are made one, two, and three years later.

When a leukosis herd is placed under public supervision, the following restrictions go into effect:

1. No animals can be sold from the herd except for slaughter.
2. No contact of animals is allowed with other herds.
3. No spread of contagious material is allowed.

Present knowledge indicates that the most practical way of eradicating leukosis in a herd consists of slaughtering all animals and replacing them with animals from leukosis-free areas. The eradication of leukosis has been attempted on an experimental basis by slaughtering only animals which showed leukemic blood changes at the time of regular examinations. However, this procedure is both complicated and expensive, and has the disadvantage of the risk that such a procedure will not eliminate the disease.

Sweet Clover Disease (Poisoning)

CAUSE. The feeding of damaged sweet clover hay or silage which happens to contain dicoumarin, a compound which prevents normal clotting of blood. The growing plants are not dangerous, and only feeding will show when the spoiled hay or silage is capable of causing trouble. The disease may appear when the sweet clover is fed alone or in combination with other feeds. Non-bitter sweet clover (Melilotus dentata) does not become poisonous with spoilage.

SYMPTOMS. Small wounds caused by castration or dehorning may cause animals to bleed to death, and cows may die of loss of blood following calving. When wounds aren't present to allow the escape of blood, large swellings may occur in various parts of the body where blood has collected under the skin following bruising. These swellings don't pit on pressure, and there is no crackling to indicate the presence of gas. Animals may appear depressed and reluctant to move, although there are no early symptoms of general illness as shown by abnormal pulse, temperature, or respiration. However, the heart rate is likely to be increased as greater amounts of blood are lost. The mucous membranes become progressively paler and weakness finally causes affected animals to go down. Loss of blood may cause abortions, particularly during the latter stages of pregnancy. Opening a dead animal reveals evidence of excessive bleeding, with no other known disease causing such an accumulation of unclotted blood. Animals of all ages are susceptible, and one attack doesn't give future immunity to the disease. Most untreated animals eventually die after a few days time, with cows sometimes calving at night and being found dead the next morning.

DIAGNOSIS. Usually on the basis of typical symptoms in connection with a history of feeding on spoiled sweet clover. May be confused with anthrax, lightning stroke, blackleg, or malignant edema at various times.

TREATMENT. Vitamin K has proved to be effective if given in large doses, but prompt recovery usually follows the intravenous transfusion of a pint or quart of blood that has been taken from a normal animal and defibrinated. This is true even when animals have gone down and are practically dead. Blood is defibrinated by shaking or stirring it for a few minutes and then straining it through gauze or cheesecloth. An alternative consists of mixing 50 cc. of 2.5% sodium citrate with every pint of whole blood to keep it from clotting. It can then be strained and used instead of defibrinated blood. The disease is not transmitted by the blood of sick animals getting into the systems of normal animals. Blood transfusion represents emergency treatment, but the removal of dangerous feed is necessary as an accompanying measure. Animals must be carefully watched even then, for new cases may develop a week or more after the feed has been changed. This is probably because damaged body tissues require a few days for making necessary repairs. Changing the feed alone will not be enough to save animals that are already bleeding to death, since experience has shown that about three fourths of them will die unless they are given blood transfusions.

PREVENTION. A matter of checking all spoiled sweet clover before it is fed to animals for very long periods. It may be given to rabbits or a less valuable animal for a couple of months and a few tests made then to see if the blood is still capable of clotting in a normal manner. If it is, the sweet clover is probably safe to feed.

Cut Tendons

Tendons of the leg are sometimes cut when cattle meet with various kinds of accidents, with the tendons running down the backs of the hind legs being most frequently involved. The accompanying photo shows a tendon that was cut when the cow kicked into the edge of a shovel while the gutter was being cleaned behind her. In such cases the entire pastern region is then allowed to drop so it touches the ground and causes difficulty in walking. There is no practical treatment, and injured cattle are likely to be left permanently deformed

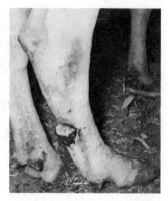

Cut tendon in hind leg from kicking edge of shovel at barn cleaning time.

Fescue Foot (Fescue Poisoning)

CAUSE. A toxic substance resembling ergot which is present in fescue grass. This trouble was first reported from New Zealand in 1949, and from Colorado during the 1951–1952 winter. In 1952 it was reported from Kentucky, and from other states since that time.

The New Zealand cases involved tall fescue grass, and those in Colorado were caused by Festuca arunincea, also known as reed, giant, king, or ditch bank fescue. Trouble in Kentucky and Virginia has been reported as due to Kentucky fescue 31. Fescue grass is usually found in wet, poorly drained areas, and is not likely to be eaten by cattle when other feeds are available.

SYMPTOMS. The poisonous factor usually affects only the hind feet, although sloughing of the tail end has been reported. Lameness and stiffness are the first signs, developing within two or three weeks after cattle have eaten 150–300 pounds of the grass. Animals lose weight rapidly, the lameness grows worse, and the affected feet grow cold with rotting away of the flesh. In some cases entire feet have been sloughed off just above the tops of the hoofs.

DIAGNOSIS. On the basis of typical symptoms appearing in cattle that have had access to fescue grass. The condition might be confused with ergot poisoning.

TREATMENT. None can be recommended, although it has been reported that mildly affected animals may recover if the causative grass is removed from the ration.

PREVENTION. Entirely a matter of either eradicating the fescue from pastures or feeding cattle well so they will not be likely to eat the grass.

Ear Ticks

CAUSE. The spinose ear tick (*Otobius megnini, Ornithodorus megnini*), the only soft tick of importance occurring in the United States. Once largely limited to our southwestern states, they now can be found almost anywhere, largely because of the movement of infested animals to feed lots. The parasites invade the ears to cause inflammation and irritation following their blood-sucking activities. Secondary infection by bacteria often causes pus formation and discharging from ears. They prefer cattle, but will attack other animals, including horses and dogs, and people.

LIFE CYCLE. The ticks lay eggs under stones and in protected places around buildings, fences, and feed lots. Larvae (seed ticks) begin hatching from the eggs in about ten days, and may live without food for several months. When an opportunity presents itself, they crawl into the ears of animals and fill up on blood a couple of times before they leave the ears as so-called nymphs. The nymphs hunt out dry protected places like cracks and crevices in buildings and fences, and in a few days they shed their skins and become adults. Soon after mating the females begin laying eggs to start the cycle all over again. When egg-laying is completed, the females die, although unmated females may live for as long as a year.

SYMPTOMS. Animals appear dull, lose weight and go off feed. Continued growth by the ticks may eventually completely block the ear canal. Animals may then shake their heads or hold the head low and tipped sidewise as described under sinusitis after dehorning. The irritation and itching may become so bad that injuries result from scratching and rubbing, and these wounds may then become flyblown. Accumulations of pus and tick discharges may cause pressure that results in all kinds of crazy actions and even death. A waxy or oily discharge is often seen from infested ears.

DIAGNOSIS. Made by first cleaning the ear of foreign material and then bringing out some the ticks. A cotton-tipped applicator stick dipped in something like olive oil or mastitis ointment can be used for this purpose.

TREATMENT. The USDA recommends a mixture of 0.75% lindane in xylene-pine oil. About a half-ounce is injected deep into
each ear with an oil can. The lower ears are thoroughly massaged
immediately after injection to help penetration. Good results have
been reported following use of EQ 3-35, originally developed for
use against screw-worms, and containing 3 parts of lindane and
35 parts of pine oil in a mineral oil, silica gel base. Practically any
preparation with the approved amount of lindane will kill the ticks.
Beef cattle may have the inner ear canal and adjoining head areas
dusted with 5% coumaphos or sprayed with a 0.5% malathion
solution or a 2.5% solution of ronnel. Treatment may be repeated
as required.

PREVENTION. Since eggs are laid around buildings and corrals,
preventive measures are largely concerned with surroundings. Infected premises may be left unused for two years in order to starve
the ticks to death. An alternative method consists of disinfecting
the premises and applying pine tar to poles, boards, and feed racks
found on them. Involved premises can also be sprayed with a
half-and-half mixture of used crank case oil and kerosene, which
is both effective and cheap.

Foreign Objects in the Eye

Cattle frequently get foreign objects like oat hulls in their eyes.
Filming, severe watering, and swelling may cause the trouble to
be confused with cancer, pinkeye, or injuries to the eyeball. In
cases of long standing the foreign body may be almost completely
imbedded, while secondary infection may set in to make the condition even worse.

Treatment begins with removal of the object. This can sometimes be done by using vaseline or penicillin ointment such as is
used for mastitis treatment. A fair amount is introduced into the
eye after the lids have been turned back, and the organ is then
gently massaged for a few minutes. This often serves to loosen the
material from the eyeball and coat it with oil so it can be easily
wiped out with a soft cloth or piece of cotton. Imbedded materials
may call for surgery and the anesthetization of the eye so movements are prevented while work is being done.

Cancer Eye (Ocular Epithelioma)

This condition is pretty much limited to Herefords, and generally involves the lower lid or false eyelid at the inner corner of

the eye. It is a true cancer and will eventually grow until it destroys the entire eye and even spreads to the brain and other parts of the body. The growth is best removed surgically in the early stages, with the animal being disposed of later as soon as practical. This is because it is likely to recur as in the case of other types of cancer. Old and neglected cases may require removal of the entire eyeball before the animal can be fattened satisfactorily. Symptoms are much like those of pinkeye or a foreign object, but a careful examination will reveal the typical angry-red growth on the eyelid.

The dye described under Pinkeye has also been used for painting around the eyes of breeding animals to decrease the glare of sun rays in the hope of preventing this trouble to some extent.

Corns (Interdigital Fibroma)

This condition may have several possible causes, including foot rot, interdigital dermatitis, or practically any other infection or irritant of the space between the claws. Predisposing factors include overconditioning that causes pouching of the cushion in the front part of the space between the claws, graveled yards, neglected trimming of the hoofs, and inherited poor foot conformation. Regardless of the exact cause, growths develop between the hoofs and produce varying degrees of lameness, depending largely on the size of the growths and whether or not they come in contact with the ground. The most practical treatment consists of surgical removal. When the growths are small, an alternative procedure calls for using copper sulfate under a bandage as described in this book for the treatment of foot rot. In addition to being painful, these growths may also pave the way for attacks of foot rot, especially during wet periods in the fall and spring. Older bulls seem particularly susceptible to this trouble.

When Cattle are Lame

There are at least 17 possible causes of lameness in cattle.

1. Some kind of foreign body may have become wedged between the toes.
2. Deep cuts or punctures may have been made, and the cause of injury may or may not have remained in the foot.
3. The soft bulbs at the heel of the hoof may have been painfully bruised.
4. Infection with *Actinomyces necrophorus* may have caused foot rot.

5. Fescue foot may be to blame in some sections of the country.

6. Various types of rusts and molds found on growing legumes like clover and alfalfa are also capable of causing lameness and sloughing of flesh from the feet of cattle.

7. There's always the chance that lameness may indicate the early stages of some older contagious disease like blackleg or anthrax or malignant edema, while lockjaw can also be expected to cause difficulty in walking. While on the subject of contagious diseases, it is well to remember that lameness could also be the first sign of a foot and mouth outbreak on a farm.

8. Similarly, a combination of lameness and slobbering by cattle might indicate the presence of vesicular stomatitis.

9. The same thing holds true in regard to diseases belonging to the mucosal disease complex.

10. Then there's always the possibility that a toe has been broken by a sudden twist on a stone or frozen ground or edge of a gutter.

11. If a toe isn't broken, such twists may cause the spraining of various tendons in the fetlock region or other parts of the legs. A cow that is "riding" others may injure ligaments of the shoulder when dismounting, or sudden slips and stretches may injure nerves to result in various forms of paralysis.

12. Lameness that appears shortly after calving may be due to injury of the obturator nerves.

13. Bones are sometimes injured by falls or kicks or blows or thrown objects. Although usually resulting in broken bones or painful bruises, such injuries may be followed by abscesses or blood clots which press on important nerves.

14. The feet may have been neglected so that hoof edges turn in like ingrown toenails on a person. Again, the hoofs may have grown so long that animals are compelled to walk back on their heels in an abnormal manner to place severe strain on muscles and tendons of the legs.

15. Selenium poisoning will cause severe lameness, and appears in many parts of the Western United States.

16. Poor feeding and mineral deficiencies may be to blame for soft bones, joint deformities, contracted tendons, and lameness, especially in young animals that are susceptible to rickets.

17. Corns may have developed between the toes of one or more feet.

Treatment of any one particular case is naturally dependent on the primary cause, and you may or may not be able to supply a remedy. You can start out by making a careful examination of the affected foot. If it isn't cut or overgrown, and if there's nothing lodged in it, you may be able to figure out which of the other possibilities is causing lameness. If you can't make a diagnosis, you'll probably do well to get a veterinarian. A lot of lame animals get worse instead of better with the passage of time, so you'd better not wait too long before getting help, either.

Interdigital Dermatitis (Bovine Thrush, Stable Foot Rot)

CAUSE. Not definitely known, but the germ *Spherophorus necrophorus* can usually be isolated from infected feet. This is the same germ that is considered the cause of foot rot, but the two diseases are not the same. In the case of interdigital dermatitis, *S. necrophorus* is usually considered as a secondary invader. This is because fungi are also recovered from most of the infected feet, and the appearance of lesions suggests that they are more likely to be the cause of trouble than any kind of germs. Moisture and filthy stabling conditions are predisposing factors.

SYMPTOMS. Lameness of some degree is usually the first one noticed. Lesions are likely to start on the skin between the claws at the back part of the foot near the bulbs of the heels. These appear as moist, raw sores with an offensive odor. As time goes on the lesions spread to the skin in the pastern area. The top of the hoof at the heel becomes undermined, and raw areas form at the bulbs of the heels. Eventually the horny wall of the hoof may be undermined.

DIAGNOSIS. Likely to be confused with foot rot, but the two diseases can usually be told apart because in interdigital dermatitis:

1. Lesions remain localized in the back part of the hoof.
2. The severe swelling associated with foot rot does not occur.
3. Channels for drainage do not develop in the deeper tissues of the foot as they do in foot rot.
4. Interdigital fibromas (corns) often accompany interdigital dermatitis, which is unlikely in foot rot.

TREATMENT. Local treatment is recommended because intravenous and intramuscular administration of drugs used for foot rot is of little value. The first step consists of thoroughly cleaning the lesions and paring away all undermined horny tissues of the hoof. Astringent and antiseptic packs should then be applied, but should be changed every 48 hours because it is important that the lesions be kept clean and reasonably dry. Drugs that are commonly used for packs include formalin, sulfa powders, copper sulfate, alum, and various tinctures. Many parings and dressings are likely to be required, for healing may take several weeks. An important part of treatment is represented by the provision of clean dry quarters.

PREVENTION. Almost entirely a matter of management to provide sanitary surroundings. When trouble has been occurring on a herd scale, feeding and watering areas should be surveyed to make sure that they are kept clean and well-drained. When lots are in particularly bad shape it will often pay to have them paved in order to get away from mud and filth. The construction of copper sulfate foot baths or hydrated lime boxes as described for the treatment of foot rot may also prove helpful in preventing interdigital dermatitis.

Sarcocystosis (Sarcosporidiosis)

CAUSE. Parasites of the protozoan genus *Sarcocystis*. More than 50 species have been named, but some of them may be identical, for the same one may look different in different animals. The one affecting cattle is generally known as *Sarcocystis fusiformis*. Typical lesions are due to cysts of the parasites which are formed in muscles. These cysts are cylindrical or spindle-shaped, run lengthwise in the muscles, and are easily seen with the naked eye in some cases.

Sarcocystosis is very common in cattle throughout the world. A recent survey showed it in 75 per cent of 48 Illinois cattle, 90 per cent of 60 cattle from a Baltimore slaughterhouse, and in about 0.33 per cent of cattle slaughtered in California. Microscopic examination will show the parasitic cysts in a great many cattle whose muscles appear completely normal under routine examination.

MEANS OF SPREAD. Through swallowing an early stage of the developing protozoan that is known as a trophozoite. This can be either in an unbroken cyst in muscle tissue or free in the droppings of infested animals. After being swallowed, the trophozoites are believed to pass through the intestinal wall into the bloodstream which carries them to the muscles where they enter the cells. About a month later, a one-celled parasite can be found in the invaded cell. This divides repeatedly, forming a many-celled cyst that contains many trophozoites, which continue to multiply by division and are then given off in droppings to be eaten by other animals.

SYMPTOMS. Light or moderate infections are not likely to produce any noticeable signs, but heavy ones may cause lameness, loss of weight, weakness, paralysis, and even death. Opening a dead animal may show the typical cysts. If they are large enough to be seen with the naked eye, they appear as yellowish-green spindle-shaped structures about the size of a wheat grain. They are most likely to be found in the heart, cheek, tongue, esophagus, and diaphragm muscles. The main losses occur through the condemnation of carcasses or parts of carcasses on postmorten examination in slaughterhouses.

DIAGNOSIS. Either by actually seeing the characteristic cysts in muscles, or finding them under the microscope in a laboratory.

TREATMENT. None recognized.

PREVENTION. Believed most practical through following good sanitary practices that lessen the chances of animals swallowing the trophozoites. Preventive measures suggested for coccidiosis control will also be effective against sarcocystosis. Since this disease may also affect human beings, the meat from possibly infected cattle should be thoroughly cooked before being eaten.

Sordelli Infection

CAUSE. An organism called *Clostridium sordella.* This is a comparatively new disease which has become increasingly important in recent years. It gives off poisons and forms spores like the other *Clostridia* germs. It is known to exist in Argentina and the western part of the United States. *C. sordella* is considered to be a soil-borne germ that enters the body through skin wounds, and has usually been found with other types of *Clostridia.* It has been found a number of times in feed lots, but is rare when compared with other types of clostridial infections which it resembles.

SYMPTOMS. Much like those of other clostridial diseases like malignant edema, black disease, red water disease, and blackleg. Affected animals may be dull, run fevers, and show a swelling at the site of infection which gives off a bad-smelling odor. Other symptoms range from bloody urine to gas gangrene, and death may occur in 24 to 48 hours after animals are first noticed as being sick. Opening a dead animal will usually show swelling, bleeding, and gas formation in the throat and on the tongue. Such lesions resemble those formed by malignant edema, but are more bloody.

DIAGNOSIS. Definite only in the laboratory through isolation of *C. sordella,* either by culture or fluorescent antibody testing.

TREATMENT. Massive doses of injectable penicillin appear to be the treatment of choice, as in the case of other clostridial infections.

PREVENTION. A mixed bacterin including *C. sordella* is available and seems reasonably effective. Bacterins have been used at feed lots, but as the disease is rare, the value of such use is questionable. There is no doubt that it is dangerous, but it may not be enough of a threat to warrant routine vaccination.

Tumors (Cancers, Neoplasms)

CAUSE. Not definitely known, although there are several theories. The words "tumor" and "neoplasm" mean practically the same thing, but the word "cancer" is usually reserved for malignant growths. The word "neoplasm" literally means "new growth." Two classes of neoplasms are recognized: malignant and nonmalignant (benign). Both are characterized by the abnormal and seemingly purposeless growth of formerly normal body cells.

A benign tumor does not endanger the life of an affected animal unless it happens to exert pressure on an important nerve, blood vessel, or body organ. In contrast, a malignant tumor infiltrates adjoining tissue of all kinds, destroys it, and spreads to other parts of the body to interfere with essential functions and eventually cause death. Several different kinds of both benign and malignant tumors are recognized, usually being classified according to the tissue of origin, as lipoma (fat tumor), osteosarcoma (bone tumor), lymphoma (lymphoid tumor), etc.

SYMPTOMS. Dependent on the type of tumor and its location. Thus a visible swelling of a bone might indicate an osteosarcoma, while a swelling in muscular tissue might indicate a fibroma or hemangioma, and enlargement of one or more lymph nodes might indicate lymphoma. A raw and angry looking ulcer might indicate a carcinoma like cancer of the eye. In all cases a swelling or enlargement or new growth on some part of the body signals the beginning of a tumor. This may be due to something like a bruise, an abscess, a hematoma, a hernia, or an infected wound, but when a swelling occurs in a place where it cannot be explained or when a wound fails to heal normally, it will be wise to suspect a neoplasm. Some of the commoner malignant tumors of cattle are cancer eye, malignant melanoma, carcinoma, and malignant lymphoma. Some of the commoner benign tumors of cattle are fibroma of the penis, lipoma, hemangioma, and osteoma. Tumors that occur inside the body may not be detected until a postmortem examination is made, but they may be suspected when abnormal or bloody body discharges are noted. In my own practice I once discovered a cancer of the uterus in a cow while making a rectal examination for pregnancy.

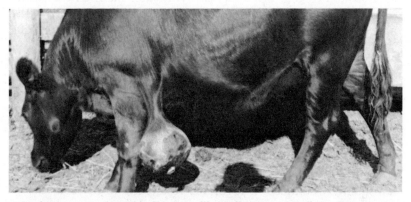

A benign tumor such as this fibroma will usually respond well to surgery.

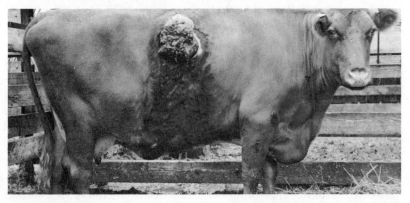

A malignant tumor such as this carcinoma has advanced too far to make the animal a good surgical risk because of the danger of spread afterward.

DIAGNOSIS. Definite only in the laboratory through examination of tissues under the microscope to show the type of cells involved in the tumor. However, a tentative diagnosis can sometimes be made on the basis of appearance, feel, location, rate of growth, and evidence of spread. Tumors might be confused with such things as abscesses, hernias, hematomas, or bruises, but an exploratory puncture with a hypodermic needle to reveal the contents can sometimes be used to identify them.

TREATMENT. Surgery is recognized as the only practical treatment for all kinds of tumors. Benign neoplasms can usually be removed without too much trouble because they tend to remain as distinct structures and to push surrounding tissues aside instead of becoming part of them. They often occur as pedunculated structures that are attached by a small base. There is little danger of recurrence, but if one does recur, there is the possibility that surgery has caused a benign tumor to become malignant.

The malignant tumor has a tendency to infiltrate surrounding tissues so they become part of the tumor and are difficult to remove completely. Because of this fact, the apparent edges of the tumor may not be its true border, and an operation may leave some of the malignant cells. When this happens the remaining cells act as "seeds" and the growth recurs, along with spread to other parts of the body. Accordingly, if a malignant tumor is to be removed, surgery should be done early, and removal should be painstakingly complete if favorable results are to be secured.

Jaundice (Yellows, Icterus)

CAUSE. Several are possible, for this is a symptom, not a specific disease. One cause is liver damage by flukes. A more common one is inflammation of the gallbladder and bile ducts, usually in connection with various kinds of digestive troubles. The condition may also be caused by pressure on bile ducts by tumors or abscesses of the liver. Jaundice from such causes is primarily due to blocking of the bile ducts, and therefore is appropriately called "obstructive" jaundice.

Another form of jaundice is known as "destructive" jaundice because it results from the destruction of red blood cells. It results from either poisoning or infection. Chemical poisonings which may cause jaundice include lead, arsenic, copper, and phosphorus. Plant poisonings which may cause jaundice include species of Crotalaria, loco weed, lupines, rattleweed, and several of the Senecio species like ragwort. Jaundice may also appear in connection with light sensitization resulting from eating damaged forage or certain plants as described under Light Sensitization and Allergic Stomatitis. Infections which may cause destructive jaundice include red water disease, anaplasmosis, leptospirosis, and piroplasmosis.

SYMPTOMS. First noted as a yellowing of the whites of the eyes and the lining of the mouth and nostrils. In female cattle this yellowing can often be seen best in the lining of the vulva. A high degree of yellowing must be reached before it can be noticed in the skin. In such cases the discoloration can usually be seen first in the white skin areas around the eyes and over the udder. Sometimes the jaundice will appear only as a "muddy" coloring instead of a distinct yellow. Other symptoms will depend on the primary cause of the trouble.

DIAGNOSIS. The discoloration is obvious enough for a diagnosis of the condition, so the big problem lies in determining the primary cause. The degree of jaundice can be established in the laboratory through the so-called "icteric index" of blood serum. A simple test (Hay's sulfur test) may be used on urine for the determination of bile salts and may prove helpful.

TREATMENT. Depends on the primary cause. Once this is corrected, the jaundice will disappear.

Pregnancy Disease (Pregnancy Toxemia)

CAUSE. Basically a matter of underfeeding during the last two months of pregnancy. Predisposing factors are the drain of glucose by the developing calf, and the lessening of abdominal space as the calf grows in the uterus. This cuts down on both digestive ability and the rumen capacity for food. It has been reported that every kilogram of calf weight results in a decreased food intake of 100 grams daily of dry matter. Such underfeeding eventually leads to a decrease of blood sugar at the same time that the blood ketone level is rising. A continuation of this condition results in kidney trouble, poor circulation of blood, liver coma, and toxemia from poisonous body wastes that are absorbed by the blood.

SYMPTOMS. Dullness and a tendency to leave the rest of the herd are likely to be the first ones shown, and there may be excessive watering from the eyes. A little later on there may be twitching of the muscles around the eyes and ears, together with apparent blindness and inability to swallow. Temperatures will range from normal to as high as 106° F. Breathing becomes increasingly difficult, and animals often grind their teeth. They finally go down in a paralyzed condition and die quietly, usually within a week or less after symptoms are first noted. Opening a dead animal is likely to reveal a friable, enlarged, and yellowish liver, while the lungs may show evidence of pneumonia.

DIAGNOSIS. Often difficult, but any poorly fed cow in advanced pregnancy which shows suggestive symptoms can be suspected of having pregnancy disease. A positive Ross test such as used for acetonemia will support a diagnosis of pregnancy disease. Under field conditions it may be impossible to tell it from milk fever occurring before calving unless a test for low blood calcium is available. It might also be confused with circling disease, displacement of the abomasum, hardware trouble, pneumonia, acetonemia, or various kinds of poisoning.

TREATMENT. The most effective probably consists of a Cesarean operation to remove the calf, for medical treatments have not been consistently satisfactory. At various times compounds like ACTH, dextrose, molasses, and fluoroprednisolone acetate have been used with only temporary benefit. In the early stages of an attack it will often help to feed palatable feeds like crimped oats, and such feeding can be supplemented with glycerin or propylene glycol for better results. The intramuscular injection of glucocorticoids has been reported as of value in some cases.

PREVENTION. Generally believed to be a matter of management. It has been recommended that the ration be restricted during the first two-thirds of pregnancy so that animals gain little, and do not become fat. Then the ration is increased during the final third of pregnancy by allowing access to good pastures or supplying grain supplements. Since it is likely that the daily bulk intake of feed will not increase with advancing pregnancy, the protein level of the ration may need to be increased. Animals should receive plenty of exercise, especially during the last third of pregnancy.

Nosebleed (Epistaxis)

CAUSE. Several different possibilities, including:
1. Foreign objects in the nasal passages.
2. Tumors in the nasal passages.
3. Severe head injuries like kicks by horses, heavy blows, etc.

4. Water belly or urinary calculi.
5. Blood poisoning associated with diseases like red nose, malignant catarrhal fever, blackleg, septic metritis, etc.
6. Poisoning by plants like sweet clover and bracken ferns.
7. Poisoning by chemicals like nitrates, mercurials, etc.
8. Rupture of blood vessels in the respiratory tract in connection with abscesses, larval damage, or aneurism.
9. Lightning stroke or electrical shock from short circuits.

SYMPTOMS. Obvious enough, but should be observed as to whether the bleeding is from one or both nostrils, and whether or not the nosebleed is accompanied by bleeding from the mouth or ears. When nosebleed is due to infection with septicemic diseases, animals may refuse to eat, be reluctant to move, and appear dull. The body temperature may be normal, subnormal, or high, depending on how long the disease condition has existed. Bleeding from both nostrils in connection with bleeding from the mouth usually occurs quite suddenly. Large quantities of blood may be coughed up, and some of it may be in massive clots.

DIAGNOSIS. Important only in regard to determining the cause and source, for the nosebleed is quite evident, of course. Bleeding from only one nostril is generally caused by a foreign object or tumor in the nostril, or injury to that side of the face. Bleeding from both nostrils is likely to be associated with poisoning, septicemic disease, or injury to the full face. Bleeding from one or both nostrils in connection with bleeding from the mouth generally indicates a ruptured blood vessel in the lungs or upper part of the respiratory tract.

Puffing of the cheeks when air is being forced out of the lungs may indicate a nasal growth or mechanical obstruction. If the mouth is held open with a stick or the hand, this will stop. When blood comes from both nostrils, a bad smell like rotting flesh may indicate an infection like mucosal disease or malignant catarrhal fever. In such a case other cattle in the herd should be examined for signs of illness. If bleeding from both nostrils occurs in connection with water belly or urinary calculi, swelling of the abdomen and an odor of urine on the animal's breath can probably be detected. Nosebleed due to electrical shock or lightning stroke will generally be accompanied by other symptoms like a lack of muscular coordination and apparent blindness. Bleeding from one or both ears in association with nose bleed is apt to indicate a fractured skull.

TREATMENT. Mechanically useless unless the bleeding occurs in the front end of the nasal passages where the area can be reached. Blocking the nostrils with packs of various kinds may actually cause damage by forcing the blood back into the throat where it may be drawn into the lungs to cause pneumonia. Tumors of the nostrils may be removed surgically or reduced in size by daily intramuscular injections of antibiotics at the rate of 1 gram per 100 pounds of body weight for about a week. Such treatment will prove effective only when the growth has become infected with susceptible organisms.

When bleeding is due to injuries or rupture of blood vessels, the injection of blood-clotting agents may be desirable. These include cephalin and lecithin in dosages of 10 cc. each. Oxalin and malonic acid solutions may be given intravenously or intramuscularly at the rate of 5 cc. for every 100 pounds of body weight. In severe cases blood transfusions may be indicated to save the life of an animal.

Animals should not be excited, and in many cases it will be best not to attempt treatment. Instead, animals should be allowed to remain quiet until the blood clots normally stop bleeding.

When severe bleeding is from the lungs, feedlot animals are best slaughtered immediately. When hemorrhage has been due to a ruptured lung abscess, the carcass will probably be condemned. When due to a ruptured blood vessel, it has a fair chance of proving salvageable.

12.

CALF TROUBLES

Care of Calves at Birth

With a calf safely delivered, an attendant's first duty is to see that breathing is properly started. It is recommended that the calf be grasped by the hind legs and raised so fluid will be drained out of the respiratory tract. Swinging or shaking the animal will help in this job as well as stimulating the beginning of lung movements. It's sometimes surprising how much fluid can be poured out of a new-born calf's mouth by such a procedure. The calf is then laid down and the mouth cleaned of any remaining mucus by using the fingers. A sharp slap on the ribs or across the rump may start breathing through reflex actions. If other methods fail, artificial respiration may be given by regularly raising the front part of the body at the same time that the ribs are gently compressed and then releasing the pressure as the body is lowered.

With breathing satisfactorily started, the calf can be thoroughly dried with a rough towel or gunny sack and briskly rubbed to promote the circulation of blood. Allowing the cow to lick the calf will have a stimulating effect on the circulation, too. With everything going as it should, the navel cord should be disinfected with iodine. The job is best done by using a wide-mouthed container like an ink bottle. The calf is laid down, the entire navel cord is fitted into the iodine, and the bottle is then quickly turned upside down against the belly so the whole umbilical region is disinfected. This procedure insures a good job with no mess or staining of fingers. An ounce of iodine is enough; a fresh dose used on each calf.

The next step consists of seeing that the calf is permitted to suck. Some of these wobbly-legged chaps will need help in this respect, and it's well to be around so they're sure to get a lunch a short time after birth. An early meal on that first milk or colostrum will do good in several ways. In addition to providing energy and warmth it will also supply vitamins and antibodies needed for fighting different types of infection.

Feeding Recommendations

Opinions vary greatly on the matter but it is generally believed that calves should be removed from the dam after the first twenty-four hours. There is little question but what a great many calf troubles start with overfeeding, and letting calves run with cows is certainly a good way of letting them get more milk than they

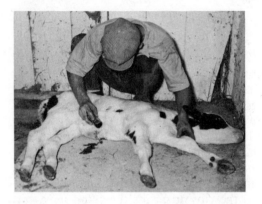

The navel of a new-born calf can be easily disinfected by using a little iodine in a wide-mouthed bottle.

should. This sort of thing was all right in Grandpa's day, but most of our present-day dairy cows give too much milk to be offered calves on a help-yourself basis. Under such conditions the animals usually suck until they're no longer hungry, and by that time they've had far too much. In addition to causing immediate sickness, it seems likely that running cows and calves together may be a means of infecting the young animals with Johne's disease or parasites, with symptoms showing up much later. Disregarding the calf entirely, it is probable that many cases of milk fever result from letting calves suck as they please to remove large quantities of milk from the udder during those critical first few days after freshening.

Once the calf has been removed from its dam, the diet can be carefully regulated to prevent overfeeding. The weight of the calf can be used as guide in determining the correct amount of milk it should have. Most authorities consider that feed for the first week should equal about 5 per cent of the body weight daily. For example, a calf weighing 60 pounds will need 3 pounds, or a quart and a half of milk daily for the first seven days. This is best divided into three feedings, with a pint of lime water added to each feeding. The lime water is desirable for decreasing the size of curds formed by the milk in the stomach and so making it easier to digest.

It is considered best to use the milk of the dam during the first seven days, with both the milk and lime water being warmed to about body temperature before feeding. We personally favor the use of nipple pails over the conventional type that allows calves to drink. This is because they prevent gulping of milk in a hurry, and insure better digestion through slower eating.

After the first week calves can be fed twice daily and the milk allowance can be increased at the rate of a half pound daily for the next three weeks. Thus a calf that is receiving 3 pounds of milk on the seventh day will get 3½ the eighth, 4 the ninth, and so on until it is getting 13½ on the twenty-eighth day of life. There are no further increases in milk after this age, but the animals can be furnished with a little grain and leafy green hay at this time. If desired the calves can also be gradually changed over onto skim milk after they have become a month old, with the changeover taking about a week for completion. Various of the milk substitutes on the market can be used instead of the skim milk if they are more practical for the owner. At this time it will be a good idea to make salt and minerals available free choice in separate boxes, too. It is important that no spoiled, dusty, heated, or moldy feeds be furnished, for they can easily upset the delicate stomachs of calves. The mention of spoiled feeds is a reminder that owners must constantly watch for calves that may acquire the habit of eating straw or filthy bedding. Young animals don't have stomachs fitted for digesting such roughage, and the

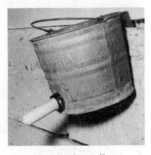

A nipple pail.

diet may cause scouring, unthriftiness, and general symptoms of ill-health. Sometimes it is necessary to place basket-type wire muzzles on calves to keep them from eating harmful materials.

Housing Recommendations

Calf pens are mighty important during the winter, since the right kind can prevent a lot of trouble. This is true regardless of whether they are in a conventional or loafing shed type of barn. In planning them, there are six major points to consider, for they should be:

1. Cool.
2. Approximately the same temperature at all times.

3. Located so they are free of drafts.
4. Located so they are easily kept clean and dry.
5. Numerous enough to permit grouping of calves by size.
6. Large enough to prevent overcrowding.

An ideal calf barn temperature runs around 50 degrees Fahrenheit, but it can be cooler. We've never known of a calf freezing to death in a dairy barn, but overheated quarters kill hundreds of calves every year. The degree of cold doesn't make much difference as long as it stays well above the freezing point. Calves will get shaggy in cold quarters, but they are usually healthier than those reared in warm barns. However, certain requirements have to be met if cold pens are to be satisfactory for calves.

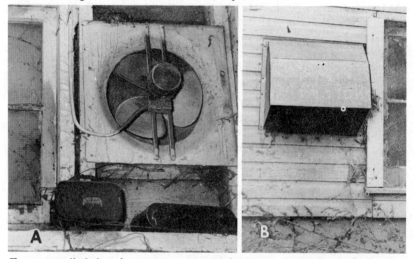

Fan controlled by thermostat to control temperature automatically and provide fresh air in barn. A. Inside View. B. Outside View.

First of all, they should be protected against frequent changes from cold to warm or from warm to cold. The matter of temperature control can often be taken care of pretty well by installing a ventilator in one of the barn windows. This consists of a suitably sized electric fan coupled to a thermostat which can be set at the desired temperature. When the building gets too warm, the fan starts automatically, drawing in fresh outside air and forcing out the damp inside air. The fan cuts off again after the temperature gets down to where it belongs.

Also, the pens shouldn't be exposed to bad drafts through open hay chutes or broken windows. Neither should they be located next to outside doors that are frequently opened in bad weather.

If they must be located in such places, the pens can be boarded up four or five feet high as shown on page 301. Concrete floors should be covered with plenty of bedding and concrete walls should be protected at floor level by boards. Otherwise the calves may be chilled by contact of their bodies with the cold cement.

It is important that pens be located where they are easily cleaned and bedded with the rest of the barn, for those that are tucked away in out-of-the-way corners are likely to be neglected. This is bad, for filthy pens encourage many kinds of calf diseases.

Overcrowding must be avoided at all costs if calves are to be thrifty and healthy.

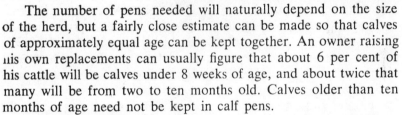

The number of pens needed will naturally depend on the size of the herd, but a fairly close estimate can be made so that calves of approximately equal age can be kept together. An owner raising his own replacements can usually figure that about 6 per cent of his cattle will be calves under 8 weeks of age, and about twice that many will be from two to ten months old. Calves older than ten months of age need not be kept in calf pens.

When calves under weaning age are kept in separate pens, these pens should be about 4x8 or 6x6 feet square. A single pen for 4 older calves should be at least 10x10 feet. Another way of figuring proper pen size for older calves is to allow 25 to 35 square feet per calf, depending on size.

Weak Calves

CAUSE. Usually one or more of the following:

1. Dams are infected with some contagious disease like Bang's or vibriosis. Such troubles may cause a form of blood poisoning that affects the health of calves even when they are carried full time.

2. A lack of vitamin A in the ration of the pregnant dam as described later in this section under the title of "three day scours."

3. General nutritional deficiencies of cows that are "roughed through" the winter on poor feeds like corn fodder and marsh hay. Unborn calves need plenty of protein for development and a lack of it in the dam's feed is hard on them.

4. A lack of iodine in the rations of pregnant cows may be involved in certain sections. Such a deficiency can sometimes cause weak calves that show no evidence of being affected with goiter.

SYMPTOMS. Calves are weak and sickly at birth, usually undersized, and many of them come a few days earlier than expected. They often need help in order to stand and suck. Some refuse to suck at all, appear to be in a sort of stupor, and a great many die within a few days after birth. Animals that live usually develop slower than normal calves, and may seem stunted a few weeks later when compared with animals of a similar age.

TREATMENT. Feeding can be done oftener than the recommended three times daily, but the total amount of milk should be decreased in order to prevent scouring. Sometimes the animals can be helped by adding an ounce or two of olive oil to the regular milk fed in a day. A teaspoonful of the APF (Animal Protein Factor) or antibiotic compounds given daily may also prove helpful. Seriously weak calves may be given blood transfusions of 50-250 cc. either intravenously or subcutaneously. The APF and antibiotic compounds can be obtained through your veterinarian and many feed stores.

PREVENTION. Largely a matter of doing something about the causes already listed.

1. Herds can be regularly blood-tested for the detection of Bang's and vibriosis. If the diseases are discovered, control measures can then be instituted before many of the weak calves are born.

2. Preventive measures can be followed as suggested for "three day scours" in this section.

3. Dry cows can be fed liberally on balanced rations of good quality feeds so that unborn calves will be supplied with plenty of protein. Suitable feeding practices are discussed in the Practical Pointers section of this book under the heading "Care of the Dry Cow."

4. Both iodized salt and a complete mineral mixture can be supplied free-choice at all times. These are best furnished in separate boxes so cows can get whichever they want without being compelled to eat the other. In addition it won't hurt to mix a couple of pounds of the salt with every hundred pounds of the grain ration. In iodine deficient areas the cows may be given two or three grains of sodium iodide in their drinking water every week during the last three months of pregnancy as suggested for the prevention of goiter. This practice is recommended because the use of iodized salt alone cannot always be depended on to prevent a deficiency of iodine.

"Three Day Scours"

CAUSE. Not definitely known, but apparently due to a deficiency of vitamin A in the feed that is responsible for a lowering of reserves generally stored in the livers of pregnant dams. This vitamin protects the lining of the digestive tract and is highly important in getting calves off to a good start in life. Being transmitted through the uterine "buttons," a lack of it in the dam may mean the start of intestinal infection before calves are even born. Vitamin A is normally formed from carotene, a compound that is present in green feeds or leafy, well-colored hay. Cows on pasture ordinarily store up reserves during the summer that are sufficient to insure healthy calves at the next freshening. However, there is considerable variation from year to year because of the difference in growing seasons that may affect the quality and vitamin A content of forage.

SYMPTOMS. Trouble is commonest during the late winter or early spring, with calves dying within three or four days after they are born. They may be born at night, appear perfectly healthy, be strong enough to stand and suck within a short time, and still be found dead the next morning. In such cases the owner is likely to believe that they have been laid on or crushed by the dam. At other times the calves may seem healthy for the first day or two, and then suddenly go off feed, appear severely ill, and die within a few hours. The word "scours" is sometimes confusing, for many animals die without showing any signs of scouring whatever. Those that live for a day or two commonly show evidence of diarrhea before death in addition to appearing droopy, listless, and sunken-eyed. If a dead calf is opened, nothing at all may be found or there may be varying degrees of inflammation shown by the stom-

ach and intestines. Sometimes evidence of diarrhea may be found
in the first few feet of the intestines, with fecal matter in the rest
of the digestive tract appearing perfectly normal. In such cases it
is reasonable to assume that a little longer life would have permitted the scouring condition to travel the full length of the intestines and finally appear at the anus. There are few recoveries.

DIAGNOSIS. Usually on the basis of deaths that occur for no
apparent reason within three or four days after birth of normal
calves. When animals live long enough for scouring to appear the
trouble may be confused with diarrhea or white scours.

TREATMENT. None has been demonstrated as effective, with
serums, sulfas, other drugs, vitamins, and blood transfusions all
being tried at various times with discouraging results. Treatment
after birth is evidently too late in most of these cases, and control
is pretty much a matter of prevention.

PREVENTION. Evidently a matter of supplying vitamin A to
the cows during the last weeks of pregnancy. This can sometimes
be done by feeding plenty of leafy green hay during the critical
winter months when cows have been off pasture for a long time
and their body reserves have been seriously depleted. However,
this isn't always enough, since feeds that look green may still be
low in vitamin A. Such a condition is due to the fact that both
carotene and vitamin A are easily destroyed by oxidation and may
be lost through drying for hay or long storage of feeds. Consequently, it is sometimes desirable to supply vitamin A in capsules
to the cows. It is recommended that it be given in 500,000 unit
doses twice a week during the last three weeks of pregnancy. Vitamin A capsules of this size may be obtained from your veterinarian.

Nutritional Diarrhea (Common Scours)

CAUSE. Usually overfeeding, but almost any kind of sickness
can also be to blame. In addition, such things as navel ill, the eating of bedding, feeding from dirty pails, sudden changes of temperature, and chilling can be involved. Overcrowding, sudden
changes of feed, and confinement in filthy pens can also be contributing factors.

SYMPTOMS. Calves sometimes appear perfectly healthy except
for being afflicted with a watery diarrhea. At other times they
may also refuse to eat while showing signs of weakness and general
droopiness. In older calves the diarrhea may be so dark that the
disease is sometimes called black scours, but the feces are usually
white and sometimes tinged with blood. In uncomplicated cases

the temperature usually remains about normal. The scouring may persist for several weeks and finally cause death, but with proper feeding and good nursing most calves can be expected to recover within a short time. When diarrhea persists for any length of time in young animals it is likely to be followed by pneumonia, probably because of lowered resistance and weakening of the body. Calves that recover after a serious siege of scours are often seriously retarded in growth and in later life seem subject to various kinds of breeding troubles. Once started in a herd, an epidemic of white scours often shows signs of being contagious, with trouble evidently spreading directly from animal to animal.

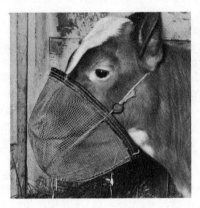

Calf wearing wire muzzle to keep it from eating filthy bedding and making itself sick with diarrhea.

DIAGNOSIS. Usually made on the basis of a diarrhea that appears in overfed and poorly managed calves without causing many deaths. A definite diagnosis is sometimes difficult, as nutritional diarrhea can easily develop into infectious diarrhea so that nutritional diarrhea today can be infectious and even contagious tomorrow. In addition to infectious diarrhea and three day scours, this disease might be confused with worm infestation, coccidiosis, and diseases like pneumonia where the diarrhea develops as a symptom of some other trouble.

TREATMENT. Begins with removal of the cause, since no medicines are effective against such things as drafts, overfeeding, unsanitary conditions, chilling, and overcrowding. When milk is being fed it is wise to skip one meal entirely. Castor oil in a dose of 2-4 ounces may be given instead for the purpose of cleaning rotting materials out of the digestive tract where they are fermenting to cause a form of blood poisoning. A teaspoonful of powdered alum can be dissolved in a half pint of warm water and given orally for its astringent effect on the stomach and intestines. Such a dose may be repeated in twelve hours. Equal parts of salol and bismuth subnitrate can be given at the rate of a half ounce four or five times daily, while a half ounce of vinegar well diluted with water and given three times daily may also prove beneficial. After skipping one meal, feeding can be resumed with rations being reduced by half the amount formerly fed. Boiling of milk may prove helpful, and including a well-beaten egg in it will help to supply energy without contributing to the scouring. When the diarrhea has been stopped the feed may be gradually increased to an amount in keeping with feeding recommendations made earlier. Increases in feeding amounts should not exceed a half pound daily.

When infection is involved, various drugs may be indicated in combination with the treatment already mentioned. Various of the sulfas are commonly used nowadays, with sulfathaladine being especially good. This can usually be given at the rate of a grain per pound of body weight daily for not over five days at any one time. The time limit is mentioned because all of the sulfas may cause kidney damage through prolonged use, and it is desirable to discontinue their use as early as possible in outbreaks of any kind. The effectiveness of these drugs is evidently increased by giving the recommended amount in several divided doses a few hours apart rather than all at once.

Severely weakened calves may require blood transfusions or injections of glucose in 250-500 cc. doses. These may be given either intravenously or subcutaneously, with intravenous administration giving faster results. The use of various calf scour serums and other biologics is often recommended, but results following the use of such products are likely to be disappointing.

PREVENTION. Entirely a matter of following suggestions made under Feeding Recommendations and Housing Recommendations for calves earlier in this chapter.

White Scours (Infectious Diarrhea, Calf Septicemia)

CAUSE. Generally a germ called *Escherichia coli,* although viruses, yeasts, molds, salmonella, and other types of bacteria have been involved in outbreaks. The various causes listed for nutritional diarrhea in this book can also act as contributing factors.

SYMPTOMS. Sudden death may be the only indication of trouble when calves do not receive colostrum within a few minutes after birth and are exposed to a highly virulent type of infection. In the worst of these cases calves may appear sick within a few hours after birth and die during the first day, sometimes without even showing evidence of a diarrhea. At the other extreme, properly fed and well managed older calves may show no symptoms other than bowel movements which are slightly softer than normal. In between, calves may look healthy at birth, sicken the second day, get worse the third, and die on the fourth day.

The first signs generally include loss of appetite, dryness of the hair coat, and more frequent bowel movements. As time goes on the manure changes from a yellow color to white, and becomes watery in consistency. Slobbering that wets the lower jaw is often seen, and the buttocks become smeared with filth. Continued dehydration results in sunken eyes and general dullness. Affected animals may stand in a humped back position with the head extended or stretch out flat on the floor. During warm weather the buttocks may become flyblown, and larvae may even invade the rectum. When calves are forced to move, they are likely to show weakness by staggering. The body temperature drops in the final stages, and the body becomes cold and clammy to the touch. Breathing becomes increasingly shallow, and calves go into a coma shortly before death. Opening a dead animal is unlikely to show anything more than a reddening of the stomach and intestines, and even this may be absent if it has died suddenly of septicemia or bacterial poisoning. Once started in a herd, an epidemic of white scours often shows signs of being contagious, with the disease evidently spreading directly from animal to animal. Heifer calves that recover from a severe siege of white scours are often seriously set back in growth, and in adult life seem subject to various kinds of breeding troubles.

DIAGNOSIS. Usually made on the basis of typical symptoms in combination with the age of affected calves and a history of previous trouble. The biggest job consists of differentiating infectious diarrhea from nutritional diarrhea and three day scours. However, animals with nutritional or common diarrhea usually are not so sick, the death rate is low, and they generally recover when the diet is corrected. Calves affected with three day scours generally die quicker, and trouble often can be stopped by supplying vitamin A to the pregnant cows as recommended in this book. Opening a dead animal that fails to show significant lesions will help in making a diagnosis by eliminating other possible troubles. In doubtful cases a laboratory examination that reveals E. coli or salmonella organisms will help establish infectious diarrhea as a cause. In addition to nutritional diarrhea and three day scours, this disease might be confused with troubles like coccidiosis, worm infestation, and pneumonia with diarrhea occurring as a secondary symptom.

TREATMENT. A combination of good nursing with measures to replace body fluids lost by dehydration, drugs and antibiotics to control infection, compounds to coat the digestive tract, and absorbents to neutralize bacterial poisons.

Blood transfusions offer the best way of replacing lost body fluids and should be given intravenously at the rate of a pint to a quart of blood as needed. The blood will also have a good chance of containing antibodies that will fight the infection. If blood transfusions are not practical, commercial antitoxins may be used that are effective against E. coli and salmonella germs. Different kinds of electrolyte solutions are also available for replacing lost body fluids. The amount to be used will depend on the amount of dehydration. For example, if a 100-pound calf has suffered 10% dehydration (10 pounds), then 5000 cc. (10 pounds, 10 pints) will be needed for replacement.

Many different antibiotics and drugs have proven effective in the treatment of infectious diarrhea, and the one of choice is usually a matter of selecting a remedy that has been satisfactory in the past. Neomycin, chloramphenicol, and polymyxin B have all been shown as particularly effective against E. coli and salmonella germs. When antibiotics are given by mouth, the first dose is usually 5 to 10 milligrams per pound of body weight, and then half this dose at 12-hour intervals for 2 days. When given both by mouth and by injection, the dosage is increased by half and divided equally between the two methods. Sulfas have been widely used in the treatment of white scours, and they are definitely indicated any time there is a suspicion that coccidiosis may be involved.

Remedies containing combinations of pectin, kaolin, and sulfas can be used to coat the digestive tract, decrease absorption of bacterial poisons, and speed up healing. Numerous commercial preparations are also available for these purposes, and the salol and bismuth subnitrate mixture described under the treatment for nutritional diarrhea in this book will also prove helpful.

The most important part of nursing consists of keeping the sick calf warm. When conditions permit, it can be placed in an empty stall between a couple of cows. Otherwise a heat lamp can be used to keep the temperature around the calf from falling below 55 degrees F. Under no conditions should the barn be overheated, for pneumonia is then very likely to develop. Blanketing the calf or securely fastening gunny sacks on it can also be used as a means of keeping the calf warm. Some owners have used a horse manure pack under a thick layer of straw as a means of supplying heat to sick calves.

Whatever is used in the way of medical treatment, all food should be withheld for at least 24 hours. After this period a pound of milk (1 pint) mixed with the same amount of water can be allowed every 12 hours. Whole milk is preferred to milk replacer, and colostrum is even better. Some owners freeze surplus colostrum and keep it on hand for such emergencies. The amount of milk is gradually increased as the condition of the calf improves. Since a beef cow may not reclaim her calf after it has been taken away, it may be advisable to let beef calves nurse for short periods every day instead of hand-feeding them.

PREVENTION. Largely a matter of good management and proper feeding as described in this book under Feeding Recommendations and Housing Recommendations. Commercially prepared antitoxins and serums are available for the prevention of this disease, but they are effective only if they contain the specific antibodies needed for protection. A pint of whole blood given intravenously to each calf at birth is often effective, and has a better chance of containing the right antibodies because it is drawn from older animals in the home herd that have developed resistance through previous exposure. Making sure that the calves get several early meals of colostrum is also recognized as an effective preventive measure.

Vaccination with various commercial bacterins has not appeared as very effective against white scours, although a bacterin made from bacteria isolated from dead calves in the home herd has been of value in some herds. The bacterins are not to be used on the calves. Instead, two or more injections should be given to pregnant cows at 2-week intervals, beginning at about six weeks before calving. Preventive measures of any kind cannot be expected to do much good in the absence of good management practices.

"Scalding" Following Diarrhea

It frequently happens that all the hair comes off the tail, buttocks, or hind legs of a calf following an attack of diarrhea. The cause is unknown, but loss of hair occurs only in areas that have been plastered with bowel movements. The bald spots frequently have a red or cooked appearance which led to use of the descriptive term, "scalding." Hairless areas grow a new coat within a short time after the diarrhea has been corrected, and the condition is not usually considered as serious. Daily application of agents like zinc oxide or wool fat may soften the skin and help to speed the growth of new hair in affected areas.

Crooked Calf Disease

CAUSE. A monster-producing agent in lupine plants. The trouble has been associated with cattle grazing ranges where a great many lupine plants were growing. Although known to occur in most of the dairy breeds and all common breeds of beef cattle, it has been a serious problem only in western areas of the U.S. and the northeastern part of Kodiak Island. Usually not more than 10 per cent of the calf crop is affected in a herd.

SYMPTOMS. Calves are born with stiff immovable joints. Although generally appearing in connection with the elbows of the front legs, any of the various body joints may be affected to cause such deformities as wryneck and abnormal curvature of the backbone. Difficult births are common, and ranchers have killed many calves shortly after birth because they were unable to stand and nurse or follow their dams. Sometimes stiffness of joints appears in combination with cleft palate and other abnormalities of the skull.

DIAGNOSIS. Based on typical stiff joints and a history of dams having run on lupine ranges during the pasture season. This trouble might be confused with contracted tendons of the legs. However, when tendons are contracted, the joints are properly lined up, which is not the case with the stiff joints syndrome. In addition, the contracted tendons can be straightened out with a little effort in most cases, or will correct themselves within a week or so. In contrast, the crooked calves grow progressively worse with age as the affected joints are subjected to more strain.

Crooked calf disease might also be confused with a similar trouble that results from an inherited trait. Practically all calves with the inherited type of stiff joints will have cleft palates, while only a few of those born with the lupine-caused stiffness will show this deformity.

The calves are different in another way, too, for those stiffened by lupines are usually carried to about full time, are born alive, and of normal size. Calves that are stiffened because of heredity are apt to be carried for some time past the due date, are about half normal size, and are either dead at birth or so weak that they die shortly afterward. Carefully controlled feeding and breeding experiments have proved that crooked calf disease is completely different from the inherited trouble that is marked by similar symptoms.

TREATMENT. None recommended, for these crooked calves are hopelessly deformed and nothing can be done for them.

PREVENTION. Entirely a matter of keeping cows off ranges abundant in lupine plants during their gestation period.

Colds

This trouble is discussed rather completely under "Catarrh" in the section on Respiratory Troubles. Doses of medicine will have to be proportionately decreased for calves. Prevention is almost entirely a matter of following the recommendations made in regard to housing.

Calf Pneumonia (Calf Influenza)

CAUSE. Not definitely known. Bacteria of different kinds were once believed to be the cause, but the disease has been transmitted with bacteria-free filtrates, indicating that this is not true. On the other hand, various kinds of viruses have been isolated from calves showing signs of this disease. At this time it is generally believed that a virus or virus-like agent is the basic cause, and that many different kinds of bacteria act as secondary invaders to make a bad situation worse.

In addition, predisposing factors are recognized as being important in bringing about an outbreak of calf pneumonia. The list includes such things as inadequate nourishment and vitamin deficiencies, and some authorities believe that all cases of calf pneumonia are preceded by enteritis and diarrhea. Other predisposing factors are wet bedding, drafts, overcrowding, poor ventilation, and infestation with parasites. Calves from 2 to 6 months old are most susceptible, but calves from 2 weeks to one year of age may be affected.

Calf pneumonia may occur either as a primary disease or as a complication of other troubles. Calves that are weak when born, those that do not get colostrum within a short time after birth, and those that are poorly fed during the first few weeks of life are most susceptible. The disease is most likely to appear during the early fall when animals are brought in and bunched in poorly ventilated quarters, particularly when calves of different age groups are placed together in a single building used exclusively for calves. If an outbreak appears on a farm one year, it is likely to recur the next year unless effective preventive measures are used.

SYMPTOMS. One or several calves become sick, followed in short order by many more so that an outbreak occurs on the order of an explosion. Temperatures may range from below normal to 107 degrees F. or higher. Open-mouth and labored breathing is shown early, and a short hacking cough is common. As might be expected, the sick animals refuse food and appear dull. Usually abnormal lung sounds are absent in the early stages, but they soon develop, and then disappear as solidification occurs in various areas of the lungs. A watery discharge from the nostrils gradually changes to a thick type, and the muzzle becomes dry and crusted. Diarrhea may either precede or follow these symptoms, and, as a result of dehydration, affected animals soon become little more than skeletons with sunken eyes and a rough hair coat. Death may occur within three days to a week, but in chronic cases animals may linger along for several months. These chronic cases seldom recover completely because of extensive lung damage and the formation of abscesses which cause toxemia. The death rate is very high for untreated animals. Opening a dead calf will usually show inflammation of the intestines and a grayish exudate in the respiratory tract. Large areas of the lungs are likely to be solidified, and abscesses of various sizes may be found in these organs.

DIAGNOSIS. Based on the typical symptoms of pneumonia—difficult breathing, high fever, diarrhea, nasal discharge, and dehydration. Under farm conditions the condition might be confused with such contagious diseases as shipping fever and mucosal disease.

TREATMENT. The most desirable is a combination of sulfas and antibiotics combined with supportive treatment and good nursing. The sulfas are best given intravenously at the rate of 1 to 2 grains per pound of body weight for the first dose. The sulfas are then given by mouth at the rate of 1 to 2 grains per pound of body weight in 3 divided doses during the next 24 hours. During the second 24-hour period the sulfas are given by mouth at the rate of 1 grain per pound in 3 divided doses. If calves are not seriously sick, the first dose of 2 grains per pound of body weight may be given by mouth instead of intravenously. Care must be used when sulfas are given intravenously, particularly when animals are weak and dehydrated, for severe reactions may occur when these drugs are given too fast, for too long, or in over-large doses.

Penicillin has not given very good results when used alone, but has been shown as fairly effective when given in combination with streptomycin. Both of these antibiotics have given better results when used in combination with sulfas. The broad-spectrum antibiotics like oxytetracycline and chlortetracycline have given satisfactory results and are used extensively.

Transfusions of citrated blood represent the best of the supportive treatments, and have saved many calves that would otherwise surely have died. If blood is not available, a pint of 5% dextrose solution given intravenously may help by applying energy at a time when it is badly needed. Small doses of stimulants like arsenic and nux vomica may help animals that are extremely depressed. A so-called "pneumonia jacket" can often be used to good advantage for keeping sick calves warm and protecting them against drafts. There is little trouble in making one of these, for an old quilt or sack is simply folded across the calf's back and tied around the body with strong cords like binder twine.

Sometimes calves are "steamed out" with compounds like eucalyptus oil and the nose drops commonly used by human beings against colds. A satisfactory "steamer" can be made by using a sack that has the bottom cut out so it forms a tube. A quart or so of hot water is placed in a small pail and a little of the compound mixed with it. One end of the sack is then tied around the top of the pail and the other is fitted snugly around the calf's nose as shown in the illustration. Under such conditions the animal has no choice about breathing the medicated steam, and treatment may be continued for as long as necessary. Such a procedure often helps considerably in loosening mucus in the lungs to aid breathing.

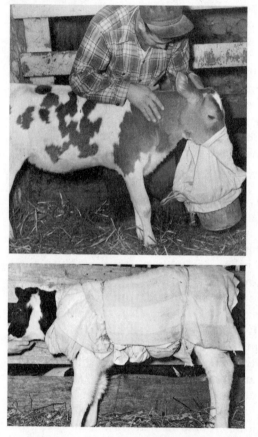

Calf being "steamed" for pneumonia.

Pneumonia jacket for use on calves.

PREVENTION. Largely a matter of management that includes:

1. Being careful about bringing infection into the home herd. Animals that have been purchased or been away to exhibitions should be isolated for at least 30 days.

2. Cleaning up buildings where sick animals have been quartered. Such buildings should be cleaned and disinfected after an outbreak, allowed to stand vacant for six months or more, and then cleaned and disinfected again before calves are brought in.

3. Following housing recommendations as given earlier in

this book under Calf Troubles.

4. Following feeding recommendations as given earlier in this book under Calf Troubles. The value of supplemental vitamin feeding is doubtful in well-managed herds where adequate nutrition is provided.

5. Grouping calves according to age so that older animals cannot act as reservoirs of parasites and disease to infect younger calves.

6. Isolating all infected animals at the very first symptoms of sickness so that the entire herd is not infected.

7. Vaccinating with rhinotracheitis vaccine or myxovirus parainfluenza-3 vaccine if one of these diseases is proved to be associated with pneumonia in a herd.

Diphtheria (Necrotic Laryngitis, Oral Necrobacillosis)

CAUSE. A germ called *Spherophorus necrophorus,* the same one that is involved in foot rot, liver abscess, and necrotic stomatitis. Some authorities consider necrotic stomatitis to be a mild form of diphtheria. The disease often occurs in connection with poor feeding and filthy housing conditions. However, these conditions are not required, for outbreaks sometimes occur in barns and feed lots where cattle are kept under excellent conditions. Predisposing factors include infections like IBR and BVD, mouth injuries from coarse feeds and plant awns, and possibly a vitamin A deficiency.

SYMPTOMS. Painful coughing is usually noticed first, and it may be accompanied by difficult breathing and a temperature of 104-106 degrees Fahrenheit. Depending on the extent of infection, feed may be taken as usual or refused entirely. Excessive slobbering is commonly seen, and examination of the mouth will usually reveal yellow or grayish spots of various sizes in the throat or on the cheeks and gums. These are generally covered with a cheesy material resulting from the necrosis and rotting away of flesh. Breathing becomes increasingly difficult, and extensive involvement of the throat that prevents swallowing causes slow starvation and weakness that eventually results in death if animals are left untreated. The disease is not usually considered as contagious, although several cases may occur in the same herd within a short time. Outbreaks are commonest during the winter, but the disease occurs the year 'round in both beef and dairy cattle. Although calves and young stock are most commonly affected, the disease has been reported in animals up to two years of age. Opening a dead animal frequently shows cheesy masses of necrotic tissue that have entirely plugged the trachea. In other cases infection can be demonstrated as having penetrated deeply into tissues of the mouth and throat.

DIAGNOSIS. Through typical symptoms and characteristic mouth lesions, particularly in regard to the yellow cheesy material that appears on the gums and lining of the cheeks. Sometimes the ulcers will be found extending into the lungs, down the esophagus, and even into the stomach. Under farm conditions the disease might be confused with "wooden tongue," bad teeth, IBR, BVD, ulcerative stomatitis, or injuries caused by foreign bodies in the mouth.

TREATMENT. None for advanced cases when the soft palate and trachea are badly damaged. Other cases may be helped by the administration of various sulfas and broad-spectrum antibiotics. Intramuscular injections of penicillin and dihydrostreptomycin have also been demonstrated as helpful. Vitamin A supplements are indicated for young calves that happen to be affected. Early treatment is recommended to prevent the development of chronic respiratory troubles.

PREVENTION. Largely a matter of management, which includes vaccination against diseases like IBR and BVD, feeding good quality roughage to eliminate mouth injuries, and keeping animals in clean, well-ventilated quarters. Supplying plenty of vitamin A in the ration will probably help, too.

Necrotic Stomatitis

CAUSE. A germ called *Speropherus necrophorus,* the same one that is involved in foot rot, liver abscesses, and calf diphtheria. As a matter of fact, some authorities consider this disease to be nothing more than a mild form of calf diphtheria. Predisposing factors are the same as those given for diphtheria.

SYMPTOMS. Animals appear dull and run moderate fevers of about 104° F. They slobber profusely and have a characteristic bad-smelling breath due to decaying tissues in the mouth. Food may be eaten or refused, depending on the soreness of the mouth. Opening the mouth will show characteristic ulcers on tongue, cheek lining, pharynx, larynx, and sometimes farther down the respiratory and digestive tracts. These ulcers have raised edges with yellow, cheesy centers. Untreated animals are apt to die in a week or so of starvation, suffocation, or toxemia, or a combination of all three.

DIAGNOSIS. Through the characteristic raised-edge, cheesy ulcers appearing in the mouth and upper respiratory tract. Under farm conditions necrotic stomatitis might be confused with the same troubles listed under the diagnosis of diphtheria.

TREATMENT. None for advanced cases if the tongue has been almost cut in two or infection has spread to the lungs to cause suppurative bronchopneumonia. Others may be helped by treatments mentioned as of possible value under the treatment of diphtheria.

PREVENTION. The same measures as suggested under the prevention of diphtheria .

Goiter

CAUSE. A deficiency of iodine in the rations of pregnant cows.

SYMPTOMS. There are a few abortions, but most calves are born alive in a seriously weakened condition. Many are unable to stand alone after being helped to their feet. The thyroid glands are usually enlarged to give the calves a swollen throat in the region between the lower jaws. The jugular veins may be distended and prominent on one or both sides of the neck. If dead animals are opened the thyroid glands are often found to be swollen and resembling clotted blood. This trouble may appear almost anywhere in the United States, although it is commonest in the Northwest and in the area around the Great Lakes. It may appear some years and not in others, probably because of a difference in iodine content of feed and water during different seasons. In some areas the deficiency is so slight as to be seen only at extremely rare intervals.

DIAGNOSIS. Through typical symptoms of weak calves with enlarged thyroids. May be confused with some of the other causes of weak calves.

TREATMENT. Calves are usually so far gone that nothing can be done for them, but some may improve rapidly if they are helped to suck a few times. The oral administration of a grain or two of potassium iodide daily for the first week or two of life may help, and daily painting of the swollen thyroids with iodine may also prove beneficial. In general, though, preventive measures are much more practical than treatment.

PREVENTION. The year-'round feeding of iodized salt free-choice may be all that is required. This can't always be depended on, though, for salt that has been stored for a long time may have

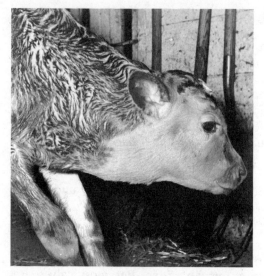

Calf with goiter.

lost most of the iodine through evaporation. When iodized salt doesn't prevent trouble the cows may be given 5-10 grains of sodium iodide in the drinking water every week during the last two months of pregnancy. Iodized salt can be mixed at home by adding one part of potassium iodide to every 3000 parts of common salt. The iodides must not be given in larger doses than recommended, for the drugs are capable of causing abortions when improperly used.

Navel-Ill

CAUSE. Infection by different kinds of bacteria which get into the body through the navel cord. Such infection may occur before birth and involve reproductive diseases like Bang's, vibriosis, trichomoniasis, and others. However, it probably occurs more often through contamination of the raw navel cord with filth after birth.

SYMPTOMS. Calves infected before birth are likely to be born weak and covered with a filthy yellow slime. They may die within a few days or recover their strength so they apparently grow in a normal manner. Animals infected after birth often show swelling of the navel with occasional dribbling of urine and discharging of pus from the region. Within a few days or weeks the calves may lose their appetites, appear weak, start scouring, and run fairly high temperatures. Owners are often puzzled by such cases and treat the calves for diarrhea with unsatisfactory results. Infection may spread all through the animal to cause swollen joints and pus pockets in various parts of the body that are discovered only after death.

Sometimes calves simply appear unthrifty and fail to do well without showing any definite symptoms of the real trouble.

DIAGNOSIS. Often impossible until examination of a dead animal shows pus in the joints and abscesses in different parts of the body. Sometimes swelling of the navel and joints in combination with other symptoms will help to indicate the nature of the ailment. A history of breeding troubles in a herd and the frequent birth of weak, yellow-stained calves that fail to do well may also prove helpful in establishing a tentative diagnosis.

TREATMENT. Not generally satisfactory, but transfusing a pint or so of the dam's blood may be of some value. Intramuscular injections of penicillin and streptomycin in million-unit doses may be tried. In some cases the transplanting of cuds seems to be of benefit, and the procedure is worth a trial in all cases when calves are vaguely unhealthy. Treatment for navel-ill may well be combined with that recommended for diarrhea, especially when calves are failing to eat properly and show evidence of scouring.

PREVENTION. Infections that occur before birth are best prevented through the elimination of reproductive diseases. Cows shouldn't be bred back in less than sixty days after calving, and only healthy animals should be mated. Infections that occur after birth can be almost entirely prevented through treating the navel cord with iodine at birth as described in this section under "Care Of Calves At Birth". Calves should be kept from sucking each other's navels, or infection may occur in this manner.

Yellow Calves

Calves are frequently noticed as being covered with a filthy yellow slime when they are born. This is evidence of diarrhea and indicates that calves have scoured before birth and then practically bathed in their own manure for some time before delivery. Such scouring can always be taken as proof of infection in the uterus. Genital diseases like Bang's and vibriosis are often involved, even though animals have had enough natural resistance so actual abortions haven't occurred. At other times it seems that a lack of vitamin A may have allowed ordinarily harmless bacteria to cause infection of reproductive tracts and scouring in unborn calves.

Bloating

At one time or another most owners have had calves of varying ages that were "chronic bloaters." This is a very serious condition, for practically all untreated affected animals either die in a short time or eventually become so stunted that they are worthless. There are several possible causes.

Ulcers of the stomach are sometimes to blame, often being started by a sudden change from roughage to grain that produces an extremely acid condition in the stomach. Trouble of this kind seems more likely to occur when barley forms a large part of the ration.

Another possible cause involves infection of the so-called *torus pyloricus,* a thickened fold of lining where the stomach connects with the small intestine. Swelling of this fold may then close off the intestinal opening to prevent normal emptying of the stomach.

Various types of stomach worms will also cause chronic bloat, probably through iritation that eventually causes swelling of the *torus pyloricus.*

Foreign bodies or indigestible materials in the rumen or abomasum frequently cause chronic bloat, with hair, feed sacks, paper, coarse hay, shavings, filthy straw, or spoiled silage being involved in such cases.

Highly fitted show calves often remain bloated most of the time due to crowding of the digestive system with fat.

Beef calves that are kept on nurse cows until they are a year old or older may bloat, probably because the milk interferes with digestive actions of the normal rumen bacteria.

The use of milk substitutes or other artificial feeds may also have the effect of changing or destroying normal stomach bacteria so that bloating results. The same thing may be caused by the prolonged oral administration of antibiotics and sulfas intended for the control of diseases. Since these rumen bacteria are absolutely necessary for normal digestion, any interference with their activities can easily show up as chronic bloating.

Pail-fed calves may bloat because they are victims of "windsucking" that occurs when they suck each other or on parts of their pens after feeding. The bloating may also be due to excessive drinking of water or greedy gulping of milk from a pail. Such gulping may have the effect of interfering with digestion because the milk then becomes large lumps of curd in the stomach.

The treatment of bloat in calves will naturally depend on the primary cause. Oral administration of an ounce of turpentine or kerosene well-diluted with milk will help in some mild cases. Intramuscular injections of penicillin or streptomycin may be tried against infection of the *torus pyloricus,* or oral administration of various antibiotics may help. Animals can be treated for removal of stomach worms that are causing the bloating. In some cases the surgical removal of indigestible stomach contents represents the only procedure that is likely to help the condition.

However, efficient management procedures will do a great deal to prevent bloating in calves, and they will generally prove more practical than treatments. The following are recommended:

1. Stanchion calves so they can't suck after getting their milk.
2. Supply them with a good mineral mix and salt free-choice.
3. Add a pint of lime water to each feeding of milk to decrease the size of the curds formed in the stomach.
4. If necessary, use basket muzzles on calves to keep them from eating filthy bedding and other indigestible materials.
5. Don't overdose with antibiotics and sulfas given orally.
6. Smear pine tar on mangers or parts of pens where calves suck or try to chew.
7. See that calves don't drink a lot of water right after feeding.
8. Stop using any milk substitutes or other feeds that show a tendency to cause bloat in calves.
9. Don't allow calves to suck cows for long periods.
10. Follow a program of internal parasite control, particularly in regard to rotation of pastures used for young stock.
11. Change gradually from roughage to grain in feed lots.

Sucking After Feeding

Calves are often wildly anxious to suck each other or anything available immediately after they've had their milk. The habit is objectionable under any conditions. It may disfigure calves through "scalding" of noses, jaws, ears, and tails. It may be responsible for "windsucking" that causes bloat and various digestive

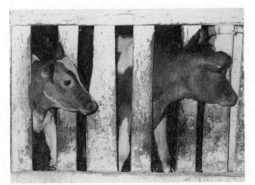

Fastening calves in stanchions will prevent udder sucking after feeding.

troubles. Chewing on teats and udders may ruin quarters that aren't noticed until heifers freshen with their first calves. Sucking on navels may lead to infection and subsequent navel-ill. The habit is extremely hard to break when it has once been established, but several methods of prevention can be adapted to various conditions. The most practical consists of tying or stanchioning calves so they can't get at each other for a half hour or so after feeding. Filling the mouths with a handful of finely ground grain immediately after meals may help to eliminate the taste of milk and make the calves forget about wanting to suck. In extreme cases it may be necessary to buckle a narrow strap around the muzzle for a few minutes after feeding so that the mouth is entirely prevented from opening.

Swollen Jaws

There are six general causes of swollen jaws in calves:
1. Bruises caused by blows or pulling back in stanchions. Resultant swellings may disappear or develop into abscesses.
2. Hematomas following injury to the jaws.
3. Occlusion of the parotid duct.
4. Actinobacillosis.
5. Diphtheria.
6. Goiter.

Lumpjaw has not been listed because it isn't likely to show up in animals less than a year old. A careful examination will usually show the true nature of trouble, and proper treatment can then be given as recommended for the various conditions.

Colic

CAUSE. Generally the excessive formation of gas from the fermentation of food in the digestive tract. This causes "griping" and pain through distension of the stomach and intestines. It usually follows the eating of roughage like bedding or corn fodder by animals that are too young to digest such materials. However, trouble may be caused by customary milk rations, particularly if the feed is gulped down hurriedly.

SYMPTOMS. Uneasiness, frequent lying down and getting up again, kicking at the belly, groaning, and bawling at irregular intervals. Animals may occasionally lie down, stretch out, even go into convulsions of pain. There may or may not be bloating.

DIAGNOSIS. Based on the typical symptoms and the elimination of other troubles causing similar evidence of pain. May be confused with calcium "tic", white muscle disease, lead poisoning, or epileptic fits.

TREATMENT. The oral administration of drugs that will serve to move the gas along and expel it from the digestive tract. A teaspoonful of ginger dissolved in a cup of warm water is good, and so is a tablespoonful of turpentine diluted with a half pint of warm milk. Peppermint or spearmint oils diluted with warm water are also good. Two or three tablespoonfuls of castor oil may be given later for the purpose of eliminating fermenting feed that caused gas in the first place. The next feed following treatment should be decreased by half.

PREVENTION. Primarily a matter of following the recommendations already made for feeding calves. The animals should also be kept from eating indigestible or spoiled feeds.

Patent Urachus

In unborn calves urine passes from the bladder through a canal called the urachus which is included with other structures in the navel cord. When the navel cord is broken at birth the urachus normally closes up and urine then passes from the bladder through the urethra. However, things don't always go according to plan and the urachus sometimes remains open so that urine continually dribbles out at the navel. Infection and swelling of the navel usually accompany the condition, and symptoms of general illness are frequently seen. At other times the calves seem perfectly healthy except for a wet and enlarged navel region. The most practical treatment consists of surgery to remove inflamed parts of the urachus and tie it off so dribbling of urine is prevented. An alternative method consists of injecting a small amount of lugol's solution or tincture of iodine deep in the urachus in the hope that resultant inflammation will permanently close the canal. Animals that show this condition are best discarded as breeding stock when young.

Inherited Deformities of the Eye

These are probably found oftener in calves than in any of our other domestic animals. Defects may range all the way from complete blindness to a simple turning in of the upper or lower lids. A common deformity is represented by a fibrous band that extends across the pupil of the eye. Abnormal coloring that produces so-called "watch eyes" and "glass eyes" is also fairly common.

Hairless Feet and Fetlocks

This is an inherited characteristic that occasionally appears in Holsteins and more rarely in Shorthorns and Jerseys. There is a total lack of skin around the fetlock region, often on all four feet. This gives the areas a raw, bloody appearance. The condition is permanent and is unlikely to be remedied in later life. In some cases there is a lack of part of the mucous membranes in the mouth,

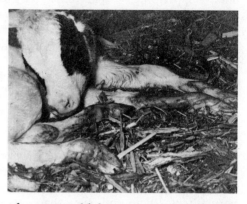

Calf with hairless feet, a hereditary defect.

too, as well as convulsions and spasms which may appear and seem to be part of the inherited characteristic. Affected animals should not be saved as breeding stock, for they have a good chance of transmitting the condition.

"Blue Baby" Calves

A calf's lungs aren't used before birth at all, since oxygen and nutrients are obtained through the buttons of the uterus, with waste products also being eliminated through them. In an unborn calf the blood circulates in this fashion:

From the left ventricle of the heart through arteries to various parts of the body. It is then returned to the right atrium or auricle of the heart by veins. Most of it then goes directly into the left atrium through an opening in the heart wall known as the foramen ovale. Only a little passes into the right ventricle, thence to the lungs through the pulmonary artery, and back to the left atrium through the pulmonary veins. Regardless of how it gets there, blood then passes into the left ventricle for another trip through the body.

A different situation exists after birth, for all the blood is then expected to pass through the lungs while circulating. The foramen ovale is supposed to close so there is no short cut from right to left atrium, and blood then circulates in this fashion:

From the left ventricle through arteries and eventually back through veins to the right atrium as before birth. With the foramen ovale closed, all of the blood goes into the right ventricle and thence to the lungs. Here it gives up carbon dioxide and other waste products and takes on a fresh load of oxygen. It then returns to the left atrium to pass into the left ventricle for another circulation.

When the foramen ovale doesn't close, much of the blood doesn't get to the lungs so it can give up waste products and absorb oxygen, and the calf really suffers from partial suffocation. Affected animals are sometimes called "blue babies" because of a similar condition that is known to occur in human infants. Calves don't really turn blue, but they do suffer from smothering and lack of oxygen.

They have little endurance, breathe fast, sometimes froth at the mouth, and spend a great deal of time lying down. When being fed they may be able to take only a few swallows of milk before needing to stop and pant for breath a few minutes. Under such conditions it may take them a long time to drink a small amount of milk. The slightest kind of exercise is likely to cause gasping and open mouth breathing. In other respects the animals usually seem perfectly healthy and normal. There is no practical way of correcting the condition, although surgery is a possibility just as it is in human infants.

Wood-Chewing

Calves sometimes show a tendency to eat wood wherever they can find it, gnawing at feed-boxes and the sides of buildings as though they were really good to eat. The cause isn't always known, but there are three likely possibilities:

1. Salt or certain minerals, particularly those of the trace variety, may be lacking in the ration.
2. Animals are instinctively trying to exercise their jaw muscles against the day when they'll need strong ones for chewing large amounts of fibrous roughage.
3. Lack of exercise may have caused them to chew wood out of sheer boredom.

Three methods of breaking the habit may be tried:

1. Salt and a good mineral mixture can be made available free-choice in separate boxes.
2. Whole oats or calf pellets can be furnished as part or all of the grain ration instead of ground feed that furnishes no opportunity for chewing.
3. Overcrowding should be avoided and facilities furnished for exercise.

Raising Twin Calves

A great deal of confusion apparently exists in regard to when it is safe to raise twin calves for breeding purposes. Some owners contend that the twins will breed when they are both heifers, but twin bulls are always sterile. Others hold an exactly opposite opinion, and say that twin bulls are breeders, while the twin heifers are sterile. Some say that all twin calves will be sterile regardless of sex, while others swear that they'll all be breeders. When twins are mixed with one of a set being a bull and the other a heifer, there are four common beliefs:

1. The bull is sterile, but the heifer will be a breeder.
2. The heifer is sterile, but the bull will be a breeder.
3. Both the bull and heifer are sterile.
4. Both the bull and heifer will be breeders.

The truth of the matter is that some calves will be sterile regardless of whether they're twins or not, but twins that are both of the same sex will have a normal chance of growing up into breeders. When one twin is a bull and the other a heifer, the heifer will be sterile about nine times out of ten. There is a good reason why this should be true.

As calves grow in the uterus, both the testicles and the ovaries eventually start secreting hormones which are emptied into the circulating blood. The testicles mature a little faster and start secreting hormones a little earlier than the ovaries, with each of the hormones having an inhibiting effect on hormones produced by the opposite sex.

When twins have the same circulatory system the male hormones get into the blood first and prevent the development of female genital organs after that time. As a result the heifer twin is born as a so-called "free-martin" which will never breed. Since most twins are on the same circulatory system, it is only natural that about ninety per cent of the heifers born twins to bulls prove to be sterile.

"Free martins" can be identified in laboratories where blood typing is done. A heifer born twin to a bull and showing a certain blood admixture is sterile. An examination of the afterbirth will sometimes show whether or not the calves have had the same circulatory system. An alternative method consists of examining the vagina with a tiny speculum and flashlight to see if it is normal. A final choice consists of keeping the heifer until she is about a year old. If she grows into a coarse, staggy-looking animal that has no heat periods, you're pretty safe in deciding that you've raised a "free-martin."

Rickets

CAUSE. A deficiency of calcium or phosphorus, and possibly faulty proportions of these minerals in relation to each other in the diet. A lack of vitamin D is often mentioned as a cause of rickets, but it is not likely to cause trouble for calves that are receiving fair amounts of good quality roughage.

SYMPTOMS. Calves appear unthrifty and rough-coated, often with heads that seem too big for their bodies. Leg joints are frequently enlarged, and bones are so soft that they are likely to be bowed out of shape. Knobby growths may appear in rows along the ribs to create a condition commonly called the "rickety rosary", and the spine may be weakened to cause "swayback". Calves occasionally show a tendency to stand on their toes, and in mild cases this may be the only sign of trouble.

DIAGNOSIS. Through typical symptoms and a history of faulty feeding. This latter fact may not be entirely dependable, for seemingly good rations may be lacking in calcium or phosphorus when the feeds have been grown on poor soils. Consequently, rickets may develop when calves appear to be well-fed.

TREATMENT. Most practical through supplying the missing minerals free-choice in addition to mixing them as one per cent of the grain ration. A satisfactory mineral mixture can be made at home by combining 200 pounds of trace-mineralized salt, 200 pounds of steamed bone meal, and 100 pounds of finely ground limestone. Small grains are generally rich in phosphorus, and legume hays will usually supply plenty of calcium, so good feeding is a helpful part of any treatment. Irreparable bone deformities are likely to keep advanced cases from being benefited, and such animals are usually considered as hopeless. Vitamin D can be supplied either by injection or by dosing orally. As much as 500,000 units per day have been fed to affected calves for a week, then followed by feeding a grain mixture containing 5000 units per pound of grain.

PREVENTION. Exposing calves to direct sunlight for at least an hour every day, feeding sun-cured roughage, and adding 1000 to 4000 units of vitamin D per pound of grain have all been demonstrated as effective.

Calf Tetany (Calcium "Tic")

CAUSE. A deficiency of magnesium which may be complicated by a deficiency of calcium in older calves that have been fed an all-milk diet. Calves usually have magnesium levels of a little over 2 milligrams per 100 cc. of blood at birth, but these decline to 0.7 mg. per 100 cc. of blood in the next two or three months when only milk is fed. Tetany can occur when the levels fall below 0.7 mg. per 100 cc. of blood. This explains why calves are usually 3 months of age or older before signs of trouble appear. The disease is most likely to occur in rapidly growing calves, and is rare in those that are getting feeds besides milk because solid feeds are apt to provide five times more magnesium than milk.

SYMPTOMS. Include such things as shaking the head, carrying the ears bent backward, exaggerated reflexes, nervousness, violent reactions to a touch, a stiff gait and, finally, convulsions. Sometimes there is twitching of various muscles, grinding of the teeth, apparent blindness, frothing at the mouth, and other symptoms suggestive of the nervous form of acetonemia as it appears in cows. In some cases calves have been known to run wildly around pens, blatting frequently, and occasionally trying to climb walls or jump over pen partitions. The death rate is high, and death often occurs within a half an hour after an attack of convulsions. Calves which survive the first attack of convulsions are likely to be killed by a later one.

DIAGNOSIS. Based on the typical symptoms of calves that have been on a straight milk diet. There is no way of distinguishing between a magnesium and calcium deficiency other than through laboratory examination of the blood. The condition may be confused with white muscle disease, epileptic fits, lead poisoning, and colic. White muscle disease should always be considered as a possibility when calves die suddenly, for both tetany and white muscle disease can cause death with few or no previous symptoms of sickness. In addition, this trouble may be confused with others such as epilepsy, lead poisoning, and colic.

TREATMENT. The most effective consists of the subcutaneous injection of 100 cc. of 10% solution of magnesium sulfate. However, improvement may be only temporary unless the milk diet is supplemented with magnesium oxide (¼ to ½ ounce daily), or magnesium carbonate (½ to 1 ounce daily). Calcium deficiency can be remedied by the subcutaneous injection of a 20% solution of calcium gluconate (50 to 100 cc.). In addition, calves should be kept in a quiet area, and may be treated with tranquilizers and a quarter-ounce of chloral hydrate well diluted with water daily for a few days to control nervous symptoms.

PREVENTION. Largely a matter of adding good quality hay and grain and calf starters supplemented with minerals and vitamins to the all-milk diet at about 30 days of age. This can often be best accomplished through creep feeding.

"White Muscle Disease," WMD, Muscular Dystrophy

CAUSE. Originally believed to be a deficiency of vitamin E, but in recent years it has been shown that a lack of selenium is related to this disease in some way, and other causes may possibly be involved in certain areas. Scientists at the Oregon State Station produced the disease experimentally in lambs whose dams received a predominant diet of ladino clover during the last two months of pregnant cows on an all-alfalfa ration. In Florida the disease has appeared almost exclusively in calves on lush clover pastures, while in other areas it has been seen in animals on alfalfa and even some kinds of grass pasture.

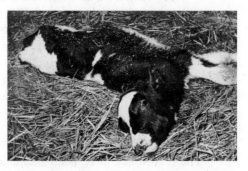

Calf with white muscle disease.

SYMPTOMS. Calves 6-10 weeks old on an all-milk diet are those usually affected. In the beginning they act sleepy, appear unwilling to stand, and assume unnatural positions. Sometimes they drop dead following a romp, or are unexpectedly found dead without any previous signs of sickness, while at other times they are noticeably sick and linger for several days. Affected animals are likely to be noticed as walking in a peculiar stiff fashion, or they may appear to be blind. Sometimes they will be thrown into convulsions by a scare or sudden loud noise, and again they will run in circles while frothing at the mouth and bawling wildly. Examining a dead animal will often show that the heart and muscles of the hind legs are pale and carry white streaks.

DIAGNOSIS. Through typical symptoms appearing in milk-fed older calves, and the elimination of other troubles producing similar symptoms. It might be confused with such things as calcium "tic," lead poisoning, and enterotoxemia.

TREATMENT. The feeding of wheat germ meal or wheat germ oil often proves helpful, and so do intramuscular injections of alpha-tocopherol. Experimental work has indicated that 60-120 mg. of sodium selenite given orally or injected subcutaneously is of value.

PREVENTION. The following measures are recommended:

1. Feed cows an ounce daily of wheat germ meal, wheat germ oil, or vitamin E concentrate during the last two months of pregnancy and for two months after calving.
2. Feed pregnant cows on a ration containing both wheat bran and linseed oil meal. The linseed meal is particularly desirable because it contains preventive amounts of selenium.
3. Feed calves wheat germ products or vitamin E concentrate.
4. Give calves, either orally or by subcutaneous injection, 1 to 8 cc. each of a sodium selenite solution made by adding 1 gram of sodium selenite to 100 cc. of distilled water.* Repeat once or twice at weekly intervals if needed.
5. Inject pregnant cows with 20 cc. of the above solution every four months.
6. Inject cows and calves with both alpha tocopherol and selenite solution at recommended levels.

Ruptures or Hernias

These troubles have been included under Skin Troubles, since they may affect older animals as well as calves.

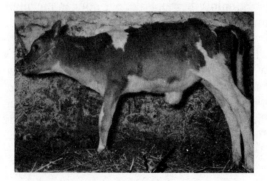

Hernia in young calf.

* Dr. F. H. Fox, Cornell University.

Hemorrhagic Enterotoxemia

CAUSE. An organism called *Clostridium perfringens* which gives off at least four different kinds of poisons which may affect cattle. These greatly resemble each other, and are known as Types A, B, C, and D. Type C was once believed to be the only one affecting cattle, but B and D have been known to cause more trouble in certain areas than C. Type A seldom shows up as a digestive disease of cattle, and is more likely to be seen as gas gangrene in any part of the body where wounds have occurred to provide entry for the germs.

SYMPTOMS. Somewhat dependent on the type of poisons involved, but death within a day or two after symptoms are first noticed is common for all types, and the discovery of dead animals that were apparently healthy a short time earlier may be the first indication of trouble. Calves less than 2 weeks of age are affected most often, but the disease can occur in older animals. Practically all cases are accompanied by a bloody diarrhea, and if it does not appear animals have a fair chance of recovery, although they may be left as unthrifty, poor gaining individuals. In addition:

Type A is characterized by dullness without fever, jaundice, bloody urine, and labored breathing.

Type B may be indicated by weakness, rapid loss of weight, and a bad-smelling, brownish diarrhea.

Type C may be announced by failure of calves to nurse, and a little later by colicky symptoms like kicking at their bellies, and straining.

Type D is apt to be shown by signs of brain involvement like walking in circles, pushing against objects, excitement, and convulsions.

Opening a dead animal will often show little other than an inflamed condition of the small intestines. Parts of them may appear to be bloody and areas of the lining may be sloughed in irregular patches. At times there will be evidence of jaundice, and considerable fluid in all of the body cavities. The kidneys may be swollen, dark-colored, and soft. Bloody spots sometimes appear on the heart, stomach, lungs, and diaphragm.

Reports indicate that calves out of high-producing cows are most likely to be afflicted with this ailment. Some such cows have been known to lose two or three successive calves from enterotoxemia. In most cases trouble appears on farms where there have been no recent changes in management or feeding practices. Herds that experience serious losses are likely to go several years before the disease appears again.

DIAGNOSIS. Definite only in the laboratory through guinea pig inoculation and fluorescent antibody tests. However, the short course of the disease and suggestive symptoms may help in making a tentative diagnosis. Under farm conditions the disease might be confused with troubles like leptospirosis, bacillary hemoglobinuria, botulism, circling disease, and BVD.

TREATMENT. It is unlikely that any kind of treatment will do much good in really bad cases, since death occurs so quickly after the first symptoms are shown. However, many calves can be saved by intravenous injection of antitoxin in 25 cc. doses. In addition, large doses of penicillin or broad-spectrum antibiotics given intramuscularly may help.

PREVENTION. Either one of two preventive programs can be followed. One consists of injecting each calf with a 10 cc. dose of *Clostridium perfringens* antitoxin within a few minutes after birth. This gives protection for about three weeks, which will carry calves through the critical period for this disease.

The other consists of giving each pregnant cow two injections of *Clostridium perfringens* toxoid. This product must not be confused with antitoxin or serum, for it is entirely different. Such vaccination is started two to four months before freshening, with the second injection being made three to five weeks after the first one. This second injection acts as a "booster" shot to increase immunity, which in turn is passed on to the calf through the colostrum in the form of antibodies. Cows that have had two of these injections at the proper time will thereafter need only one injection each year about two months before calving. Since immunity from colostrum lasts for only three or four weeks, calves in infected areas should be vaccinated with toxoid about the time that such immunity disappears. The colostrum from vaccinated cows can be used for the treatment of this disease. Both the antitoxin and toxoid can be obtained from your veterinarian.

Prevention in the feed lot is often a simple matter of management. This includes such things as:

1. Separating the animals according to size.
2. Providing plenty of feeding space at grain bunks.
3. Feeding regularly so animals have no chance to become over-hungry.

4. Being careful not to over-feed on grain.
6. Supplying plenty of good quality roughage with the grain ration.
7. Including antibiotics in the feed.

Polyarthritis of Calves

CAUSE. A virus of the psittacosis-lymphogranuloma (PL) group which appears to be the same as the one that causes polyarthritis of lambs. Although different it also resembles the agent that causes epizootic bovine abortion. It is extremely virulent, as shown by the fact that it killed every calf inoculated with it in experimental work.

SYMPTOMS. The first signs are likely to be a reluctance of the affected animals to move and a tendency to lie down most of the time. They may run a fever, and although weak, will usually suck if they are carried to the dam and helped to stand. A diarrhea soon appears. Animals become progressively duller as time goes on, and show signs of pain in their legs by standing in a humped-up position and stretching out when lying down. The joints and tendons of the legs are apt to become swollen and painful to the touch, although experimental calves died within four days after exposure without showing any signs of joint involvement. The disease has been seen in calves ranging from four days to four weeks of age.

Opening a dead animal will generally show lesions in practically all the joints, even including those in the backbone. The liver is generally enlarged, and may show evidence of nodules on its surface. An accumulation of yellowish fluid causes enlargement of the joints, and there is usually swelling of the tendon sheaths around them.

DIAGNOSIS. Definitely made only through isolation of the causative agent in the laboratory. However, if typical symptoms appear in young calves without evidence of umbilical lesions, polyarthritis should be suspected. Under farm conditions the disease might be confused with navel-ill.

TREATMENT. Experimental work has shown chloramphenicol, tylosin, and the tetracyclines to be of value if given during the early stages of an attack. Calves are apparently not helped by injections of penicillin-streptomycin combinations, and streptomycin alone does not seem to have any effect on PL agents. Even the most effective of antibiotics probably do little more than lessen the severity of attacks, and do not eliminate the causative agent. This is because treated animals often remain as carriers and spreaders of the PL organisms.

PREVENTION. No definite recommendations can be made, for little is known about the susceptibility of cattle to PL agents. It has been reported that natural attacks do not give increased resistance to experimental infection with PL organisms, so the outlook for vaccines does not appear to be encouraging.

Zinc Deficiency

CAUSE. Usually poor rations that are lacking in zinc. In addition, calcium is believed to sometimes interfere with the absorption of zinc in the digestive tract, and phytic acid in soybean proteins may also have a binding effect on zinc. Some workers believe that the zinc deficiency may sometimes be related to a lack of vitamin C in the ration. In recent years this trouble has been recognized as being much commoner than once believed to be the case.

SYMPTOMS. The first ones shown are apt to be loss of hair in patches around the head and fetlocks, accompanied by a reddening of the skin. As time goes on the animals go off feed, become dull, and tend to put in a great deal of time lying down. Other symptoms likely to be shown include inflammation of the nose and mouth, stiffness, an unthrifty appearance, thickening and cracking of the skin, and the development of scaly skin areas in various parts of the body. Borderline cases may show no symptoms other than poor growth and slow gains. This trouble is much commoner in calves than older animals that will probably get better rations.

DIAGNOSIS. Through suggestive symptoms that appear in combination with a history of faulty feeding. The diagnosis may be checked by a change in rations, for affected animals respond dramatically when zinc is made available. In such cases alertness and the appetite will often improve within 12 hours.

TREATMENT. A matter of supplying zinc in the ration. Zinc oxide, sulfate, or carbonate are all suitable sources, and can be mixed with concentrates to supply 260 ppm. zinc. Individual treatment can consist of a half an ounce of zinc oxide daily in combination with a single intramuscular injection of 20,000 units of vitamin C. A change to better rations is recommended as part of any other treatment that may be given. The skin condition will improve within a few days, and new hair will start coming in by the end of the second week. Overdosing with zinc must be avoided, for it may have damaging effects like interference with growth, and cause troubles like enteritis and arthritis.

PREVENTION. Entirely a matter of supplying a good ration, for most of our commoner feeds include adequate amounts of zinc for cattle. When feeds are of poor quality or are grown on deficient soils, the ration may be fortified as described under TREATMENT. Making trace-mineralized salt available on a free choice basis is also recommended as a preventive measure.

Lead Poisoning

This trouble is discussed earlier under Poisoning By Chemicals in the section on digestive troubles. It is mentioned here as a reminder that calves are particularly susceptible, and that a tiny amount of lead is often sufficient to cause death. Accordingly, calves that show evidence of blindness, paralysis, convulsions, or spasms must always be considered as possible victims of this type of trouble. When diarrhea appears the condition may be mistaken for various other disorders, and convulsions may cause it to be confused with white muscle disease or calcium "tic". Recommendations for treatment will be found under the condition already mentioned as appearing in an earlier section of this book.

Dwarfism

Dwarf calves are caused by an inherited character which is evidently due to a single gene or factor. Factors of this type are known as simple recessive traits. Most dwarf calves are produced by normal parents because such animals are not suspected of being carriers of the factor, and consequently are allowed to remain in a herd. These carrier animals do not always produce dwarfs, for a carrier female must be mated with a carrier bull to produce one. Even then, such a mating will not always produce a dwarf calf. This is because recessive traits are governed by a natural law of heredity which enables them to show up in only about one-fourth of the offspring from carrier parents.

When both parents are carriers, about one out of every four calves will be a dwarf that can quickly be removed from the herd. About two out of every four calves will be normal-looking carriers, while the fourth will be both normal in appearance and a non-carrier. When a carrier bull is used on a herd of non-carrier females, no dwarfs will be born, of course. However, about half of the resulting calves will be carriers, with dwarfs showing up in following generations when a second carrier bull or the original carrier sire is used on the carrier females. If one of the carrier calves was a bull that was later used on a carrier female in the same or another herd, dwarf calves could be expected, too.

Since no figures are available on the number of dwarf calves that are born every year, no one knows exactly how serious this problem really is. It is known that all of the major beef breeds are involved, and that no line of breeding is entirely immune. In addition, dwarfism is evidently on the increase all over the country.

We do not know why there are more dwarfs than there were a few years ago, but it has been suggested that the gene for dwarfism may be closely linked with those for blockiness or fast gaining or early maturity or other desirable characteristics which breeders have been emphasizing in recent years. An increase in the number of cattle with such a characteristic would naturally account for a corresponding increase in the number of dwarfs. Several methods have been suggested for identifying the normal-looking animals that are carriers of the dwarfism gene, and so are the ones most responsible for continuing the dwarfs.

Owners have been advised to test bulls by using them on cows known to be carriers because they have produced a dwarf calf. A bull should be bred to at least ten of these cows, and if no dwarfs result, it is fairly certain that the bull is not a carrier. On the other hand, siring a single dwarf is enough to convict him. It is not practical to prove cows by mating them to carrier bulls, for a single cow can produce only a few calves in her lifetime, and about three-fourths of these will be normal in appearance even when she is a carrier and is bred to a carrier bull. Although this breeding method is a positive means of identifying carriers, it is slow, difficult, and expensive.

A few years ago workers at the University of California claimed a so-called "profilometer" was a fast means of detecting dwarfism carriers. This instrument was used to measure animals from poll to muzzle in order to detect an invisible slight bulge in the forehead which is supposed to be almost always present in carriers. Opinions are still divided in regard to its accuracy.

A little later on workers at Iowa State College suggested another way of detecting carriers. They reported that X-rays of the backbone showed crowding of the loin vertebrae in dwarfism carriers.

Then in the summer of 1956 Dr. Lasley at the University of Missouri reported that beef owners might soon be able to detect dwarfism carriers with a comparatively simple and inexpensive test. It begins with an injection of insulin directly into the jugular vein. After a short interval, blood samples are taken from the animal and white blood cell counts are made. An increase in the number of white cells is claimed as a measure of the activity of the animal's adrenal glands. In non-carriers the white cell count is expected to rise much higher and within a shorter time than in carriers. In dwarfs, little change is expected in the white cell count. These results are taken to indicate active adrenals in non-carriers, medium active glands in carriers, and inactive glands in dwarfs. This method was reported as successful in tests with the University's beef cattle breeding herd, with significant differences between carriers, non-carriers, and dwarfs.

More recently, Dr. Julian of the University of California claims that the sphenoid and occipital bones that form the brain cavity floor of an animal's skull furnish an X-ray identification of dwarfs, and possibly carriers, too. These bones come together in the so-called "S-O junction" and dwarfism is indicated by the age at which they fuse permanently. In a normal Hereford bull, for example, this fusion does not occur until the animal is two or three years old. In dwarfs, such fusion may exist at birth, and certainly occurs within the first six months of life. Theoretically, at least, dwarfism carriers might also show an abnormally early fusion of the S-O junction.

Research on dwarfism is continually being carried on at many of the land grant colleges, and additional methods of detecting carriers will probably be reported as time goes on. We are confident that some practical means of handling the dwarfism problem will eventually be worked out.

INDEX

INDEX